Nursing the English from plague
to Peterloo, 1660–1820

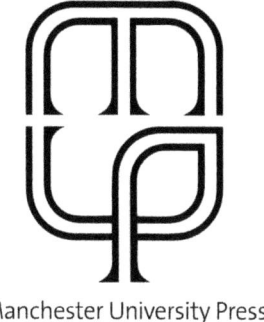

Manchester University Press

NURSING HISTORY AND HUMANITIES

Series editors: Christine Hallett, University of Huddersfield and Jane Schultz, Indiana University

The Nursing History and Humanities series is devoted both to historical approaches and humanities perspectives: work that explores nursing cultures over time and place, in moments of pandemic and public health crisis and in creative and critical contexts. The series aims to capture the current challenges facing nursing in local and global spaces, even as our books continue to document the long historical trajectories of the profession in structural and organisational terms.

The only book series devoted exclusively to nursing pursuits in the world, the editors welcome scholarly manuscripts within and across the fields of nursing history, nationally and internationally, the medical humanities and health studies of nursing practice, and the social histories of race, gender and sexuality as they pertain to the nursing profession. At the intersection of practice-based clinical nursing and rigorous cultural examinations of nursing, the series provides a forum for nurses, medical practitioners, historians, philosophers and cultural critics to present new research.

To buy or to find out more about the books currently available in this series, please go to: https://manchesteruniversitypress.co.uk/series/nursing-history-and-humanities/

Nursing the English from plague to Peterloo, 1660–1820

Alannah Tomkins

MANCHESTER UNIVERSITY PRESS

Copyright © Alannah Tomkins 2025

The right of Alannah Tomkins to be identified as the author of this work has been asserted in accordance with the Copyright, Designs and Patents Act 1988.

Published by Manchester University Press
Oxford Road, Manchester, M13 9PL

www.manchesteruniversitypress.co.uk

British Library Cataloguing-in-Publication Data

A catalogue record for this book is available from the British Library

ISBN 978 1 5261 7852 7 hardback

First published 2025

The publisher has no responsibility for the persistence or accuracy of URLs for any external or third-party internet websites referred to in this book, and does not guarantee that any content on such websites is, or will remain, accurate or appropriate.

Typeset
by Cheshire Typesetting Ltd, Cuddington, Cheshire

For the guys, who might all prove just as good at nursing as the gals: Adam, George, Harry, James, and Stanley

Contents

List of figures	viii
List of tables	ix
Acknowledgements	x
Introduction	1
1 Domestic nursing by women: ideals and experiences	41
2 Nursing the metropolis: the ancient London hospitals of St Thomas's and St Bartholomew's	87
3 Nursing provincial infirmaries 1735–1820	130
4 Nursing in the Royal Hospital Chelsea	175
5 Nursing by men: an issue of identity	219
6 Nursing in wartime 1793–1815	264
Conclusion	309
Select bibliography	315
Index	332

List of figures

1.1 T. Rowlandson, [A convalescing woman trying in vain to rouse her slumbering hired nurse], *Miseries of Human Life* (1807)   56
1.2 C. Eisen, A nurse gives a man an enema [1762]   73
2.1 J. Folkema, detail from an etching of a hospital dormitory or ward [1702–67], showing a typical eighteenth-century arrangement of hospital beds   101
3.1 A comparison of annual inpatient numbers at the Birmingham, Chester, Gloucester, Liverpool, and Salop infirmaries 1787/88 to 1816/17   135
4.1 T. Rowlandson, 'Sir Cecils Budget for Paying the National Debt' (1784)   181
4.2 Chelsea pensioner marriages by year 1699–1753   193
5.1 W. Bromley after A.W. Devis, detail from *The Death of Lord Nelson: key to the painting* (1812)   230

List of tables

0.1	Applying the 'dirty work' model to pre-professional nursing	17
0.2	Categories of pre-professional nursing activity	22
2.1	Women employed as Sisters, helpers, or nurses at St Bartholomew's Hospital for whom the onset of widowhood can be dated	115
3.1	English provincial infirmaries and their capacities 1735–1820	133
3.2	Institutional records sampled for nursing data	139
3.3	Comparative table of nurse wages and tenures in selected infirmaries	140
4.1	Status of couples at the Fleet, where the groom was a Chelsea in-pensioner, 1699–1753	194
5.1	Public asylums in 1819	236
5.2	Private licensed madhouses in 1819	237

Acknowledgements

Research for this volume has taken me to the county archives of Cheshire, Gloucestershire, Shropshire, Staffordshire, and Worcestershire, plus the city archives in Birmingham and Liverpool, in addition to the National Archives and the London Metropolitan Archives. Staff in all of these locations have been brilliant, but none more so than Kate Jarman and her colleagues at the Barts Health Archives who have been unstinting with professional hospitality, in an era when the search room was very small. I would have liked to be able to thank archivists in Manchester too, but the Manchester NHS Trust has got rid of its archival staff and have made it very difficult to access the historic records of the Manchester Infirmary. Sort yourselves out Manchester and meet your statutory obligations.

I am indebted to the suggestions and support offered by audiences for seminar and conference papers at Birmingham and Chester universities, for the Women's History Network, for the Royal College of Nursing, and at Florence 2020 just before the first lockdown. The members of the UK Association for the History of Nursing have been welcoming and encouraging from the first, even when I was entirely new to the history of nursing, and I owe them all particular thanks. The association's annual colloquium has proved a fantastic resource.

Readers of chapters have given me wise counsel at different points in the writing process: thanks to Kristen Brill, Christine Hallett, Geoff Hudson, Dominic Janes, Susannah Ottaway, Len Smith, and the anonymous readers of the book manuscript. Any errors or (more likely) unhelpful exaggerations remain my own.

Acknowledgements

Among my family and friends who have tolerated my research special thanks go to Ian Atherton who listens to me even when no one else will, to my mum Molly and my daughter Lo for genealogical research assistance, to my son Ed for laughing at my research in a salutary fashion, and Liam for everything else.

Introduction

Nurse. n.s. [nourrice, French] 4. An old woman in contempt.

Can tales more senseless, ludicrous, and vain,
By winter-fires old *nurses* entertain?[1]

Nurses at the outset of the period 1660–1820 were held in low esteem, not least because they, like their patients, had to confront a drastic epidemiological challenge.[2] The bubonic, pneumonic, and septicaemic strains of the plague appeared episodically in England up to the later seventeenth century, with consequences for perceptions of both contemporary medical expertise and the efforts of ancillary workers of all stripes. Observers of the final plague visitations in England of 1665–66 essentially spoke with one voice about plague nurses: they were damning.[3] Ignorance and indiscretion were the mildest charges to be levelled.[4] Nurses' faults were generally held to be numerous, covering their appearance, demeanour, and behaviour. They were 'the off-scouring of the city ... dirty, ugly and unwholesome Haggs' who were not only 'strange' (meaning personally unknown to the patient) but also rapacious.[5] Any customary right of nurses to claim the clothing and household textiles of their former patient was recast during plague as a callous act of overeager requisition liable to spread disease, while the interloping nature of an unfamiliar nurse aroused suspicions and literal charges of theft.[6] In their supposed pursuit of household plunder, nurses were accused of strangling their charges, or wilfully infecting healthy residents with matter from plague sores.[7] Consequently patient apprehensions were such that, allegedly, they were more afraid of their nurse than of the plague.[8] Defoe's startling extenuation – to the effect that not *all* plague nurses can have murdered their patients – came later in 1720.[9]

We might now find reasons to be sceptical about the uniformity of nurses' wickedness and consider that plague nurses suffered a form of narrative collateral damage. Authors' bitter invective might have had a broader admitted or unarticulated agenda, such as opposition to the practice of household quarantine or tacit resentment at the failure of family or neighbourly care, which meant nurse reputations fell victim to a polemic with different end goals.[10] As the first ailment to induce a serious public health response, plague was naturally the first available vehicle to inspire a backlash against community measures and personnel. Similarly, the relative independence of nurses who were not always quarantined may have been the attribute that inspired resentful male commentary.[11] These acknowledgements, though, leave us with some uncertainty about the day-to-day competency and probity of plague nurses.

Historians can be confident that treatment of plague 'was more frequently nursing-assisted than medical practitioner-assisted'.[12] Plague nurses were paid more highly than nurses in other complaints, partly owing to the greater risks they ran of contracting the same illness as their patient.[13] Plague certainly represented an economic opportunity for women willing to undergo personal jeopardy, a scenario apparently deeply resented by the patients and observers who went into print.[14] If a patient died and the nurse survived, so much the worse for the nurse's reputation. It is not surprising, therefore, that nurses became the most available target for patient anger and distress. Historical articles published very recently have gone some way to temporise these initial apprehensions. The conclusions that may be drawn from Joan Cheate's work in Haverfordwest are slim, even if the mayor characterised her as 'an instrument for good'.[15] Yet such women worked under confining circumstances if they shared household quarantines, may have offered the same varieties of care that were inherent to the role in other diagnoses, taken on a greater share of the medical initiative than was usual in cases of domestic sickness, and died as a consequence of their office.[16] They were not noticeably lauded for their sacrifice. The most recent work reinterprets nurses' behaviour on the basis that parish records can demonstrate prior relationships with patients, and a narrow/personal rather than a wide/acquisitive nursing practice. Most importantly, their seeming greed can be reconstrued as desperation following the closure of other avenues for work.[17]

The paucity of sources giving specific details about individual nurses in the seventeenth century perhaps makes the long fixity of criticisms towards plague nurses a regrettable inevitability. It is more surprising that the wider history of the 'pre-reform' nurse has remained in a similarly concrete plight. In the twenty-first century, the pre-Nightingale nurse remains something of a caricature. All histories of nursing have been written subsequent to the nursing reform movement, activated in the 1820s and consolidated from the 1850s onwards and, therefore, have been infused with low expectations for nurses' personal qualifications. Reformers including Elizabeth Fry and Mary Stanley aspired to raise the social background and work-based performance of nurses.[18] In the process, they stressed the failings of the women already in post, reconstruing nursing as a form of 'spiritual work' for which existing nurses were largely unfit.[19] Their ambitions were driven further by Florence Nightingale's advocacy for the nurse's 'calling'.[20] Nightingale's own polemic left her readers in no doubt: in describing her predecessors' activities she wrote 'I use the word nursing for want of a better.'[21] She reserved her strongest criticism for privately employed domestic nurses but, despite some praise for London hospital sisters, readers tended only to remember the critique. Not every later historian is equally dismissive of the nurses before the 1850s: Brian Abel-Smith's early history tries to be even-handed.[22] Anne Summers deconstructed the stereotype of the pre-reform nurse in the late 1980s, but a combination of the power and volume of Nightingale's own writings, plus the literary horror of Dickens's Sarah Gamp (an insanitary, self-serving tippler), have made for a powerful narrative that historians have struggled to escape.[23] Margaret Pelling has regarded as 'inevitable' the 'tendency to place over the unknown earlier terrain, a map of the battleground of the nineteenth century'.[24] At best nurses in the years before the 1850s have been dismissed as 'just servants', while at worst drink was their besetting sin.[25] Even Carol Helmstadter and Judith Godden's

Nursing before Nightingale begins as late as 1815, and exonerates the women of wilful evil (rather than hopeless incompetence).[26] Again only the most recent work, including doctoral research by Erin Spinney and Tanya Langtree, disrupts this very settled historiography.[27]

It is a relatively simple matter to contradict the impression that pre-Nightingale nurses were all equally drunken or careless of their charges. Even a single instance of a good nurse performance, such as by the 'Heroine of Matagorda' whose reputation is elaborated in Chapter 6, can destabilise such totalising generalisations. It is much more difficult to characterise nurse activity more acutely. Who were the women and men who undertook nursing work, and was there a gulf or no appreciable difference between the motivation and behaviour of paid and unpaid nurses? What were the characteristics of different employment settings, and what experiences did nurses accrue as a result? How far is it possible to calibrate the successes and failures of pre-reform sick-nurses on the existing spectrum of squalid and uneducated to ladylike and angelic? Do we need new spectra for judgement?

This book takes up the challenge laid down by Anne Borsay 'to avoid the historiographical rupture imposed by nineteenth-century reformers to strengthen the case for change, and acknowledge the deeper roots of professionalisation in the Georgian era'.[28] It charts the performances, experiences, and contexts of sick-nurses, plus the rhetorical uses to which narratives about nursing were put, from the final years of plague to the occurrence of Peterloo. This Introduction will set out the historiographies of nursing before 1820 and the parallel factors for our understanding of the social and cultural contexts of this occupation in terms of women's and men's bodies, life cycles, and the opportunities or constraints of female and male labour. It goes on to debate the methodological choices of a study in this period, and to identify definitional markers for the activity of sick-nursing. This includes a model for pre-professional nursing that permits an inclusive approach to work by men as well as women, unpaid as well as paid nurses. It concludes with a brief outline of each chapter and the place of different cohorts of nurses in constituting the professional roots of modern nursing.

The history of nursing

Margaret Pelling's foundational article about nursing in the early modern period observed 'it is quite difficult to decide whether the early modern sick-nurse existed in England at all before the late seventeenth century'.[29] Hers is the first serious attempt to identify and evaluate the sick-nurse well before the period of reform, in part by extending the terms of historians' inquiry to people recorded as 'keeping' or working as 'nurse-keepers'. Ian Mortimer's subsequent research encourages us to conclude that the sick-nurse existed, but she was not known by the title 'nurse'; the modern label is itself a product of changes in describing different types of care and medically related work between 1650 and 1700 which loosely speaking (and confirming Pelling) transitioned from keepers, to nurse-keepers, to nurses at around the same time in both London and Kent.[30] Mortimer's analysis of probate accounts is positioned to speak to the marketplace for medical services, but is even more convincing (in my view) in relation to commercialised caring services. Consequently the work of both of these historians underlies the research for this book and provides touchstones for this treatment of the long eighteenth century, traditionally set down as the 'dark ages' of nursing provision.[31] Echoing Borsay, Mortimer perceives the title nurse becoming a semi-occupational label in the second half of the seventeenth century, representing a more specialised skill set than merely attending or keeping, and one which largely excluded men, the very poor, or people who were entirely inexperienced in nursing activity.[32]

Historians from Alice Clark onwards have assumed that, lacking either spiritual inspiration or convincing material reward, recruits to paid nursing were motivated solely by their need to earn a living and thus 'did not represent the most efficient type of women'.[33] Successors to Clark have essentially characterised nurses as domestic servants, who chiefly worked as cleaners in a more than usually filthy environment.[34] Economic histories of the female labour market observe the extent of participation by women in nursing, usually undifferentiated between sick-nursing, wet nursing, and nursery nursing, and the propensity of nursing to be undertaken by spinsters, wives, or widows.[35] A focus on activity and 'doings' rather than occupational labels reveals the discrepancy between male and female 'repertoires of practices' showing the ways that behaviour could be more flexible (if only a little more flexible, in the case of nursing) than labels imply.[36] The amount of time spent on unpaid care work, and its significance for the wider economy, has been routinely undervalued by historians and economists as 'non-work'.[37]

The need to work as a paid nurse for either men or women has been seen as expressive of economic precarity; the relatively high weekly wages for plague nurses were anomalous. Nursing work for women may have become even less remunerative towards the end of the seventeenth century. Mortimer ascribes this to the decline of the plague, and the lifting of pressure to pay high wages in acknowledgment of nurses' bodily risk.[38] To this, labour historians might add that the feminisation which Mortimer also identifies was itself a driver towards lower pay, because 'hiring women meant reduced labour costs'.[39] It is not clear whether anyone before 1820 could earn a reliable weekly income from domiciliary but non-residential nursing activity. Research to date suggests that if it was possible the scope only pertained in larger towns or in London, but that if women or men nursed for a multitude of different employers, then they could acquire a relatively stable occupational identity as a nurse.[40]

There has been additional focus in the literature about the boundaries between nursing and medical work, with historians being generally keen to emphasise the validity of women's informal medical role. Mortimer and Thorpe stress the need for plague nurses to take the medical initiative in the absence of other healthcare practitioners visiting an afflicted household: was this also the case in the decades after the disappearance of plague?[41] A certain amount of medical judgement was required too by metropolitan searchers of the dead, during and after the plague years, and like plague nurses the searchers were subject to similar accusations of ignorance or worse.[42] The ongoing presences of handywomen – drawn from the ordinary labouring population rather than the educated middling or elite – were possibly as ubiquitous as they are now difficult to detect. All of this means that, if there was a 'medical revolution' in the eighteenth century, female practitioners were not noticeably part of the corresponding upswing in commercial provision.[43] That said, King stresses the diversity of women's healthcare work in the period after 1750 and finds individual women being trusted with medical procedures. Lucy Goodwin of Ardington was a surgeoness without the name.[44] This is the start of a useful corrective, in the sense that the apparent male domination of medicine in forms of training and recognition can be adjusted to accommodate an array of feminine expertise.[45] What this focus on medicine does not necessarily do, however, is to seek continuities between the pre- and post-reform sick-nurse and their delivery of *care* distinct from medicine. Nightingale and other nurse leaders were emphatic that the changes they advocated and oversaw were not concerned with turning nurses into quasi-medical practitioners. This requires us to disentangle the tasks, skills, and attitudes of people called 'nurse' to trace the foundations of the modern sick-nursing role.

Existing recent research specifically on nursing does not necessarily wield the appropriate level of authority. Tanya Langtree's research comes from her position as a twenty-first century nurse rather than her immersion in the traditions of historical inquiry.[46] Her search for continuities is therefore unique but uninformed by the historiography. She draws on a body of twenty-four texts in five different languages to chart the advice literature on nursing issued by individual and collective authors across Europe and North America between the sixteenth and early nineteenth centuries. This gives her ample opportunities to see the ways that Nightingale's recommendations summarised and digested existing expertise rather than wholly innovating in nurse practice. She does not, however, consider the scope for discrepancy between advice and lived experience, nor the impact of different cultures, contexts, and centuries on her findings. Furthermore, her work sits outside of existing debates: Pelling and Mortimer, for example, are both missing from her coverage.

One systematic, consistent, and potentially continuous way to assess the activities of nurses in the period 1660 to 1820 is to investigate their involvement with parish poor relief. Parochial welfare was the recourse of all ordinary poor people who were unable to meet the cost of their own treatment, medicines, food, care, or household assistance in times of illness.[47] It is not surprising, therefore, that records of the Old Poor Law have given rise to the fullest considerations of pre-reform nursing to date. Samantha Williams surveys the varieties of nursing on offer in the eighteenth and early nineteenth centuries, ranging from the simpler tasks of watching and cleaning to more sophisticated work such as dressing wounds or the application of treatment regimes in epidemics like smallpox. She speculates that the scope for employment and recognition of women adept at the more advanced forms of care, and the money available for any variety of parish-funded care, was in decline.[48] If correct, this raises (for the first time in the literature) the possibility that nurses in the 1820s and onwards had not always been uniformly reprehensible. Instead, nurse reputations may have been at their nadir in the second quarter of the nineteenth century. This does not necessarily require there to have been anything akin to a golden age at any earlier date: rather, it begins to suggest that, after the last epidemic of plague, nurses' status was uncertain, fluctuating, with sporadic development of skill and patient trust, in ways which became much less allowable as the nineteenth century progressed.

Jeremy Boulton used the overseers' accounts of the metropolitan parish of St Martin-in-the-Fields to identify three, at the time astonishing, aspects of parish provision in London in the three decades up to 1725. First, a very significant proportion of all overseers' spending, 11–18 per cent, was devoted to the cost of nurse care. Second, large sums of money were paid annually to a small cohort of women, who with the help of staff delivered broad-spectrum care to numerous children and to older people, as well as to the sick: they were community-based nurse coordinators running houses for treatment and recovery. Third, settlement examinations reveal some fine detail about the life experiences of selected women, confirming their profile as older women with experience of running households and the capacity to specialise in different types of care while still enduring financial marginality. The prominence of female-run nursing establishments was relatively short-lived, though, being superseded by the parish workhouse (specifically in 1725 within St Martins, and perhaps pervasively across London).[49]

This localised pattern of nursing the parish poor by semi-institutional means had equivalents across numerous counties in the English provinces in the late eighteenth and early nineteenth centuries, albeit at a smaller scale than was required for overcrowded London parishes. Steven King has given an authoritative account spanning seven counties. The patchier presence of workhouses in particularly rural areas was perhaps one of the factors which saw nursing provision after 1750 become a 'discrete service': in other words, the amount spent on nursing was independent of parish welfare for strictly medical relief such as payments to practitioners or on medicines.[50] That said, the proportion of spending on nursing services by parishes fell overall but concealed different styles of parish commitment to nursing care. In one model, characteristic of rural parishes, 'nursing was clearly written into the very fabric of poor relief' routinely comprising the most prominent form of relief after cash.[51] Elsewhere, spending dedicated to nursing was either substantial but intermittent, or low level and very patchy. Even so, parish opportunities are found to have comprised 'a formidable opportunity for female labour force participation'.[52]

Little of this work has had much impact on re-evaluations of sick-nurses as precursors to their trained descendants of the nineteenth century and later, despite King's determined use of the word 'professional' to describe the women (not the relatively few men) he finds in parish employment. There is a prima facie case for querying this pre-emptive professional label on the grounds of training, which was casual and experiential rather than organised or systematic (although we might not now perceive ad hoc training for women in this period as a negative feature of their background). Jacques Carré has pointed to the absence of formal training for hospital nurses.[53] Nonetheless, the coincidental commentary available from the records of St Bartholomew's Hospital in London (discussed in Chapter 2) and provincial infirmaries (in Chapter 3) suggests that aptitude and cumulative experience were likely to be badged in ways we do not immediately now recognise as comprising training. If nurses in eighteenth-century hospitals picked up their skills as they went along, their capacity was likely to be recorded as 'good behaviour' rather than increasing expertise.[54] Similarly searchers of the dead could acquire skills over many years as 'searcher-sextonesses' in London while also being castigated by male medical authors.[55] Instead of their acquiring proto-professional characteristics, any women identified in the majority of histories mentioning pre-reform nurses are characterised as 'women on the edge', in the manner of Lara Thorpe on plague nurses, as alternative medical practitioners, as aberrantly independent women in line with Margaret Pelling's reading of contemporary mores, or as part of the pattern of women's work under the auspices of parish welfare provision where the focus remains largely on the benefits available to poor recipients rather than on the nurses. Men as pre-reform nurses have not made any noticeable appearance in the historiography (within or beyond the context of poor relief).[56]

Research on naval nursing (rather than parish nursing) comes the closest to offering a reassessment of nurses in the long eighteenth century with the scope to establish pre-professional norms. Geoff Hudson's examination of nurse behaviours at the Greenwich Hospital is being augmented by Erin Spinney's extensive work on nurses at Haslar, in other naval hospitals such as at Plymouth, and on hospital ships.[57] The latter in particular evades 'a traditional nursing history narrative' to see nurses as individuals with careers, capabilities, and personal concerns.[58] Their reward might have been seen in their contractual remuneration, with pay rises, or in alternative indicators of esteem such as the award of superannuation for long service.[59]

The fine-grained prosopographical approach used by Spinney enables her to challenge the unfortunate conclusion that low pay must have entailed unremittingly low-grade work: women may have acquired extensive experience, or even performed with expertise and accomplishment, and nonetheless be paid relatively poorly. The commission of nursing work by poor women need not, ultimately, have condemned either the work or the women. It frequently had this effect for contemporaries, but the same responses need not be accepted uncritically by nursing histories any longer. This is particularly the case if historians can accept that nurses might sporadically have been highly regarded even in the context of reactions to poor, older women more broadly, and to the conditions of nursing service in this period.

The social context of the pre-professional nurse

Nurses working in any capacity, in domestic, institutional, or emergency nursing, were all subject to contextual criteria relating to their gender, age, income, and social status.[60] At the same time the circumstances of their care work created a localised context which was difficult to escape. These factors combined to create a mesh of negativity and ideological contradiction which beset women and men.[61]

Nurses were predominantly women in a context where household medicine was the first recourse in all but the most urgent cases. Wives, mothers, daughters, and sisters were expected to be ready and competent to nurse adult men, children, and each other when the occasion required.[62] So far as we can surmise from the literature to date, these expectations were relatively constant over the period, and only lightly differentiated by status.[63] These background assumptions arguably posed difficulties for any men who either wanted or were compelled to care for others. A feminised occupation that was relatively undifferentiated by social background was an inherent challenge to normative masculinity and opened the way for self-conception incorporating (or for external allegations of) effeminacy.[64] The predominant masculine role among the sick and wounded was as a practitioner of medicine.

There is also a body of evidence, reinforced throughout the forthcoming chapters, that across the period women who nursed were predominantly over 35–40 years of age. Women appointed as nurses in institutions were often (or necessarily) widows, in their forties or older.[65] There was a concomitant connection between denigration of nurses and their age or life cycle stage, as indicated brusquely in the quote at the start of this Introduction.[66] These negative judgements had specifically medical connotations within the Aristotelian scientific tradition: in the sixteenth century, and at its most extreme, old women were even thought to be capable of poisoning children with just a glance.[67] There is no indication that anyone believed this in the period after 1660 and, as Pelling observes, post-menopausal women could be seen as possessing useful attributes: nonetheless, an antipathy to older women remained on a number of grounds, perhaps because, as Elizabeth Delaval remarked in 1664, 'our aged body puts them in mind of their own mortality'.[68] Elderliness was susceptible to additional markers for women, because widowhood has been described as a 'social version of old age'.[69] Widows at the point of their bereavement potentially lost household income at the least, and at worst they were deprived of home and possessions in such a way as to damage all hopes of remarriage. Widows with property were an attractive marriage prospect; poor widows much less so.[70] In less tangible ways they may have felt undermined by a loss of identity, and have been encouraged to take up nursing from a desire to contribute to community requirements, although this would be difficult to prove in this period. There is no equivalent life stage perceptible for male nurses, not least because finding men in numbers for any nursing context has proved challenging. Instead, the emphasis among those recruiting men to nursing or equivalent roles (asylum keeper, military hospital orderly) was on physical strength for the purposes of lifting or restraint. This entailed another fundamental mismatch between the women and men who nursed, and one which spoke to the supposed physical capacity of each gender in potentially detrimental ways. If women were older widows, in physical and mental decline such that their attention to patients was undermined, men were muscular and therefore at risk of too much energetic intervention in patient care.

Negativity around age was probably exacerbated by lack of material worth.[71] Despite Mortimer's sanguine conclusion that skilled nursing excluded the very poor in the later seventeenth century, nurses frequently experienced absolute or relative poverty. They were either explicitly trying to make ends meet (as in the case of parish nurses, wherever their pay was supplemented by relief, or where parish work was succeeded by parish relief) or they were paid by employers at a level that they could not have afforded themselves (i.e. the nurses would have struggled to pay other people at the same rates to nurse *them* in illness).[72] Firm evidence is sparse, but generally points in the same direction. Thorpe confirms, for example, that plague nurses in St Margaret's parish London were drawn from among the poorest; remaining in the early part of the period Thomas Firmin estimated that nurse-keeping was something which might offer women wages for just three or four months in each year.[73] Nursing in the later seventeenth century, we might assume, was casual or intermittent, especially when working in homes or at least beyond institutions, while hard evidence about their pay is patchy. In 1712 'a nurse could not be had under 4s a week & victuals' for the Quaker workhouse at Clerkenwell.[74] Towards the end of the eighteenth century, Eden's review of the Shopkeepers' Friendly Society found that 5s 6d per week was allowed to pay a nurse in the suburbs of London.[75] This would have been just about adequate, particularly if accommodation was included, but offered no buffer against weeks of unemployment. The wider European scene provides additional circumstantial confirmation. Research on Sweden between 1550 and 1820 has found that heavy, repetitive, unpleasant and time-consuming work was generally taken by people of low status in subordinate positions.[76]

Nurses' remuneration was essentially uncertain despite the fact that nurses' services were sometimes in high demand and had to be paid for more generously at times of pressure on the flexible participants in the workforce.[77] The extent of nursing capacity might therefore have been modest. Nurses in Kentish probate accounts were drawn from a finite, relatively small labour pool, and after 1780 parishes in Berkshire, Norfolk, Northamptonshire, and Wiltshire only employed between one and two nurses each per year.[78] 'Professional' parish nurses were prominent in selected counties 1750–1834 which, contradicting Williams, implies some maintenance or enhancement of recognised 'extra-parochial' nurses' skill set over time.[79]

It is difficult to detect whether the racial background of nurses was an additional factor in their denigration, in the way that racist abuse has plainly been a factor in the treatment of nurses from the second half of the twentieth century onwards.[80] In the historical records, the presence of distinctive surnames, or descriptions of the women and men which might have identified them as, for example, Irish or people of colour, is very rare. Consequently, racial diversity will be noted below only occasionally. Small sections in Chapters 1 and 5 reveal a positive set of responses to nurses, both women and men, with African and Caribbean heritage.[81]

Nurses definitely experienced a problematic social position beyond their markers of gender, poverty, and race, because nurses were constantly required to act as intermediaries. Most obviously, nurses were deputised by physicians during their absence meaning that Thomas Tryon, at least, described nurses in the late seventeenth century as the doctors' 'Tutor'd Creatures'.[82] A contributor to the *Gentleman's Magazine* in 1752 took the unusual step of placing himself in the nurse's shoes to endorse their deference to male expertise: 'If I was a nurse, I think I should like to have some superior to receive orders from' he wrote, neatly avoiding the question of what a nurse should do under changing circumstances, or in the absence of the superintending medical man.[83] A nurse also acted as a go-between for the patient with the outside world (their relations, employers, employees, and others) where scrupulous attention to one party might well entail neglecting the interests of the other.[84] In extremis, they might have to act in the patient's best interests without reference to the unconscious or incapable patient's own immediate views.[85] Patients feared the consequences of devolved responsibility and the associated loss of control and risks of helplessness.[86] Furthermore, if one of the tasks of nursing attendance was 'barring inappropriate visitors from the sick room', the nurse might have to contradict the preferences of both patient and visitor at the same time.[87] Like searchers of the dead, sick-nurses struggled with a position which was simultaneously 'authoritative but marginal'.[88] Nurses could thus find themselves 'caught within a net of competing demands' in common with low-level employees (women and men) in other contexts.[89] The problems of a role which combines the inherent need for a measure of deference with the exertion of authority (of a kind which may preserve health and save lives) have been flagged for twentieth-century workers.[90] There has also been recent recognition of the emotion work entailed in taking account of multiple sources of social pressure, a recognition that formed no part of the perception of nurses' tasks in the period 1660 to 1820 but which – it will be argued throughout this book – were a tangible component of nurses' experience nonetheless.[91]

Despite their relative poverty and the liminality of their standing, 'history from below' has leapfrogged the nurse so far. The desire to witness change over time from the perspective of the working classes, the 'crowd', or in France the sans-culottes, which was pioneered in the early 1960s, had a profound influence on histories of social relations, gender, and race. This intellectual driver made itself felt in the history of medicine when researchers turned away from the 'great men' who had identified diseases or devised innovative interventions and towards patients of all classes.[92] The significance of nurse experience was left behind, perhaps because Nightingale already appeared to secure recognition for women's work in the field and gave the impression that nursing histories had become so settled as to be unchallengeable.

Rebuttal of uniform negativity about the pre-reform nurse is both possible and urgent on the basis of gender and social history models to date, which draw on the dynamics of power and concepts of agency to restore the reputation of – respectively, for instance – older women and the parish poor. The grounds on which to address nurses' identities and experiences are legion, not least given the recent weight given in historiography and elsewhere to identity politics. In a cultural history sense, for example, female nurses in this period might now be seen as women in a medical context that were not available as legitimate objects of the male or the medical gaze and were denigrated accordingly.[93]

The position of nurses as servants, too, can be recast by turning the slur on its head: in a prosperous household, the first source of nursing other than family members was from the servants, female and male, already resident in the household.[94] To paraphrase Jane Whittle, the most common way for care work to be commercialised was via the domestic service sector.[95] The people who sought employment in nursing by advertisement in the late eighteenth century exploited the connection between service, housework, and care when they characterised themselves as suited to either (for instance) a housekeeper or sick-nurse role.[96] Nursing as a consequence of being a domestic servant conferred experience, and this experience was desirable among patients seeking attendants.[97]

Servants' prominence among domestic nursing for their employer's family was ubiquitous and probably little remarked upon if they worked well.[98] For example, the servants in the household of Faith Grey in 1813 were willing and reportedly anxious to nurse Grey's daughter Lucy when she fell ill. Lucy was 25, and able to express a preference, so she rejected their offer on unexpected grounds: 'Lucy said they would be too indulgent to her and if she was delirious, which she often was, a nurse would do better', presumably because a nurse based outside of the house and unfamiliar with the family would be better at her work for being *less* kind.[99] Consequently a nurse was recruited, and apparently not unduly blamed for Lucy's death less than a week later. Other households, too, appointed nurses 'to relieve the servants'.[100] Such shreds of evidence point to a very positive, if piecemeal, response to the servant as nurse.

The whole context of the pre-reform nurse can be seen in quite a different way in light of twentieth-century sociological and ethnographical research on 'dirty work'.[101] Margaret Pelling pointed in this direction when she flagged the degrading nature of aspects of early modern caregiving such as nappy changing, and the 'corrosive' consequences of nurses' contact with some illnesses.[102] It is now possible to push the analysis further, in ways that help to explain the fragile state of nurse reputations before 1820. Refining early work by Everett Hughes, Blake Ashforth, and Glen Kreiner have elaborated the nature of 'dirty work' to delineate categories based on occupational stereotypes.[103]

At first sight, this table supposes that there is unproblematic continuity between sociological definitions at the end of the twentieth century and nurse experiences from the seventeenth to the nineteenth centuries. Agreed norms around dirt and cleanliness, or the nature of work as unpleasant, will have changed significantly between 1660 and 1999.[104] It also takes to extremes the admission that the boundaries between the stigmatising criteria are blurred, and that 'many occupations appear to be tainted on multiple dimensions', conferring opprobrium on nurses at every turn.[105] Nonetheless, the chapters in this book will demonstrate that there are strong justifications for mapping contemporary commentary about dirt/repugnance/taint and the historic activity of nurses on to these criteria.

Furthermore, pre-reform nurses had only variable and unreliable access to what we might now term a 'status shield'.[106] This comprises a set of personal attributes or social resources that protect against stigma or emotional damage, initially construed by Arlie Hochschild as afforded by masculinity.[107] In the twentieth century,

Table 0.1 Applying the 'dirty work' model to pre-professional nursing

Hughes (from 1951 on)	Ashforth and Kreiner (1999)	Nurses 1660–1820
Physical taint	Direct contact with rubbish, effluent, or death such as mortuary attendant or	Contact with spoiled dressings, pus, vomit, urine, faeces, corpses and
	Polluting conditions such as sweatshop labour.	Rooms or wards containing the sick, dying, or dead.
Social taint	Regular contact with stigmatised people such as prison guards or	Contact with infectious, miserable, suffering patients and
	A relationship of servility to others such as receiving customer complaints.	Subordinate to doctors, patients, patient families, visitors, matrons, others.
Moral taint	Activity which could be construed as of doubtful virtue, such as erotic dancing or	Any individual behaviour in post which might include drinking alcohol and
	Methods which are deceptive/intrusive such as telemarketers.	Any actions which take initiative away from the practitioner or patient.

women's work was rendered more open to attack if in their role they were construed as distillations of femininity.[108] The predominance of women in nursing in the years before 1820 encourages a tentative application of the gendered shielding concept, and failures of shielding, to the rhetorics surrounding women's activity. It is plausible that unpaid nurses were guarded against the full range of deprecation posited by Ashforth and Kreiner because their work was conducted within the family for no obvious material reward as a daughter, wife, mother, or sister; in other words, they were aligning with expectations for quintessential femininity in an environment that conferred a status shield on occasions of external observation.[109] Their payment was presumed to derive from the gratification or pleasure they experienced at offering succour to a relation and thereby doing their duty.[110] This shield did not necessarily always pertain within the family, leaving women open to household or family criticism, or to self-criticism if they did not feel the caring emotions they were required to espouse.[111] In contrast, the 'common nurse' who was paid for her work in coin rather than kinship affection was denigrated as a 'hireling stranger' (in ways that probably intensified towards the end of the period).[112] She had to secure protective prestige in other, less convincing ways, perhaps through endorsements by medical practitioners, testimonials from former patients, or less tangibly the confidence conferred by valued work performance in a familiar setting.[113] In the absence of external reinforcements of nurses' authority, and if Hochschild's analyses had purchase in an earlier century, they were at greater risk of becoming scapegoats: this was clearly the case for the plague nurses.[114] The chapters which follow draw emphatically on Ashforth, Kreiner, and Hochschild as offering a means to interpret the experiences of pre-1820 nurses, and on the work of subsequent sociologists and historians who have refined or adjusted their analyses.

The general social context for nurses between 1660 and 1820, when seen in combination with this model, offers a checklist of reasons why nursing, whether by women or men, was at constant risk of denigration under different domestic and institutional circumstances. In addition, the model provides further insight into the way that narratives of reform functioned. Ashforth and Kreiner envisage three ways in which workers in 'dirty' occupations might evade the different varieties of taint to secure more favourable conceptions of themselves and their pursuits: 'reframing' transforms the meaning of stigmatised work; 'recalibrating' adjusts the criteria invoked to assess dirty work; and 'refocusing' draws attention away from the dirty aspects of work to prioritise other less problematic parts of the job. Reformers' achievement in conferring high prestige to nursing in the second half of the nineteenth century can feasibly be understood as a 'reframing' of nursing tasks as a 'mission', whereby 'The "dirty particulars" are wrapped in more abstract and uplifting values'.[115] This was explicitly the goal for the Protestant nursing sisterhoods which aimed at social and spiritual elevation for their trainees.[116] Alison Bashford has made a strong case for the differentiation between 'old' and 'new' nurses having been made on the grounds of dirt and chaos supplanted by cleanliness, 'ethereal spirituality and purity'.[117] In the late twentieth century, such reframing has permitted group cohesion and very positive constructions of identity for otherwise 'dirty' workers. Before 1900, though, the act of reframing involved an overemphasis on the failings of pre-reform nurses.[118]

This book supplies a history of nursing which acknowledges negative preconditions for contemporary commentary on nurses, and for subsequent dismissals of nurses in the pre-reform phase, which in common with Boulton, King, and Spinney seeks evidence of actual nurse practice in sick-nursing. For the first time, it inserts the activities of acute and chronic sick-nursing as far as possible into the life experience of the women and men who undertook care work. In this way, it places pre-professional nursing within our understanding of 'the place of work in identity formation of women'.[119]

Methodological approaches to nursing the English between 1660 and 1820

This history begins in 1660 in recognition of a number of milestones. Nursing during the English Civil War has been addressed somewhat by Eric Gruber von Arni.[120] The war and Interregnum represent a clear break with the past which influenced bodily fortunes and the need for care across disparate communities and throughout all social ranks. Therefore, to start in 1660 is to recognise the anomalous nature of nursing, and the distinctive military characteristics of the national need for nurses *c.*1640–60, and to reserve them for discrete treatment elsewhere. It also allows a short approach to the final major epidemic of plague in England, an outbreak which engendered a particularly negative stereotype for nurses, plus a longer entrée to the conflation of the occupational descriptor 'nurse' with the activity of sick-nursing identified by Mortimer.[121] The year 1820 has been chosen as the point to stop, for two reasons. Firstly, 1820 was the year of Nightingale's birth, and is therefore taken as a significant marker in the history of nursing per se. By ending in this year, the analysis also avoids any remote chance that Nightingale had an influence over perspectives on nursing up to this time. Secondly, it was the year when the revival of the Protestant deaconess movement, which so influenced Nightingale and others, was first mooted in continental writing.[122] The deaconesses were established in imitation of the Catholic Sisters of Mercy, whose devotion to nursing impressed international commentators during the wars of 1793–1815.[123] Admittedly the call for vocational Protestant nurses was initially published to little immediate, practical effect, but the same impulse motivated Pastor Fliedner of Kaiserswerth to establish his institution in 1836, which Elizabeth Fry and Florence Nightingale subsequently visited.[124] It seemed appropriate that any discussion of nursing before Nightingale should stop before the major narratives of nurse reform were activated.

The person who claimed the title 'nurse', despite any consolidation of the word away from children and towards illness, may have meant to signal a number of different skills, employment backgrounds, or life cycle roles between 1660 and 1820. 'Nurses' became attendants on the sick, yet the same label continued to be attached to the main carers for young children. The label was also conferred on women who had once looked after children and were now superannuated, but maintained an affectionate relationship with their now-adult charges. Therefore, the simple appearance of the word 'nurse' among primary materials does not inevitably refer to an attendant on the sick, injured, or dying. Consequently, any reference to a 'nurse' in the sources used here had also to be qualified as clearly distinguished from children's nurses. Phrases such as 'common nurse', 'sick-nurse', 'day nurse' and 'night nurse' were taken as reasonable synonyms for those given charge of ill or injured persons, while 'monthly nurse' or 'wet nurse' flagged people who were chiefly concerned with children and parturient mothers who were otherwise in good health.[125]

Attention to terminology does not get around the fact that the same women might be employed as both sick-nurses and children's nurses, depending on context, opportunity, age, or other factors. Personal writings reinforce this sense of occupational instability where, for example, Ellen Weeton indicated her own confusion over the difference between the two sorts of employee, and in fiction Sarah Trimmer's Nurse Wilden points to sick- and children's nurses being one and the same.[126] What is the value of separating nurses for the sick, if they were not regarded as separate in the minds of contemporaries?

I argue here that the historiography demands some separation of sick-nurses from children's nurses, given the dominance of the professionalising hospital nurse in the literature to date. Child-minding and nursery provision acquired no such authoritative status until the final third of the twentieth century. This disaggregation of sick nursing and childcare after 1820 requires us to search for the roots of each activity as somewhat distinct.

A similar sort of concern accounts for the omission of matrons – i.e. institutional housekeepers – from this analysis. Borsay points to their 'managerial role' and lower-middling status, and across the research for this book no examples emerged of nurses who went on to secure permanent appointment as an institutional matron in either London hospitals or provincial infirmaries.[127] Consequently, the only matrons discussed below are the women who were appointed to the Royal Hospital at Chelsea, denominated 'matrons' from its earliest foundation but patently with a working profile nearer to that of a nurse. The post of superior female employee at Chelsea was called the 'housekeeper', and that female role is not examined in any depth in Chapter 4.

Patricia D'Antonio has urged us to give attention to the prereform tensions between physicians and nurses as each type of practitioner 'sought to assert the centrality of their alliance with the sick patient'.[128] The nature of this relationship for nurses as sitting between medical practitioners, patients, and others can be further delineated depending on settings for the delivery of care, and where that care falls on the spectrum of moral to contractual responsibility.

Table 0.2 of necessity simplifies the context of nursing, given that, for example, one-to-many nursing could look rather like many-to-many nursing in a large urban institution. Similarly, an ordinary household might effectually offer many-to-one nursing to children whose high status depended on parental tenderness owing to their juvenile age and/or on status secured from their family position such as via birth order (since they would generally be too young to hold high status as a result of worldly success). Nonetheless this stylised model enables us to differentiate normal from emergency activity, and household from institutional arrangements, in the pre-professional era. One-to-one nursing comprised

Table 0.2 Categories of pre-professional nursing activity

	Typical	Atypical
Patient is priority	One-to-one care, offered chiefly in domestic settings (for example adult children to elderly parents, employees to employers, etc).	Many-to-one care, offered when there is an excess of resource or a high-status patient (for example royal or aristocratic households, during crisis such as death-bed illness, etc).
Staffing is priority	One-to-many care, offered in institutions (for example hospitals, workhouses, gaols or asylums divisible by ward).	Many-to-many care, offered in large-scale emergencies (for example during riot, war, epidemic, famine, etc).

the status quo. Nursing in this context was sub-professional and to some extent ahistorical given norms of human behaviour between close relations. Such nursing took place at all periods in recorded human history before 1820 and thus far in all decades afterwards. Many-to-one nursing was and is the elite ideal, being supra-professional in the sense that nursing reform made little difference to the balance of multiple practitioners for one patient. While not entirely ahistorical, this activity has been resistant to change and seems likely to persist wherever social superiority (however gauged) promotes a concentration of nursing personnel around a high-status individual. One-to-many nursing involves one nurse being responsible for multiple patients, typified by the nurse working on an infirmary or hospital ward. This generated the environment in which proto-professional nursing emerged, both a little before 1820 and after, to meet the demands of a new therapeutic approach.[129] Many-to-many nursing saw large patient cohorts such as multitudinous soldiers being attended by numerous formal or informal nurses, and it was coincidentally warfare in the 1850s which accelerated the movement for professional nursing by women.[130]

This model assumes that any form of care, whether inside the home or beyond it, whether remunerated or unpaid, 'counts' as nursing.[131] It enables, at last, a systematic response to Margaret Versluyson's call of 1980 to this end and contradicts the inequity of economic histories that are incurious about aspects of unpaid care work.[132] It conflates nursing work and work undertaken by nurses rather than differentiating between them, in order to compose a history of nurses as well as a history of nursing.[133]

Anne Borsay's chapter of 2012 provides a partial road map for this research.[134] In the chapters below, nurses are identified through personal, institutional, and public records, making extensive use of digital and genealogical sources, to reveal a more subtle history of nursing by women and men than has been achieved to date. The result of this approach is a compilation of hundreds of references to nurses by occupational label and by activity, in London and the provinces, across sixteen decades. The data have been organised partly on the basis of gender, partly by source type, and partly by institutional structure.

The personal, literary material is drawn from letters, diaries, and memoirs. Personal sources vary widely in their composition, typical content, and therefore application in this research. Letters were written with an immediacy and attention to the everyday which is not typically found in the other two genres, but which is self-censored by writers depending on the recipient and the likely circulation of the letter. Diaries by definition record those parts of life which are different to the days which become before or after, to note the distinctive features of a day. This means they are not well purposed to capture repetitive aspects of nursing work, but are more fruitful for the duration of a nurse's attention and its beginning or end. Memoirs are more heavily edited than either letters or diaries, giving rise to writers being prey to influences other than the events they describe, such as the conventions of their peers (by gender, age, status or race) and of the evolution of the form. A memoir written in 1850 will have been guided by different models to one written in 1800. These different variations and limitations are noticed and accommodated in Chapters 1, 5, and 6. A quality common to all of these narratives, however, was their capacity to incorporate reference to the emotion work demanded from nurses. Emotional labour was only considered by observers of nursing at this time in the crudest terms, as the discussion of ideal and antithetical nurses in Chapter 1 implies, but it is a part of twenty-first century sociological understandings of the role.[135] Wherever possible, this book gives priority to evidence of feelings among carers rather than solely those reported for patients.

The literary chapters draw too on sporadic examples of medical advice literature and on fiction including stories for children as offering theoretical or ideal perspectives on nurses. They do not, though, feature much engagement with the personal papers of medical practitioners. This is surprising, on the face of it, since practitioners were among the people who gave direction to nurses in terms of patient medicine, care, and the need for information about changes in patients' condition. Why were these men apparently blind to hospital nurses, as servants if they were not construed as coworkers? In a different century, another country, and a lower social context than that to which these medical men belonged, Merry Wiesner found that men's acknowledgement that they worked alongside women risked reputational damage, namely a reduction in their ownership of skill.[136] Was medical masculinity tainted by proximity to female workers as has been argued for men's occupational experience in the early modern period more widely? Or were nurses seen as competitors for expertise? Practitioners' sentiments may have been a complex mix of these two factors and more. Nurses were certainly reproached for usurping male medical territory, as at St Thomas's Hospital in 1704 when Deborah Covell or Cowill, the nurse of Susannah ward, was dismissed for usurping male medical functions when she prepared medicines and bled patients.[137] Whatever the considerations, medical letters, diaries, and memoirs are generally not the place to find evidence of nurse experience.

Hospitals are central to histories of the trained nurse and are no less significant for her predecessors, even when acknowledging the huge but unquantifiable gap between the demand for nursing care in the pre-reform period and comparatively slim hospital capacities.[138] Institutional records left by hospitals in this period rarely contain documents exclusively related to nursing staff. They do, however, feature the minutes of management meetings which observe the recruitment, behaviour, and dismissal of nurses to some extent. The governors of the Chester Infirmary, for example, began well but quickly learned to omit day-to-day evidence of nurses' employment in among the minutes. Their counterparts in Stafford were more punctilious, alluding to named nurses consistently from the time of the Stafford Infirmary's opening until 1820. The minutes kept for the governors of St Bartholomew's Hospital in London offer the most voluminous evidence of nurse engagement, since they recorded over six hundred women appointed as ward staff between 1660 and 1820. The name lists generated by routine recording, including the hospital musters held at Chelsea, provide the underlying data for Chapters 2, 3, and 4. The names of the women (very rarely men) retrieved by these means for institutions have been cross-referenced with the digitised materials characterised below.

By the end of the period, workhouses probably formed the most pervasive institutional option for ordinary working people who did not align with the admissions criteria for voluntary hospitals. Nonetheless, they are discussed only lightly here. This apparent omission relates to research capacity and source survival: records of the Old Poor Law are ubiquitous in county archives, and the distribution of workhouses across England by the later eighteenth century would appear to make them the ideal focus for a consideration of institutional nursing. The problem lies in the detail available about either the women and men who performed the nursing work, and in the labour context of buildings that aspired to set the able-bodied poor to work but rarely did so reliably/continuously in practice. We may have lists of workhouse inmates, and know that in theory they were set to nurse each other in illness or when frail or dying, without possessing any specifics. Even where dedicated workhouse workbooks survive, they may simply record the occasions when paupers were sent out of the house to work, and account for the wages that the parish received on the paupers' behalf, rather than the mundane daily routines performed within the workhouse itself.[139] Therefore, workhouses and indeed charitable almshouses (residential settings for older people funded by voluntary charity) are mentioned briefly at the outset of Chapters 2, 3, and 4 respectively without their currently offering sufficient material for a discrete chapter.

Both literary and institutional sources are augmented throughout by reference to sporadic appearances by nurses in digitised sources of records in the public domain. Chief among these are the Burney collection of newspapers, the wills left by institutional employees and inmates and supplied via the National Archives website, parliamentary reports containing publications on prisons hosted by Proquest, and, in imitation of Anne Borsay, the Old Bailey Sessions Papers online. Beyond these cohorts of defined source materials, I have added recourse to the London Lives website which acts as a hub providing access to diverse manuscript sources, and the subscription service Findmypast as a source of amassed genealogical data. The personal and literary printed sources, and archival hospital records, have been read exhaustively, with references to nurses collected throughout. The additional digital sources have been annexed selectively for keywords around nursing and care. The perils of keyword searching are well known, particularly given the differential reliance of websites on (variously) optical character recognition, rekeying original texts, or calendaring, plus the absence of a uniform dictionary for either terminology or surnames in the long eighteenth century. These collective caveats mean that the connections made between nurses identified in one source whose personal histories are elaborated by reference to other sources comprise a reliable minimum of examples, rather than an aspiration to full coverage.

The array of viable sources raises questions about the nature of nursing. What activities and demeanours did nursing in this period ideally comprise? Tanya Langtree adopted the division of pre-professional nursing care set out in 1846 by Jonathan Waddy under the three headings of restoring health, preventing complications, and promoting comfort.[140] The effect of Langtree's focus on advice literature, though, means that medical authors and interventions are given prominence in her research, and the quotidian aspects of care are de-emphasised.[141] Therefore, while recognising many of the same activities as included in the acts of nursing, I prefer a more pragmatic categorisation of watching and regulating, feeding and administering, or cleaning and removing waste where the nurse rather than the patient is of central concern. Care under these headings gave rise to a multitude of typically small but repetitive tasks involving both physical and emotional supports. Regulating, for example, could relate equally to opening and closing windows to control the flow of fresh air, or to the amelioration of distress. Each of the categories of nurses considered in the chapters below will elaborate on a subset of these tasks. My analysis is less concerned with nurses taking the medical initiative, or with identifying folk healers at the boundaries of medical and nursing care, than with employment and activity quite tightly defined, and critically situated wherever possible in the life-course of the women and men concerned.

The presence of the antithesis of the ideal nurse is conceived here in the concept of the anti-nurse, the person with an ostensible, nominal, or humanitarian duty to care, who does not merely neglect the sick and injured but who predates upon them. This might be committed by theft or removal of goods, actively withholding requirements like food/water/medicine, denigrating or stigmatising a person (for the nature of their ailment, or on other grounds), or who can be judged cruel in their treatment occasioning undue pain or actively delaying recovery. The anti-nurse is a useful device for framing the contemporary criticisms levelled at nurses and differentiating between a failure to deliver care versus occasioning harm. The phrase is deployed in such a way as to challenge existing historiographical stereotyping of nurses rather than confirm it. Both the ideal and the anti-nurse stereotypes will be given consideration in Chapters 1, 5, and 6.

This is a coherent research project, but so far one which leaves the problem of change-over-time untackled. Margaret Pelling talks about the apparent 'sameness of low-status women's work' between the fourteenth and the eighteenth centuries as a trap that other authors have fallen into, and as a temptation that should be resisted if at all possible.[142] The limited available data about the take-up of paid nursing services across the eighteenth century suggest a narrow range of fluctuation in (specifically) nursing for the dying. Between 20 and 35 per cent of probate accounts, in London and the provinces, reference payments to nurses with slightly higher uptake around 1730 than either earlier or later.[143] It is not clear from the chapters which follow that there is a linear model to discern in nursing experience over the long eighteenth century. Instead, I will make an argument for ebbs and flows of opinion towards nurses between plague and Peterloo that do not constitute any kind of either concrete progress or decisive regression. The social history research material supports a different sort of account, one which charts the oscillations and reputational frailties for both female and male nurses that prefigure a decisively negative turn in the years after 1820.

Outline

Chapter 1 offers a survey of both advisory and fictional literature about the female domestic nurse, from the negativity towards plague nurses onwards. The ideal nurse is contrasted with women's lived experience, including testimony from literary spinsters whose life circumstances periodically required them to be nurses. The difficulty of separating sick-nursing from nursery nursing requires a shift in subsequent chapters to institutional settings. Chapter 2 focuses on England's most long-standing hospitals, namely St Bartholomew's and St Thomas's hospitals in London. The practices of nursing, and the experiences of postholders, span the period under study and underpin an argument for these paid women's adequacy or better under pre-reform expectations. The newer hospitals founded by subscription in the eighteenth century, fanning out into provincial England, expanded nurse employment and bring into view the challenges facing women who worked in settings lacking the grandeur and longevity of the ancient metropolitan hospitals. These infirmary nurses are the focus of Chapter 3. The origins of geriatric and state nursing are considered in Chapter 4, concentrating on the Royal Hospital at Chelsea. Chelsea's 'matrons' were employed for each residential ward and for the internal infirmary ward, giving rise to women's experience of nursing disability, chronic ill health, and at the end of life. Chapter 5 turns attention to the early history of nursing by men. This historiography is notably thin, dominated by male attendants of the mentally ill. The chapter will gain a view of men's domestic and institutional nursing and discuss the barriers which men faced if they became carers. Finally, Chapter 6 will move beyond England but not beyond the English, to evaluate nursing during wartime from 1793 to 1815. Men and women found themselves compelled or coerced into nursing tasks in emergencies, and particularly during conflict. Women who followed baggage trains held a pernicious reputation as plunderers of the dead, and men's military foes might be well placed to fulfil the role of stereotypical anti-nurse alluded to above; nonetheless, when faced with ghastly injury or mortal epidemics, nursing activity could become notable for its compassion, if under insanitary and understaffed circumstances, even across the lines of military conflict. The chapter will conclude by flagging up the significance of nursing in Brussels after the Battle of Waterloo, and the way that this nursing, plus the many succeeding literary reminders of the battle's aftermath, laid cultural groundwork for the ready acceptance of Nightingale's 'lady nurse'.

Notes

1 S. Johnson, *Dictionary* (1755), available Open Access (hereafter OA) at www.johnsonsdictionaryonline.com (accessed 15 June 2022).
2 S. Watts, *Epidemics and History: Disease, Power, and Imperialism* (New Haven, CT: Yale University Press, 1997), p. 1.
3 These judgements were a continuation of those aimed at nurses in earlier epidemics; see the frankly histrionic T. Dekker, *English Villainies* (London: Nicholas Gamage, 1648), chapter 15. Scientific misogyny was a feature of the Aristotelian traditions of medicine: H.R. Lemay, *Women's Secrets: A Translation of Pseudo-Albertus Magnus's De Secretis Mulierum with Commentaries* (Stoney Brook, NY: State University of New York Press, 1992), p. 47.
4 V.J., *Golgotha ... Against Cruel Shutting Up* (London: printed for the author, 1665), pp. 10, 13; G. Thomson, *Loimotomia* (London: Nath. Crouch, 1666), pp. 76, 116.
5 *The Shutting Up Infected Houses* (London: [no details], 1665), p. 9.
6 M. Pelling, *The Common Lot: Sickness, Medical Occupations, and the Urban Poor in Early Modern England* (London: Longman, 1998), p. 197; Essex Record Office, Q/SR 406/82–4, 106–7 recognisance, letter, and examinations relating to the petition against Ann Taylor, 1665. For the contested subject of servants' rights to cast-off clothing see T. Meldrum, *Domestic Service and Gender 1660–1750: Life and Work in the London Household* (Harlow: Longman, 2000), p. 199.
7 N. Hodges, *Loimologia: Or, An Historical Account of the Plague in London in 1665* (London: E. Bell and J. Osborn, 1720), p. 8 [composed by Hodges during the events of 1665 and of necessity before his death in 1688].

8 T. Vincent, *God's Terrible Voice in the City* (London: [no details], 1667), p. 34.
9 D. Defoe, *A Journal of the Plague Year* (London: E. Nutt at the Royal Exchange, J. Roberts in Warwick Lane, A Dodd without Temple Bar, and J. Graves St James Street, 1722), p. 98.
10 L. Thorpe, '"In the middest of death": Medical responses to the Great Plague of 1665 with special reference to John Allin' (PhD thesis, Royal Holloway, University of London, 2017), p. 227; Pelling, *Common Lot*, p. 183.
11 Pelling, *Common Lot*, p. 197.
12 I. Mortimer, *The Dying and the Doctors: The Medical Revolution in Seventeenth-Century England* (Woodbridge: Royal Historical Society, Boydell Press, 2009), p. 193.
13 Mortimer, *The Dying and the Doctors*, p. 156.
14 Pelling, *Common Lot*, p. 195.
15 S. Hancock, 'A plague nurse at Haverfordwest in 1652–3', *Pembrokeshire Historical Society Journal* (2017), available OA at www.pembrokeshirehistoricalsociety.co.uk (accessed 8 March 2018).
16 Mortimer, *The Dying and the Doctors*, p. 195.
17 L. Thorpe, 'At the mercy of strange women: Plague nurses, marginality, and fear during the Great Plague of 1665', L. Hopkins and A. Norrie (eds), *Women on the Edge in Early Modern Europe* (Amsterdam: Amsterdam University Press, 2019).
18 R.G. Huntsman, M. Bruin and D. Holttum, 'Twixt candle and lamp: The contribution of Elizabeth Fry and the Institution of Nursing Sisters to nursing reform', *Medical History* 46: 3 (2002), 351–80.
19 M. Stanley, *Hospitals and Sisterhoods* (London: John Murray, 1855), pp. 8, 15.
20 K. Williams, 'Ideologies of nursing: Their meanings and implications', R. Dingwall and J. McIntosh (eds), *Readings in the Sociology of Nursing* (Edinburgh: Churchill Livingstone, 1978), p. 39.
21 F. Nightingale, *Notes on Nursing – What It Is and What It Is Not* (London: Harrison, 1859), p. 6.
22 B. Abel-Smith, *A History of the Nursing Profession* (London: Heinemann, 1960), pp. 4–5.
23 A. Summers, 'The mysterious demise of Sarah Gamp: The domiciliary nurse and her detractors, c.1830–1860', *Victorian Studies* 32: 3 (1989), 365–86; C. Helmstadter, 'A third look at Sarah Gamp', *Canadian Bulletin of Medical History* 30: 2 (2013), 141–59. As Barbara Mortimer bluntly put it, 'The history of nursing has been dominated, overshadowed, and at times swamped by the iconic figure

Introduction 31

of Florence Nightingale'; B. Mortimer, 'Introduction', S. McGann and B. Mortimer (eds), *New Directions in Nursing History: International Perspectives* (London: Routledge, 2005), p. 2. Revisionism which tackles the 'holy imperatives' of nursing history around the centrality of Nightingale's role is a separate historiographical matter, discussed briefly in S. Nelson, 'The fork in the road: Nursing history versus the history of nursing?', *Nursing History Review* 10: 1 (2002), 175–88, quote on p. 178.
24 Pelling, *Common Lot*, p. 180.
25 C. Helmstadter, *Beyond Nightingale: Nursing on the Crimean War Battlefields* (Manchester: Manchester University Press, 2020), p. 31.
26 C. Helmstadter and J. Godden, *Nursing Before Nightingale 1815–1899* (Farnham: Routledge, 2011).
27 E. Spinney, 'Servants to the hospital and the state: Nurses in Plymouth and Haslar Naval hospitals, 1775–1815', *Journal for Maritime Research* 20: 1 (2019), 1–17; T. Langtree, 'Notes on pre-Nightingale nursing: What it was and what it was not' (PhD thesis, James Cook University, 2020). Nightingale's negative judgements about hospitals, in contrast, were challenged long ago: E.M. Sigsworth, 'Gateways to death? Medicine, hospitals and mortality, 1700–1850', P. Mathias (ed.), *Science and Society* (Cambridge: Cambridge University Press, 1972).
28 A. Borsay, 'Nursing 1700–1830: Families, Communities, Institutions', A. Borsay and B. Hunter (eds), *Nursing and Midwifery in Britain since 1700* (Basingstoke: Palgrave, 2012), p. 36.
29 Pelling, *Common Lot*, p. 180.
30 Mortimer, *The Dying and the Doctors*, chapter 5. A similar hardening of definition may also have been taking place at about the same time in Wales: A. Withey, *Physick and the Family: Health, Medicine and Care in Wales, 1600–1750* (Manchester: Manchester University Press, 2011), p. 178.
31 M.A. Nutting and L.L. Dock, *A History of Nursing* (New York: Putnam, 1907), volume I, chapter 14: 'The Dark Period of Nursing'.
32 Mortimer, *The Dying and the Doctors*, p. 169. M. Ågren, *Making a Living, Making a Difference: Gender and Work in Early Modern European Society* (Oxford: Oxford University Press, 2016), p. 138 also detects skill among women treating wounds.
33 A. Clark, *Working life of women in the seventeenth century* (London: Routledge, 1919), p. 244.
34 P. Williams, 'Religion, respectability and the origins of the modern nurse', R. French and A. Wear (eds), *British Medicine in an Age of*

Reform (London: Routledge, 1991), p. 233; Helmstadter and Godden, *Nursing Before Nightingale*, p. 8. L. McDonald, *Florence Nightingale at First Hand: Vision, Power, Legacy* (London: Continuum, 2010), pp. 104–6. The boundaries between nursing and domestic service have remained permeable; L. Hart, 'A ward of my own: Social organisation and identity among hospital domestics', P. Holden and J. Littlewood (eds), *Anthropology and Nursing* (London: Routledge, 1991), pp. 95–8, 106.

35 H. Barker, *The Business of Women: Female Enterprise and Urban Development in Northern England, 1760–1830* (Oxford: Oxford University Press, 2006), pp. 63, 186; P. Earle, 'The female labour market in London in the late seventeenth and early eighteenth centuries', *Economic History Review* 2nd ser. 42: 3 (1989), 328–53, on pp. 337, 339; P. Sharpe, 'Literally spinsters: A new interpretation of local economy and demography in Colyton in the seventeenth and eighteenth centuries', *Economic History Review* 44: 1 (1991), 46–65, on pp. 60–1; A. Shepard, 'Crediting women in the early modern English economy', *History Workshop Journal* 79: 1 (2015), 1–24, on pp. 9, 11–12, 14.

36 Ågren, *Making a Living*, p. 18.

37 J. Whittle, 'A critique of approaches to "domestic work": Women, work and the pre-industrial economy', *Past and Present* 243: 1 (2019), 35–70, on p. 54; for a very recent corrective see also A. Shepard, 'Care', C. Macleod, A. Shepard and M. Ågren (eds), *The Whole Economy: Work and Gender in Early Modern Europe* (Cambridge: Cambridge University Press, 2023), pp. 53–83.

38 Mortimer, *The Dying and the Doctors*, p. 170.

39 D. Simonton, *A History of European Women's Work 1700 to the Present* (London: Routledge, 1998), p. 170. Feminisation continues to mean a lower wage burden in the twenty-first century: E. Murphy and D. Oesch, 'The feminization of occupations and change in wages: A panel analysis of Britain, Germany and Switzerland', *Social Forces* 94: 3 (2016), 1221–55.

40 S. Williams, 'Caring for the sick poor. Poor Law nurses in Bedfordshire, *c.*1770–1834', P. Lane, N. Raven, and K.D.M. Snell (eds), *Women, Work and Wages in England, 1600–1850* (Woodbridge: Boydell, 2004), p. 156, for earnings by women in rural Bedfordshire; Borsay, 'Nursing 1700–1830' uses the Old Bailey sessions papers to this end. For a similar profile in Edinburgh see E.C. Sanderson, *Women and Work in Eighteenth-Century Edinburgh* (Basingstoke: Macmillan, 1996), p. 47. Susan Wright speculates that

nursing in eighteenth-century Ludlow did not necessarily supply a regular income: S. Wright, '"Holding up half the sky": Women and their occupations in eighteenth-century Ludlow', *Midland History* 14: 1 (1989), 53–74, on p. 56.
41 Mortimer, *The Dying and the Doctors*, p. 177; Thorpe, 'At the mercy', pp. 33, 38–9.
42 R. Munkhoff, 'Searchers of the dead: Authority, marginality, and the interpretation of plague in England, 1574–1665', *Gender & History* 11: 1 (1999), 1–29; W. Henry, 'Women searchers of the dead in eighteenth- and nineteenth-century London', *Social History of Medicine* 29: 3 (2016), 445–66.
43 P. Wallis and T. Pirohakul, 'Medical revolutions? The growth of medicine in England, 1660–1800', *Journal of Social History* 49: 3 (2016), 510–31, on p. 525.
44 S. King, *Sickness, Medical Welfare, and the English Poor, 1750–1834* (Manchester: Manchester University Press, 2018), p. 163.
45 Williams, 'Caring', p. 164.
46 Langtree, 'Notes'.
47 For an early and still excellent integration of Poor Law and charitable options for medicine and nursing, see M. Fissell, *Patients, Power, and the Poor in Eighteenth-Century Bristol* (Cambridge: Cambridge University Press, 1991).
48 Williams, 'Caring', pp. 164–7.
49 J. Boulton, 'Welfare systems and the parish nurse in early modern London, 1650–1725', *Family and Community History* 10: 2 (2007), 127–51.
50 King, *Sickness*, p. 160.
51 King, *Sickness*, p. 162.
52 S. King, 'Nursing under the Old Poor Law in midland and eastern England, 1780–1834', *Journal for the History of Medicine* 70: 4 (2014), 588–622, on p. 618.
53 J. Carré, 'Hospital nurses in eighteenth-century Britain: Service without responsibility', I. Baudino and J. Carré (eds), *The Invisible Woman: Aspects of Women's Work in Eighteenth-Century Britain* (London: Routledge, 2005).
54 This description of Poor Law nurses as 'professional' can be challenged further on numerous grounds, however, relating to the absence of an occupational framework, or any collective identity. I am grateful to Sue Hawkins for her observations on this point at the UK Association for the History of Nursing (UKAHN) colloquium, 5 July 2022.

55 Henry, 'Women searchers', pp. 457–9.
56 See A. Tomkins, 'Male nurses in England and Europe before 1820: Beyond the madhouse', *Nursing History Review* 31 (2023), 150–70.
57 G. Hudson, 'Internal influences in the making of the English military hospital: The early eighteenth-century Greenwich', G. Hudson (ed.), *British Military and Naval Medicine 1600–1830* (Amsterdam: Rodopi, 2007).
58 Spinney, 'Servants', p. 3.
59 Spinney, 'Servants', pp. 9–10.
60 M. Carpenter, 'The subordination of nurses in health care: Towards a social divisions approach', E. Riska and K. Wegar (eds), *Gender, Work and Medicine: Women and the Medical Division of Labour* (London: Sage, 1993), pp. 96–7. These contextual factors have more readily been examined for the reform era or later, and for literary sources, than for real women in the period up to 1820: see for example C. Judd, *Bedside Seductions: Nursing and the Victorian Imagination, 1840–80* (Basingstoke: Palgrave Macmillan, 1998).
61 Ideological contradiction is observed repeatedly in histories of nursing for the twentieth century: A. La Torre, '"Vast science and difficult art". The nurse in medical journals under fascism in Italy' and K. Roberts, 'An ambiguous presence: Wartime constructions of the body of the nurse', both in *UK Association for the History of Nursing Bulletin* 10: 1 (2022).
62 L.M. Beier, *Sufferers and Healers: The Experience of Illness in Seventeenth-Century England* (London: Routledge Kegan Paul, 1987), chapter 8: A. Vickery, *The Gentleman's Daughter: Women's Lives in Georgian England* (New Haven, CT: Yale University Press, 1998), pp. 117–20. This was also the case in Europe – see M. Stolberg, *Experiencing Illness and the Sick Body in Early-Modern Europe* (Basingstoke: Palgrave Macmillan, 2011), p. 56.
63 See, among a large literature, E. Leong, *Recipes and Everyday Knowledge: Medicine, Science, and the Household in Early Modern England* (Chicago, IL: University of Chicago Press, 2018), p. 61.
64 Discussed at more length in Chapter 5.
65 Earle, 'Female labour market', p. 343; King, 'Nursing', p. 614.
66 For changing understanding of the menopause, see R. Knoeff, 'Science, medicine and health', R. Brannon and S. Ottaway (eds), *A Cultural History of Old Age in the Era of Enlightenment and Revolution* (London: Bloomsbury, forthcoming).
67 Lemay, *Women's Secrets*, pp. 47, 129–31.

68 Pelling, *Common Lot*, p. 194. Delaval quoted in T. Reinke-Williams, 'Physical attractiveness and the female life-cycle in seventeenth-century England', *Cultural and Social History* 15: 4 (2018), 469–85, on p. 480.
69 C. Phythian-Adams, *Desolation of a City: Coventry and the Urban Crisis of the Late Middle Ages* (Cambridge: Cambridge University Press, 1979), p. 91.
70 S. Wright, 'The elderly and the bereaved in eighteenth-century Ludlow', M. Pelling and R. Smith (eds), *Life, Death, and the Elderly: Historical Perspectives* (London: Routledge, 1991), p. 126.
71 Positive readings of the menopause came from medical men in relation to their search for prosperous patients rather than from people with nothing to gain from the 'climacteric': Knoeff, 'Science'.
72 Williams, 'Caring', pp. 151–2 found that between 47 and 60 per cent of the people employed by parishes as carers needed poor relief at some time in their lives; a much smaller proportion required parish relief in the same years they were paid to care. M. Dresser (ed.), *The Diary of Sarah Fox nee Champion: Bristol 1745–1802* (Bristol: Bristol Record Society, 2003), pp. 30, 63, 114 for nurse Marsden, who in 1785 (after periods of employment in the diarist's family) seemed 'old, feeble, and appearing to be much neglected'.
73 Thorpe, 'At the mercy', p. 39; T. Firmin, *Some Proposals for the Employing of the Poor* (London: Brabazon Aylmer at the three Pigeons in Cornhill, 1678), p. 18, quoted by Earle, 'Female labour market', p. 342.
74 T.V. Hitchcock (ed.), *Richard Hutton's Complaints Book* (London: London Record Society, 1987), pp. 37–8.
75 F.M. Eden, *The State of the Poor*, volume I (London: J. Davis, 1797), p. 620.
76 Ågren, *Making a Living*, p. 140.
77 King, 'Nursing', p. 616 for nurses paid more at harvest time; Sharpe, 'Literally spinsters', p. 61 for nurses recruited by parish overseers sometimes being paid more than domestic servants.
78 Mortimer, *The Dying and the Doctors*, p. 139; King, 'Nursing', p. 605.
79 King, *Sickness*, p. 164.
80 See for example M.A. Shields and S.W. Price, 'Racial harassment, job satisfaction, and intentions to quit: Evidence from the British nursing profession', *Economica* 69: 274 (2002), 295–326.
81 The implications of race in parallel literatures, such as wet nursing in America, provide valuable context and scope for reflection to

an otherwise thin field for the pre-1900 period: S. Jones-Rogers, 'She could spare one ample breast for the profit of her owner: White mothers and enslaved wet nurses' invisible labour in American slave markets', *Slavery and Abolition* 38: 2 (2017), 337–55 and R.J. Knight and E. West, 'Mothers' milk: Slavery, wet-nursing, and black and white women in the Antebellum South', *Journal of Southern History* 83: 1 (2017), 37–68.
82 T. Tryon, *A Way to Health, Long Life and Happiness, or, A discourse of temperance* (London: Baldwin, 1691), p. 179.
83 *Gentleman's Magazine* volume XXII (1752), p. 405. The problematic nature of nurses deputising for doctors is discussed for the twentieth century in M. Jolley and G. Brykczynska, *Nursing: Its Hidden Agendas* (Suffolk: St Edmundsbury Press, 1993), p. 49.
84 'Anecdotes', *Oracle and Public Advertiser*, 24 September 1795 for Lord Northington ordering his nurse to exclude his female relations from the sickroom.
85 This exercise of nursing power over patients is also noted by twentieth-century sociology: Carpenter, 'Subordination of nurses', p. 98.
86 Pelling, *Common Lot*, p. 202, and reflected in the twentieth century by Williams, 'Ideologies of nursing', p. 43. Leong, *Recipes*, pp. 62–3, 66 makes the point that housekeepers liked to make their own medicines from a similar desire for control.
87 Borsay, 'Nursing 1700–1830', p. 25. The tension between deference and authority was also perceptible in institutional rather than domiciliary nursing: Carré, 'Hospital nurses', p. 90; Spinney, 'Servants', pp. 11–12.
88 K. Siena, 'Searchers of the dead in long eighteenth-century London', K. Kippen and L. Woods (eds), *Worth and Repute: Valuing Gender in Late Medieval and Early Modern Europe: Essays in honour of Barbara Todd* (Toronto: Centre for Reformation and Renaissance Studies, 2011), p. 125. By the twentieth century this tension had evolved into the untenable requirement for nurses to be simultaneously bold and passive: L. Stein, 'The nurse–doctor game', R. Dingwall and J. McIntosh (eds), *Readings in the Sociology of Nursing* (Edinburgh: Churchill Livingstone, 1978), p. 109.
89 S. Ottaway, '"A very bad president in the house": Workhouse masters, care, and discipline in the eighteenth-century workhouse', *Journal of Social History* 54: 4 (2021), 1091–119, on pp. 1092, 1096.
90 A.R. Hochschild, *The Managed Heart* (Berkeley, CA: University of California Press, 2012), p. 177.
91 K. Townsend, 'Do production employees engage in emotional labour?', *Journal of Industrial Relations* 50: 1 (2008), 175–80; C. Mansell,

'Reconstructing the labour of care in early modern England', *Historical Journal* 67: 1 (2023), 1–21.
92 J.C. Burnham, *How the Idea of Profession Changed the Writing of Medical History* (London: Medical History Supplement, 1998), pp. 42, 113–14.
93 This problem is not necessarily overcome by construing the nurse as a functionary of the gaze: Carpenter, 'Subordination of nurses', p. 102.
94 Meldrum, *Domestic Service*, p. 151 on the relationship between sick-nursing and employers' children; see also Pelling, *Common Lot*, p. 200; Mortimer, *The Dying and the Doctors*, p. 184; Wallis and Pirohakul, 'Medical revolutions?', p. 516.
95 Whittle, 'Critique', p. 65.
96 *Oracle and Daily Advertiser*, 9 April 1799.
97 See for example the value placed on a nurse's prior experience given in L.J. Clark (ed.), *The Letters of Sarah Harriet Burney* (Athens, GA: University of Georgia Press, 1997), p. 201.
98 In the period 1500 to 1700, 5.1 per cent of female servants' time and 2.7 per cent of male servants' time was taken up with care work, broadly defined: Whittle, 'Critique', p. 67.
99 A.V. Gray, *Papers and Diaries of a York Family, 1764–1839* (London: Sheldon Press, 1927), p. 200.
100 Bedfordshire Archives L30/14/333/49, Wrest Park [Lucas] Archive correspondence, letter to Thomas Robinson 20 October 1769.
101 E.C. Hughes, 'Work and the self', J.H. Rohrer and M. Sherif (eds), *Social Psychology at the Crossroads* (New York: Harper & Bros., 1951), pp. 313–23.
102 Pelling, *Common Lot*, pp. 185, 193, 198, 202.
103 B.E. Ashforth and G.E. Kreiner, '"How can you do it?": Dirty work and the challenge of constructing a positive identity', *Academy of Management Review* 24: 3 (1999), 413–34.
104 Ågren, *Making a Living*, p. 140 for a characterisation of some caring work in this way, where her dataset concerns Sweden 1550–1820.
105 Ashforth and Kreiner, 'Dirty work', p. 415.
106 For the application of 'status shield' theory to twenty-first-century nurses, see M.D. Cottingham, R.J. Erickson and J.M. Diefendorff, 'Examining men's status shield and status bonus: How gender frames the emotional labour and job satisfaction of nurses', *Sex Roles* 72: 7–8 (2015), 377–89.
107 Hochschild, *Managed Heart*, pp. 174–81.
108 Hochschild, *Managed Heart*, p. 175.

109 For the resources which have developed for twenty-first-century professional nurses, see also the 'virtue script': M. McAllister and D.L. Brien, 'Narratives of the "not-so-good nurse": Rewriting nursing's virtue script', *Hecate* 41: 1–2 (2016), 79–97.

110 The difficult ideological position of poorer people who were paid by parishes to nurse their relations is not noticed in the observational literature: King, 'Nursing', p. 613; S. Ottaway, *The Decline of Life: Old Age in Eighteenth-Century England* (Cambridge: Cambridge University Press, 2004), pp. 233–4 sees the payment of relatives as evidence of family and community working together to deliver welfare.

111 P. Smith and M. Lorentzon, 'Comment: Is emotional labour ethical?', *Nursing Ethics* 12: 6 (2005), 638–42, on p. 638. This point is discussed further in Chapter 1.

112 S. Nicklin, *Address to a Young Lady on her entrance into the world* (London: Hookham and Carpenter, 1796), pp. 171–2. See discussion of nurses in the context of 'separate spheres' ideology in Chapter 1.

113 Hart, 'A ward of my own', pp. 101, 107.

114 Hochschild, *Managed Heart*, p. 177.

115 Ashforth and Kreiner, 'Dirty work', p. 421.

116 M. Vicinus, *Independent Women: Work and Community for Single Women 1850–1920* (Chicago, IL: University of Chicago Press, 1985), chapter 2.

117 A. Bashford, *Purity and Pollution: Gender, Embodiment, and Victorian Medicine* (Basingstoke: Macmillan, 1998), pp. 28–34.

118 Carré, 'Hospital nurses', p. 89.

119 Nelson, 'Fork in the road', p. 178.

120 E.G. von Arni, 'Who cared? Military nursing during the English Civil Wars and Interregnum, 1642–60', G. Hudson (ed.), *British Military and Naval Medicine* (Amsterdam: Rodopi, 2007).

121 Mortimer, *The Dying and the Doctors*, p. 145.

122 J.A.F. Klönne, *On the Revival of the Deaconesses of the Ancient Church* (Leipzig: [no details], 1820). There was perhaps a groundswell of continental opinion on this topic across the usual congregational divides, as Abbé Gregoire, the former Bishop of Blois, also recommended nurse training in this year: *Christian Observer* 19 (1820), pp. 519–20, cited by Williams, 'Religion, respectability', p. 236.

123 S.D. Broughton, *Letters from Portugal, Spain & France 1812–1814* (Stroud: Nonsuch, 2005), p. 134; C. Jones, *The Charitable Imperative: Hospitals and Nursing in Ancien Regime and Revolutionary France* (London: Routledge, 1989).

124 C. Winkworth (trans.), *Life of Pastor Fliedner of Kaiserswerth* (London: Longmans Green & Co., 1867).
125 Digital searches for sources for 'nurse' must also winnow out those people whose surname was Nurse, particularly prevalent in East Anglia.
126 E. Hall (ed.), *Miss Weeton: Journal of a Governess 1807–1811* (London: Humphrey Milford and Oxford University Press, 1936), p. 146; S. Trimmer, *Instructive Tales* (London: Hatchard et al., 1812), 'Tale XV: The good nurse'.
127 Borsay, 'Nursing 1700–1830', p. 32.
128 P. D'Antonio, 'The legacy of domesticity. Nursing in early nineteenth-century America', *Nursing History Review* 1: 1 (1993), 229–46, on p. 230.
129 Helmstadter and Godden, *Nursing Before Nightingale*, p. 4 and *passim*.
130 See, among many, Abel-Smith, *A History*.
131 A question raised but not decisively answered by C.E. O'Lynn, 'History of men in nursing: A review', C.E. O'Lynn and R.E. Tranbarger (eds), *Men in Nursing: History, Challenges and Opportunities* (New York: Springer, 2007), pp. 6–7.
132 M.C. Versluysen, 'Old wives' tales? Women healers in English history', C. Davies (ed.), *Rewriting Nursing History* (London: Croom Helm, 1980); Whittle, 'Critique', p. 55.
133 In the process, I respectfully contradict R. Dingwall, A.M. Rafferty and C. Webster, *An Introduction to the Social History of Nursing* (London: Routledge, 1988), p. 4.
134 Borsay, 'Nursing 1700–1830'.
135 See for example P. Smith, *The Emotional Labour of Nursing* (Basingstoke: Macmillan, 1992) and P. Smith and H. Cowie, 'Perspectives on emotional labour and bullying: Reviewing the role of emotions in nursing and healthcare', *International Journal of Work Organisation and Emotion* 3: 3 (2010), 227–36.
136 M. Weisner, 'Wandervogels and women: Journeymen's concept of masculinity in early modern Germany', *Journal of Social History* 24: 4 (1991), 767–82.
137 St Thomas's Hospital minutes of the court of governors 21 June 1704, London Lives reference LMTHMC552020157; www.londonlives.org (accessed 29 November 2022).
138 C. Davies, 'The regulation of nursing work, an historical comparison of Britain and the USA', *Research in the Sociology of Health Care* 2 (1984), 121–60, on p. 124; S. Tesseyman, 'Complex alliance: A study of relationships between nursing and medicine in Britain and

the United States of America 1860–1914' (PhD thesis, University of Manchester, 2013), pp. 23–4.
139 Staffordshire Record Office, D 880/2/6–7 Brewood Workhouse work books 1822–25, 1825–28.
140 Langtree, 'Notes', p. 218; J.M. Waddy, *On the Education of Nurses: An Address to the Subscribers and Friends of the Lying-in Hospital, Birmingham* (London: Sherwood et al., 1846).
141 A problem she sometimes identifies but does not interrogate: Langtree, 'Notes', pp. 148–9.
142 Pelling, *Common Lot*, p. 201.
143 Wallis and Pirohakul, 'Medical revolutions?', p. 516.

1

Domestic nursing by women: ideals and experiences

[Nurse Rooke] is a shrewd, intelligent, sensible woman ... Women of that class have great opportunities and if they are intelligent may be well worth listening to.[1]

Like the plague nurses before them, the paid domestic nurse has her literary equivalents. Many of the depictions are ambivalent or humorously indicative of venal sins, but Jane Austen's Nurse Rooke stands out as a sympathetic portrait of a competent if gossipy woman. Histories of nursing have acknowledged her as such.[2] Yet *Persuasion* contains not one but three vignettes of nursing. Anne Elliott cares for her nephew to enable the child's mother to go out for dinner, at some emotional cost to herself: the unpaid family member as nurse. Later in the novel Louisa Musgrove is nursed after her famous fall from the Cobb at Lyme by Mrs Harville, the wife of a naval captain and 'a very experienced nurse' who 'left nothing for anybody [else] to do', albeit her manners were 'a degree less polished than [those of] her husband'.[3] No money changed hands but the Harvilles were paid in other ways, namely in the childcare offered by the Musgroves during Louisa's convalescence. In this way, Austen works up to her heroine's favourable report of Nurse Rooke, the nurse who is paid in cash for her care, by way of finding trustworthy nurses elsewhere among unmarried aunts and friendly hosts.

This chapter adopts a similar approach to consider domestic nursing as spanning the voluntary-contractual divide, by first considering the nursing tasks common to both. It debates the templates for ideal versus demonised nurses, in both fiction and advice literature, before focusing on descriptions of actual nursing work.

Accounts of work written by the nurses themselves cluster in the second half of the period covered here and generally represent the perspective of unpaid spinsters. Discussion homes in on the significance of the nurse's attentiveness to their patient in physical and emotional terms, and the conditions which threatened to leach that attention away. The risks of nursing to the nurse were not entirely appreciated by those who had not themselves nursed. Yet risks, like tasks, were common to both paid and unpaid nurses. The chapter concludes that domestic nursing by women was both an unquestioned resource and the target of stereotyped misogyny, sometimes simultaneously. The first person testimony of literate and literary women who reflected on their nursing activity provides essential context for otherwise well-worn caricatures.

The tasks of the pre-professional nurse

The tasks of the nurse in this period can usefully be summarised as watching and regulating, feeding and administering, cleaning and removing waste.[4] Nurses watched patients and symptoms with a view to recognising and reporting changes to, for example, skin, temperature, pulse, and evacuations. Regulating the patient's environment involved (among other things) controlling heat, managing air flow, light, and noise, plus adapting the patient's interaction with that environment, perhaps by helping them to change their position, to move, or to exercise. These practical matters were frequently joined by management of patient emotions via the offer of comfort and encouragement which may perhaps have included prayer, or helping the patient to procure sufficient rest/sleep. Feeding and administering encompassed preparation, provision, and delivering appropriate food and drinks to the patient, plus ensuring their ingestion at the right times or in the correct sequence. Supplying and administering medicines or treatment interventions, either at the instruction of another party (physician, apothecary, the patient, patient's relations, other) or under the nurse's own initiative required a good memory and attention to the clock. Cleaning and removing waste have been the activities most commonly associated with the pre-professional nurse, given the propensity of historians to conflate nurses with domestic servants.[5] In both sickness and injury the patient's wounds, body, and environment required attention in a timely way which probably included changes of patients' clothes and bedding, and in the seventeenth century extended to laundry (although laundering became a matter of contention in eighteenth-century institutions, as Chapters 2 and 3 demonstrate).[6] Removal and disposal of soiled dressings, catarrh, vomit, excrement, and potentially body parts were smelly tasks which risked expressions of repugnance from an incautious nurse. This latter point of self-policing, that the nurse repress visible disgust, was perhaps encompassed by hospital and infirmary rules for nurses that urged them to treat patients with kindness and humanity.[7]

The boundaries that were supposed to exist between nurses and other practitioners in terms of applying medical procedures were shifting and contested. This area of nursing activity comprised just one in a series of double binds suffered by women, whereby they were expected to act competently based on experience but were nonetheless routinely denigrated for their conceit in claiming expertise they did not possess. This is discussed in more detail below, but here it is enough to observe that nurses were assumed to have facility in minor interventions such as applying blisters, plasters, or leeches throughout the period.[8]

In addition to attention during life, nurses were routinely persuaded or available to lay out and sit up with the body if their patient died. This was an important service for both practical and emotional reasons. It was not unheard of for patients to revive after seeming death, so the presence of an experienced attendant was necessary to look for signs of returning life. Similarly, families might be frightened by the presence of a corpse in the house and want the reassuring presence of a person in the same room as the body.

The ideal nurse

Health advice literature existed from the earliest days of printing and often had something to say about nurses. Therefore, when the tirades around plague nurses quieted after the 1660s there was constant, if low-level, commentary about aspirations for nursing care. Famously in the historiography, the criteria for 'good' domestic nursing (in cases of fever) were given at some length in a physician's publication of 1730, much quoted subsequently as the supposed yardstick against which eighteenth-century female nurses might be judged.[9] She was to be middle-aged but fit and healthy, a good 'watcher', quick of hearing, able to act promptly and quietly, while being cheerful and clean in her person. Continental European publications seem to have recommended a similar array of attributes across the period 1660–1820.[10]

In Britain these ideals were given an occasional boost or reminder in the mid-eighteenth century, for example in Thomas Tanner's *Treatise on Smallpox* of 1745, providing 'The Way for the Nurse to manage the Patient at every Crisis', or Robert Johnson's *Some Friendly Cautions to the Heads of Families* in many editions from 1767 containing 'ample directions to nurses who attend the sick'.[11] Recommendations could be quite granular, particularly if derived from case histories, as where William Grant recommended the nurse of Mrs Bland to scour her patient's lips and teeth with a rag dipped in vinegar in a case of 'putrid fever'.[12] The advice literature was dominated in the last decades of the eighteenth and the first decades of the nineteenth century by *Domestic Medicine*, a lengthy household advice manual for treating illnesses and injuries. This volume was first published in 1769 and was reissued until 1846 for the British market: it enjoyed even more longevity in the United States, where editions reached the twentieth century.[13] The attitude of this work has been judged uniformly hostile both to nurses of the sick and to the nurses of small children as ignorant old women.[14] Nonetheless the declared author of *Domestic Medicine*, the Scottish physician William Buchan, pursued a clear agenda to make simple medical diagnoses and procedures more open to the public. This was carried into his other (less popular) publications which ceded some ground to the judgement of women. His book on venereal disease, for example, confirmed 'Bark and Laudanum are now prescribed everywhere by nurses and mistresses of families, with safety and advantage ... I would rather trust myself in the hand of an experienced nurse than of a theoretical physician.'[15] Similarly his co-authored work on smallpox contains case studies where the attending medical man unproblematically takes cues about the patient's state from the attending nurse.[16] In this way, practice and experience among women was quietly and occasionally given its due by medical men.

As Buchan's conflation of mistresses and nurses implies, there was a background assumption across the period that women who nursed fell into one of two groups: either they undertook nursing of their relations, friends, and neighbours in unpaid performance of duty, or they left their own house to receive payment in someone else's residence by offering care for a fee. The former group were occasionally noticed for their virtue, while the latter were regarded with suspicion for being a 'hireling stranger' and will be considered further below.[17] Here it is enough to conclude that nursing *gratis* by women was an expression of the duty, reciprocity, and affection that pertained within 'settled relationships' until or unless disruption 'shifted this care role towards one of economics rather than emotion'.[18] Women nursed female and male relations, but might be compelled to hire nursing when they themselves fell ill.[19] The erosion or collapse of the ideal might therefore have relied on a failure of reciprocity as much as on the frailties of any individual nurse.

The sick-nurse was potentially rendered ideal by the perfect patient. Joseph Alleine, for example, was a seventeenth-century divine ejected from his living at the Restoration whose biography was written by his wife Theodosia. His powerful religiosity and poor health claimed and apparently received a willing array of nurses. During a stay at Dorchester in 1667 Alleine's wife could call on the four young women who lived in the same house who 'were ready night and day to help me', and a further ten young women who lived elsewhere 'that took their turns to watch with him constantly'.[20] Joseph's spiritual greatness was evident in part via the plenitude of devoted nursing he received.[21] He offers a potent example of the 'many-to-one' nursing model for high-status patients posited in my introductory chapter above.

For further evaluation of the ideal nurse, it is necessary to turn to fictional literature where she made the occasional appearance in English prose.[22] In terms of glory reflected from the perfect patient, there was no patient more idealised than Clarissa Harlowe. In a story told by protracted correspondence, Clarissa is inveigled from her parents' home, imprisoned, and raped as the precursors to a rapid and virtuous death. While still in the parental home, Clarissa cared for her mother: 'My mamma has been very ill and would have no other nurse but me'.[23] In turn Clarissa requires a paid nurse to care for her in the decline towards death. She initially describes Ann Shelburne as simply 'diligent, obliging, silent, and sober'.[24] Yet the nurse is unable to attend Clarissa without feeling the tragedy of the circumstances. She weeps somewhat when Clarissa is persecuted by her attacker, and copiously when witnessing her patient's death.[25] The emotional investment of Clarissa's nurse illustrates Shelburne's own fitness for employment but also the power of Clarissa's virtue to extract appropriate emotional responses even from hireling strangers.

The first clear indications of a changing attitude and an upswing in expectations for superlative nursing came from Sarah Trimmer, an author with a keen interest in children's moral education, active from the end of the eighteenth-century onwards. Trimmer's publications were extensive, and her comments on nursing were essentially small-scale and time-limited, but even so she comes closer to setting out an agenda for nursing reform than anyone else in the eighteenth century. She began with a brief non-fictional commentary 'On Nursing' in *The Family Magazine* edition of May 1788 addressed to women 'in all ranks of life'.[26] She referenced the frequency of patients' 'suffering from the ignorance of their friends, and the aukwardness [sic] of their attendants', emphasising 'A good nurse is one of the most useful characters in life.' Trimmer deprecated amateur 'doctoring' and instead characterised the good nurse as 'one who can lay a bed smooth, without fatiguing the patient, make the various messes [meals] which are proper for invalids, and dress blisters, &c with a light and tender hand'. She went on to give rather longer instructions for the management of the sick room which prioritised ventilation and cleanliness of rooms and beds. Trimmer also made recommendations for cleaning people: 'a sick person may have his hands and face wiped with a towel dipped in warm water with a little brandy in it, if be improper to do more' followed by instructions about caring for a patient's mouth, hair, legs and feet. These advices were teamed with guidance for nurses on self-care. The women should change their clothes daily, have access to fresh air, and exercise out of doors.

Trimmer's second and longer discussion of nursing best practice was given in the form of a children's short story, a genre she had been developing for nearly a decade. 'The Good Nurse' also appeared in *The Family Magazine* and represents a pre-professional fiction of the nursing vocation.[27] The central character, Nurse Wilden, offers a much more comprehensive portrait of the ideal nurse than Trimmer's earlier observations and her example is more notably didactic. Polly Wilden enjoyed her positive reputation because her character and upbringing had coincidentally been perfect for the purposes of a future nurse. The eldest child in a large family, she had been 'a nurse almost from her cradle' with 'a strong desire' to help her parents. In other words, the ideal nurse was someone whose experience began in extreme youth and in her own family with the care of small children. Ominously for would-be emulators of Polly Wilden, 'she was ready to work herself almost to death for their ease, if necessity had required it', although Polly's own parents ensured that the demands on her were not unreasonable. The collateral benefits of Polly's hard-working childhood were that her father and brothers did not seek the 'comforts and conveniences' of an alehouse, even during her mother's repeated lyings in. Her further induction to nursing was facilitated by a spell in service with the widow of an apothecary, who offered her an apprenticeship in all but name in 'kitchen physick' and 'the management of the sick'.[28] These experiences ensured that when Polly was widowed after seven short years of marriage, she quickly decided to hire herself out as a sick-nurse. In her first employment to a poor family she became 'mother ... friend ... adviser' to the household and at the second managed to convert both parents and children from being 'a set of heathens' to a state of spiritual reform. Thereafter requests for her service came thick and fast, particularly when she secured the favour of recommendations from local medical men and took the place of an established nurse who fortuitously died. Her life is then depicted in a series of set pieces, where Nurse Wilden always acts wisely and in her employers' best interests.

Every character trait exhibited by this good nurse throughout her life was calibrated to align with Trimmer's initial thoughts on nursing, plus her promotion of a narrow vision of life for poorer women consisting of modest deportment, practical piety, and restrained ambition. As a young unmarried woman Polly Wilden was not fond of expensive attire and was not so vain as to wear her mistress's cast-off clothing. She was so devoted to her parents that she would not move away from them even to please her indulgent employer. The beguiling opportunities of higher wages or London service, the choice of 'female adventurers', were strongly deprecated. In maturity she eschews gossip, devotes her leisure hours to philanthropic work, and defers to the greater expertise of the apothecary or physician.

These writings about nursing were consonant with Trimmer's wider agenda to promote exemplary tales for poorer children that avoided the damaging secular aspirational qualities of fairy tales like Cinderella and replaced them with improving Christian fables. Her turn to nursing as a subject succeeded a series of publications aiming to interpret scripture for children's understanding and to idealise devoted industry for girls, particularly those of the lower-middling or downwardly mobile ranks, and inculcate appropriate parameters for gendered behaviour. Nurse Wilden was not, therefore, a herald of the lady nurse but rather an early forerunner of the lower-status women who took up nurse training after 1860.

There was little or no direct response to Trimmer's recommendations for nurses in advice literature, but her story may have influenced a move towards the proper behaviour and identity for nurses being noticed in children's literature.[29] In addition to the eighteenth-century criteria of being clean, healthy, attentive, and cheerful, children's short stories added weight to the nurse being both female and feminine. Agnes Porter for instance, the daughter of a clergyman and sometime reader of Trimmer, published a story in 1791 that echoed Trimmer's direction of travel. Porter was employed as a governess to the Earl and Countess of Ilchester's children. She was devoted to her 'darlings' and volunteered as a sick-nurse during childhood illnesses 'with all the anxieties of a mother'.[30] Porter's one publication, a book aimed at the moral instruction of young girls, is valuable for its inclusion of a short tale which recognised the refocusing of ideal nursing. Sophia was described as pretty, good humoured, affectionate, and

Domestic nursing by women

compassionate but chronically inattentive to her parents, teachers, and to the needs of others. Her aunt decided to teach her a lesson by feigning illness and designating Sophia as her carer.

> Little nurse, said she, step into the closet and pour me out a medicine that is on one of the shelves; it is called a mixture for the gout: away tript Sophia, opened the closet, snatched up a vial, poured out its contents, and gave it to her aunt, who drank it, but presently remarked that it did not taste as it should do.[31]

Sophia read the label on the vial 'Poison for rats' and was agonised by guilt, until her aunt revealed that she had substituted the poison with milk and water. 'May it prove a remedy for you in a complaint that is worse than either the gout or fever!' she cautioned, and Sophia was forthwith cured of her 'defect'.

Specifically, this vignette addressed both the value for would-be nurses of early training in paying attention, and the emotional penalties of failure. More generally the layering of additional values for aspiring nurses via this writing offered intrinsically female versions of delivering care. Both qualities were frequently implicit in writings of the seventeenth and eighteenth centuries but were being given additional emphasis in the final decades under study here. This means that when Melesina Trench made a note in 1815 of 'A jesting account of women by a woman ... The best point in their character is that they are good nurse-tenders' there was no doubt that the 'good' nursing should be tightly knitted to superlative femininity.[32]

Furthermore, this quality adhered to women regardless of their race. A final literary example illustrates the presumed power of the good female nurse as a motif in the campaign for the abolition of slavery. Amelia Opie was a prolific writer of both verse and prose. She was also embedded in radical political circles and in later life adopted Quakerism.[33] Her novel of 1805, *Adeline Mowbray*, anticipated her later work (written and philanthropic) in delivering a sympathetic portrait of a Jamaican woman. This character, Savannah, is embedded in Adeline's life, being present in her household for a number of years and described by the eponymous heroine as 'my nurse, my consoler, and my friend'.[34] Details of the depiction are problematic for twenty-first century readers given that Savannah is repeatedly denoted 'the mulatto', and her speech is rendered in broken English. Her skills as a nurse are emphatic, however, since she replaces a 'heavy treading' hired nurse and attends Adeline's dying lover with quiet and unwavering devotion: 'Hers was the service of the heart; and there is none like it.'[35] It was Savannah's emotion work which made the difference. Furthermore, her character is one of 'conscious integrity' at the most critical moments, such as when she subsequently confronts Adeline's errant (white, wealthy) husband to condemn his intended bigamy.[36] The intrinsic capacity of women of any race to deliver excellent nursing is mobilised here as an endorsement of femininity held in common, and a tacit argument for the abolition of enslavement.

The negative stereotype

While health literature gave guidance for the performance of paid and unpaid nurses, the negative stereotype is wholly concentrated on the figure of the hired nurse and the separation of delivery of care from proper feeling. This was partly because, as in the twentieth century, 'Domestic work which, when performed in the home, enhances a woman's status has quite the opposite effect when performed outside it in the public realm.'[37] This sentiment underlay commentary over a long period but was worked out at length by Susan Nicklin in 1796, when considering the difference between the comfort of ageing parents nursed by their daughters versus the 'cold offices' of nursing by

> the hireling attendant ... hardened by the continual sight of sufferings and of death ... Can a daughter flatter herself with the hope of attentions, anxious and tender as those which filial piety should dictate ... that sentiments by whose influence she herself is unmoved, should soften the breast of a mercenary stranger?[38]

She presumed that the feelings of such women must be dead to pity, since others' suffering is their own insurance against poverty. This is a refinement of the abuse reserved for plague nurses in the seventeenth century, because Nicklin does not blame them for their indifference but merely notices its likely causes: 'money was not made to purchase the thousand nameless, but inestimable kindnesses which rise involuntarily from tender friendship and affectionate gratitude ... These are the wants the nurse cannot comprehend'.[39] This is an eighteenth-century expression of the capacity for nursing work to taint the carer by blunting her sympathy. It is impossible to test whether, in this respect, eighteenth-century nurses became hardened to illness in the same way as nursing and domestic staff on a modern hospital ward, but the assumptions expressed by Nicklin in theory were echoed by others with practical experience.[40] Author Mary Lamb's letter to her friend Sarah Stoddart of November 1805, concerning the latter's mother in illness (possibly insanity), stressed

> let your whole care be to be certain that she is treated with *tenderness*. I lay a stress upon this, because it is a thing of which people in her state are uncommonly susceptible, and which hardly any one is at all aware of: a hired nurse never, even though in all other respects they are good kind of people.'[41]

Lamb had herself nursed her own mother and had undergone treatment in a madhouse (episodes treated at more length below), so she was apparently well-informed. These comments provide a distant echo of the twentieth-century ambition for the nurse to 'maintain the integrity of the patient' in the face of challenges to identity from both illness/injury and medicine.[42] The paid nurse of 1660–1820 was bound to fail if she could not commit to the required intensity of emotion work: 'They serve, but cannot soothe'.[43]

It is telling that these detailed critiques are most readily available towards the end of the period studied here, at a time when the separation between unpaid and paid work by women was apparently becoming more ideologically fraught. The assumption of their low pay and casual commitment has seen sick-nurses excluded from the historical research on 'separate spheres' applied to middling women. This is unfortunate, in that the experiences of labouring women employed as sick-nurses have been largely neglected in an important literature for gender history, and historians of nursing in the revisionist vein have missed the chance to underscore just why the stereotype of the drunken, insanitary, and incompetent nurse became so potent a threat. Perry Williams has argued that rising evangelicalism among the middling sort concentrated attention on the low moral standing of nurses, and draws on the parallel development of domestic femininity to explain the appeal of and support for the new 'ideal' nurse.[44] He does not turn this around, though, to unpick all of the ways in which 'unreformed' sick-nurses lost out in the significant ideological shifts affecting women between 1750 and 1850. They automatically breached emergent separate spheres injunctions because they did not solely attend their own family members. At first sight this was a negligible risk, because women who nursed outside the home were of necessity not middle class.[45] But the employment and observation of nurses by middling householders (whether as private individuals, parish officers, or infirmary trustees, for example) meant that the women's activity risked carrying increasing cultural negativity. At the same time, the domestic ideology that developed to underpin the justification for separate spheres rendered suspect all nursing activity not undertaken by a relative.

Aside from blanket assumptions of disengaged or inappropriate care from paid nurses, ideas in both advice literature and fiction across the period take a jaded view of these women's performance on the grounds of their behaviour and character. For medical men, the worst aspect of their conduct was their tendency to usurp medical authority. Walter Harris MD wrote for many when he scorned the 'fantastical *Nurses*, and conceited *Attendants*, who will needs mix [sic], and often prefer their little skills, to very Rational and Advised Prescriptions'.[46] This attitude was maintained throughout the period. William Brownrigg, for example, could hardly bear to use the word nurse in his mid-eighteenth-century casebook, preferring to denote attendants on the sick as 'old wives' or 'bystanders' rather than nurses.[47] Unlike Buchan writing a generation later, Brownrigg did not take the view that women could be trusted to dose themselves and others. Instead, he was sarcastic about his pregnant patient Mrs Taylor, for example, for her independent 'recourse to her sacred sheet anchor, laudanum'.[48] Buchan's *Domestic Medicine* of 1769 and onwards 'repeatedly denigrates the medical knowledge of nurses, midwives, and old women' according to existing readings of his work.[49] On closer inspection, however, this judgement relies largely on his indictment of nursery and wetnurses rather than sick-nurses. The medical critiques of nurses' independence were eventually endorsed by Trimmer's fiction, wherein Nurse Jessep, the antithesis of the ideal Polly Wilden, combined ignorance with quackery.[50] Medical writers throughout the period were perhaps making an early attempt to impose the 'handmaiden' role among the women who nursed and were frustrated when they did not comply.[51]

The conflicted nature of Buchan's attitude, however, points towards a modicum of fluctuation in opinion over time if not categorical change. There is a period, between approximately the 1710s and the 1790s, when it is possible to detect a partial remission of physicians' criticisms of nurses, paid or unpaid, and occasional recognition of the shared nature of care. This attitude differs from the ideal nursing characterised above because it is matter of fact and attempts to draw lines of responsibility between the nurse and medical practitioners without undue prejudice, yet in chronological terms it coexists with the negative stereotype.[52] *Medicus Novissimus; or, the Modern Physician* of 1712, for example, commented in relation to smallpox: 'I could write several Observations on this disease, but 'tis needless, seeing every Skillful Nurse can cure this distemper without a physician'.[53] The sporadic admission by doctors that nurses could be skilful gives an uneasy and contradictory quality to these works, even if we assume that practitioners' attitudes to nurses varied according to the condition the women were recruited to attend (i.e. if doctors granted more latitude to nurses specifically in cases of dangerous diseases like smallpox). Medical writers were on steadier ground when they reverted to critical mode.

Members of the medical faculty might also be concerned about nurses' fitness for their job on the grounds of physical fragility if not stubborn opinion. One author from the first half of the eighteenth century alludes to prescribing medicine in such a way as to obviate mistakes 'if a NURSE, through Drowsiness, or Carelessness, or a shaking Hand, should happen to let a few Drops fall into the appointed Vehicle, more than was ordered'.[54] If an error of this type occurred, it fitted seamlessly with the stereotype without any apparent need for concern about mitigating circumstances.[55]

Household managers, in contrast, might concentrate instead on poor practices. Hannah Woolley was an early advocate of clean linen for the sick, and anticipated opposition from 'some old Dotard of our sex' on the grounds that changing attire and shifting about weakened the sick and disposed them to catch cold. Woolley had no truck with these arguments and wrote as some length about the value of removing foul linen 'to let Gentlewomen see how much they are abused by their credulous and ignorant nurses'.[56]

Paid nurses were suspected of being dubious characters even where nothing concrete was known against them. A satire in circulation from 1761 onwards (and reprinted into the mid-nineteenth century) sees the former nurse of a deceased patient working alongside a London searcher, both women showing a prurient interest in the physique of the naked male corpse as just one of the first indignities of death.[57] A more common complaint about the personality of nurses was that they were too talkative, and likely to share melancholy anecdotes with patients, to the detriment of their recovery.[58]

The recoil from paid nurses moved from generally dubious practice to specific vices, prominently their supposed tendency to drink alcohol. Drink was deprecated on moral and practical grounds if it rendered nurses inattentive to their patients. The spectre of the drunken nurse was present throughout the period, in muted form. Samuel Bamford, for example, retrospectively described a night nurse attending himself and his father as callous and unfeeling when sober, but verbally threatening when drunk (on the wine intended for consumption by her patients).[59] The antithetical 'drinking' nurse can be seen in retrospect as offering a template for what the attentive nurse should not have been.[60] As might be expected, an upswing in ideals at the end of the eighteenth century contributed to bringing the literary prevalence of the drunken nurse to the fore. Trimmer's Nurse Wilden had her antithesis in an unnamed monthly nurse who 'was generally in a state of intoxication from morning till night', a woman quickly discharged at the youthful Polly Wilden's insistence.[61] A collateral risk to the patient occurred if a nurse was open to bribery with drink. Laetitia Pilkington's son recruited a woman to look after his mother in her final illness but reported that on the promise of half a pint of rum the nurse had admitted the landlord (to whom the family owed rent) to the sick room.[62]

Nurses' poverty was not a very prominent feature of the negative stereotype, not least because information about poverty might have mitigated the nurses' failings. Nicklin assumed in 1796 that it must be poverty which compels women 'to seek the residence of pain', but aside from this, economic pressure was reconstrued as a tendency to extort presents or extras from the family they served. This was explicitly a component of Trimmer's critique, because her story 'The Good Nurse' contained several depictions of poor practice, such as attempting to extract perks from families of the dying or dead.

It would have been logical to suppose that nurses might be feared for their possibly acting as a conduit to disease, infecting the next patient with the contagion of their last. This could have fitted neatly with the assumption of taint by association, posited in my Introduction. Nonetheless, little confirmation of this sort of criticism has been found. Instead, the nurse became a target for patient fears around ceding their autonomy. If patients could not dictate their own choice of nurse, particularly in the absence of female relations, the strangeness of a stranger might emanate from the nurse not being selected directly by the patient, as well as from the nurse being personally unknown to them. It has long been observed that illness converts homes to prisons, repeated in the early part of this period by prolific medical writer Everard Maynwaringe.[63] The risks to patients from unregulated domestic nurses of virtual imprisonment was similarly recognised in the early twentieth century.[64]

This leaching of patient control and transfer of power to nurses was neatly portrayed in 1807, in an illustration which imitated Thomas Rowlandson's popular series 'The Miseries of Life'.

This cartoon is accompanied by a narrative which betrays the fears of the disempowered patient at the turn of the nineteenth century, namely that the nurse will be inattentive, neglectful of her employer's home and property, ignorant as to the best actions to take, and more interested in her own comfort than the patient's recovery. She even injures her patient in body and spirit when she 'stamps about the chamber like a horse in a boat – slops you as

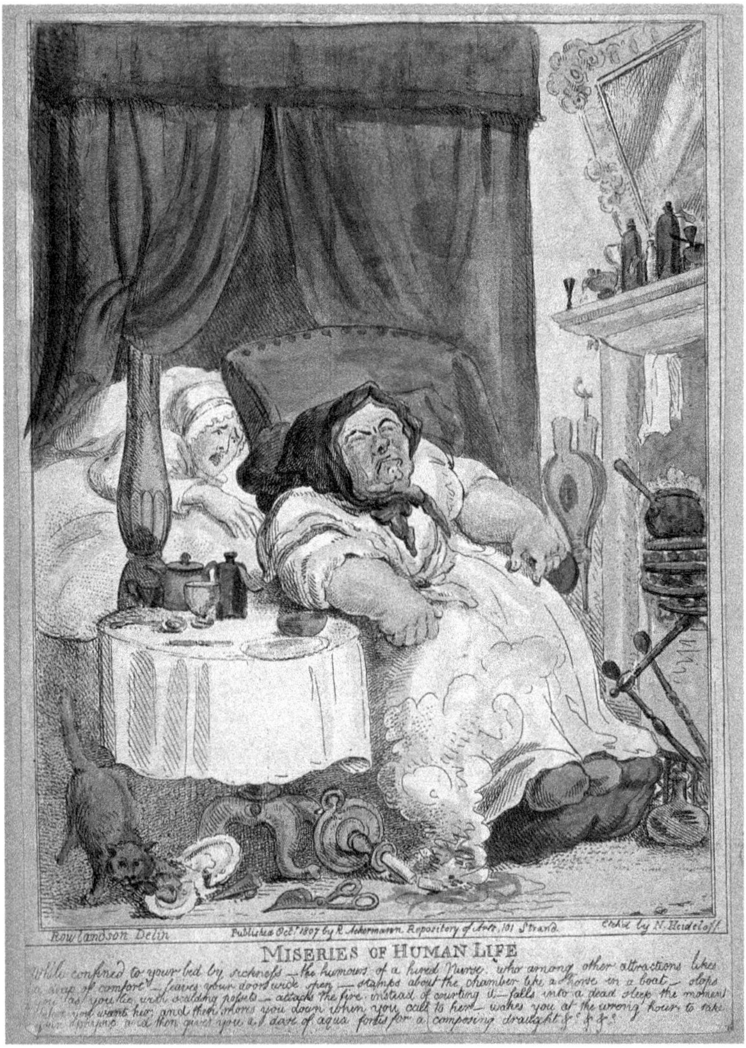

Figure 1.1 T. Rowlandson, [A convalescing woman trying in vain to rouse her slumbering hired nurse], *Miseries of Human Life* (1807): etching courtesy of the Wellcome Trust

you lie with scalding possets'. A patient, the engraving implies, was partially or wholly defenceless against careless demeanour.

The most acute form of risk came from the potential of the nurse to commit intentional harm. Violence is the polar opposite of care, and a person disposed to inflict it is characterised throughout these chapters as an anti-nurse. Acts of violence by nurses can be seen on a spectrum from the violence of wilful inaction, including the intentional withholding of medicines, through to easy murder of a vulnerable victim.[65] This extreme position is not well represented in the literature on domestic nursing until the end of the period, and then is identified most decisively in accounts where the practice of nursing is aggravated by additional factors such as war.[66] It is notable that the few allegations of anti-nursing found in the British press in the eighteenth century emanated from beyond England, suggesting that such drastically aberrant behaviour could only be perceived through the lens of racial prejudice.[67] In 1796 Dublin, for example, it was alleged that the women attending a female patient, dubbed 'witches of death', purposefully ignored the doctor's orders, pronounced the patient's death, then failed to notice the remaining signs of life.[68] The patient was only saved when unidentified others revived her. The patient was not named and the description of the nurses' behaviour was blatantly informed by an animus against uneducated Irish women, so the anecdote is nearer to the negative stereotype than it is to actual evidence of anti-nurse behaviour.[69]

Descriptions of 'real' nursing by female nurses, patients, and others

The fixity of ideas about different types of nurse, and the entrenched opinions about them, were at odds with more heterogenous experience in practice. Paid nurses, servants, and unpaid relations worked together (i.e. at the same time, in the same house, attending in turns on the same patients).[70] Their views of each other, and of the tasks required, were similarly varied. This means that it is much easier to characterise a range of narratives than it is to pinpoint change or fluctuation over time.

Lady Hannah East made extensive note of the nursing required by her husband during an attack of gout in 1791.[71] Lady Hannah dressed Sir William's foot and hands with flannel and plasters, and refreshed poultices. She also rubbed or massaged his head, shoulder, and chest which has been interpreted as a form of pain-relief: 'presumably the therapeutic value of such action when dealing with aches, pain and stress was self-evident', or perhaps attendants still employed counter-irritation to alleviate pain by inducing awareness of feeling in other parts of the body.[72] She acknowledged her husband's frequent low spirits, but was uniformly sympathetic rather than irritated (despite her sometimes taking a different and more positive view of his progress towards recovery).[73] The couple seem to have been exceptionally close and companionate. Even so Lady East shared the tasks of nursing with her stepson, unmarried sister, and servants.[74]

Women who themselves possessed experience of nursing were likely to be attentive to snippets of personal information about other nurses. Agnes Porter, cited above as responsible for disseminating one of the portraits of an ideal nurse, had the task of recruiting a live-in nurse for her widowed mother. She found someone 'who had an excellent character – lived fifteen years in her last place ... liked her appearance'. The passing of time did not diminish her faith in the 'good' nurse Mrs Betty.[75] A nurse's good character could derive from either patients or from professional witnesses to her work. This means that any decision about a nurse's fitness for duty could be delegated among higher-status observers. Diarist Abigail Gawthern, when suffering a fever in London, recruited Nurse Smith at the recommendation of the apothecaries Messrs Hingeston & Devaynes.[76] Apothecaries were therefore a pathway for nurse employment in eighteenth-century London, even as in this case apothecaries to the royal court.[77]

Detailed experience of nurses recommended by an apothecary is given by a series of letters in early 1733 written about John and James Collier, the sons of the town clerk of Hastings. The boys were born in 1719 and 1721, and by the later months of 1732 were at school in London, living in the house of their maternal uncle William Cranston. In the final days of December John caught smallpox, was removed to lodgings with a Mrs Canham (a mantua-maker who was presumably willing to take contagious patients) and died within a week. The family was devastated, yet the death was not in any way blamed on the attending nurse, who was described as 'recommended by the apothecary and seemed to me [William Cranston], for I carefully examined her motions, to be a person of judgement and humanity and very diligent in attending upon him'.[78] Both this nurse and 'nurse Davis who sat up with him' were given a pair of white gloves at the time of John's funeral. Davis's service was of particular value to Mrs Canham 'so long as the corpse remained at her house; for without somebody's being in the roome at nights, her children, she and her servants would be afraid to go by it', presumably fears arising from proximity to death rather than from the continued risk of contagion.

When James also fell ill with smallpox in January the family was grieving and desperate to secure him every form of attention. They sought another lodging, trying three or four places, before finding that Mrs Canham was willing to take James. Perhaps surprisingly then, James was carried to the same lodging that had proved so unfortunate for his brother and from which John's body was swiftly removed, 'for what could have been a more melancholy thought than to have one child dead and another in a doubtful condition in the same house?'[79] James was given a bed in the parlour, 'a handsome warm, quiet room', and his case was quickly pronounced by the physician to be more favourable than his brother's, but he still needed a nurse. The letters which flew between London and Hastings in the January and February of 1733 illustrate the family's satisfaction with this nurse, yet also indicate their susceptibility to the negative stereotypes.

From the outset of James's care, his nurse's character was approved and her experience acknowledged. She was judged 'a good, understanding, careful woman and I verily believe indulgent and kind', and well-liked by the young patient. When the doctor ordered a form of enema, William Cranston consulted with both his friend William Page and the nurse before concluding 'we thought very happy [sic] and concluded to send to forbid the glyster'. The nurse's voice was thus allowed to join those of a male relation and of an attorney who was a friend of the family in contradicting the recommendation of the attending physician. The trust placed in her did not change, because she did not allow her attention for her patient to slip: she 'has taken a great deal of care of him; she's the same as at first'.

Her activities included some which might be anticipated, and others of a more distinctive nature. She was trusted to have drugs at hand, specifically a 'paragorick' to administer in case James could not sleep, and boiled chicken for him when he was hungry. Slightly unusually, when convalescent James was found to have lice in his hair, it was the nurse who was asked to procure a fine comb to try and remove them. The nurses to both John and James were assisted in all of their tasks by other household members including Mrs Canham's two female apprentices, and the maids in both Mrs Canham's and William Cranston's houses who 'have upon all occasions been very handy'. James himself, when able to write, was flippant about this array of attendants (despite or perhaps because of his brother's death) telling his father 'one body or another are mostly with me and divert me'.

There was a substantial social difference between the nurses employed to care for John and James and the family household in Hastings. The boys' father, also John, was a lawyer who was to be elected mayor five times and who has been credited for his professional talent and social influence in the town. It is unsurprising therefore that John senior was rather sneering about James's nurse. He reported: 'I went today to the house and saw the old nurse who is just such a piece as one would imagine'. In other words, the first characteristics that he noted were the woman's age and her imaginable traits, by implication the negative nursing stereotype. Even John senior, though, was compelled to add 'but I believe very carefull and humours him [James] very much'. This emotionally invested father did not otherwise remark on the inherent contradictions in his reaction to a lowly sick-nurse.

This is entirely consonant with the genre, because writing by non-medical men about female domestic nursing was typically scant.[80] Clergyman William Holland is unusual in offering a rare example of a male diarist who took careful note of nursing activity (at least in terms of its commission, if not its mundane details). He remarked on nursing work across his parish and within a wide circle of acquaintance, including among the parish poor.[81] His feelings were particularly engaged in the topic in 1805 when his only surviving son William suffered a riding accident. Two women and one man rushed to the scene to help, and the child was carried to a bed in a nearby cottage where he stayed for the next week before being carried home. The nursing was conducted by Holland's servant Sally, who stayed with him overnight, as well as the two women on site called Sarah Styling and Mrs Rich. At Christmas in the same year, Holland gave Styling and Rich half a guinea and invited the two women to dine with him every Christmas day in future in recognition of their 'care, kindness, and humanity'.[82] Holland was sometimes an acerbic commentator on parish life but did not find any particular fault with the nurses whom he knew best, and whom he had most reason to surveil.

It was also the case that female commentators on nurses could be committed to the negative stereotype on the basis of social difference. Gertrude Savile was an unmarried woman on the fringes of the British elite whose diary is that of a touchy and critical personality.[83] In 1756, she employed a nurse for a month who was 'neither a drunkard nor saucy', but still judged 'bad is the best of them' [sic].[84] Savile later admitted that she had chosen her subsequent nurse, Mary Robinson, on the basis of Mary's being accustomed to care for sick and infirm women, but found her uncongenial on social grounds: 'being only used to Trades-folks' Families, which made her very vulgar and too Familiar' Savile thought her 'no good nurse to me'. She still thought Robinson cruel, though, when the latter gave notice.[85] Employers thus encountered a contradiction if they wanted experienced nurses but also demanded social subtlety.

As Savile's longer account made plain, female servants routinely nursed their mistresses.[86] She also implies that, in a time of household emergency, mistresses nursed servants.[87] Sick servants who required nursing might give rise to pungent commentary from employers or worse. Servant Catherine Newman, sometime nurse of the Witt family, made her employer Agnes Witt's day 'vexatious & tiresome by Catherine being both ill, helpless, & hopeless' in May 1794.[88] Charles Lamb railed intemperately against his sick servant 'a stupid big country wench' who now lies a dead weight upon our humanity ... she seems to have made up he[r] mind to take her flight to heaven from our bed ... O the Parish, the Parish, the hospital, the infirmary, the charnel house, these are places meet for such guests.[89]

He seems to have been serious rather than reaching for comic hyperbole. Elizabeth Freke, an unhappy or even depressed memoirist, moved from words to actions. She had to care for a grandson with smallpox in December 1712 and accommodate female servants who caught the same infection but ran out of patience in early 1713: 'my man Isack fell sick of the small pox, whom I putt out of my house, being very ill my selfe and quitt tired with doctters and nurses for above two monthes'.[90] Other employers were more generous. When William Holland's servant John feared he was dying, Holland paid a woman to sit up with him.[91] Abigail Gawthern called a doctor for her servant Michael after a fall, as well as sitters up.[92]

Nurses, whether paid or unpaid, were credited with rescuing the lives of people thought to have died, but in whom the nurse detected signs of life. In a rare example of a medical man ceding credit to a nurse, Thomas Sydenham recounted a patient's anecdote from the mid-seventeenth century to the effect that he had been saved from death in smallpox. The patient's apparent death and the heat of the season meant that he was taken out of bed and placed on a table under a sheet. When his nurse saw him, however, she 'imagined she saw some small signs of life, and therefore put him to bed again directly, and using some means or other she brought him to himself'.[93] In the later eighteenth century Quaker Sarah Fox reported the revival of Martha Dallaway, by her nurse administering teaspoons of brandy after the household's supposition of her death.[94]

As these snippets of evidence imply, the flow of respect was not all one way from nurse-servants to employers, particularly in acute or dangerous cases where patients' families sought the best attendance they could muster and reassurance that nursing work would be conducted well. Sarah Hurst was the unmarried daughter of Richard Hurst, a tailor and mercer in Horsham Sussex, and she kept a detailed diary.[95] When Richard fell ill with smallpox in 1760 Sarah nursed him until he (like John and James Collier before him) was removed to lodgings, and after removal he was attended some of the time by his younger daughter Bet (Elizabeth). The family then tried to secure an experienced paid nurse or nurses to share the care work. One of the nearby Sussex medical practitioners, Doctor Smith, ran an inoculating house, and the nurse who attended the inoculation patients initially agreed to attend Richard Hurst. Sarah was naturally disappointed and distressed to discover, then, that the people having undergone inoculation were unwilling to part with their nurse. She (Sarah) rode over to beg the inhabitants of the inoculating house to allow the nurse to leave, whereupon they reluctantly consented. This made Sarah very happy, suggesting she perceived the unnamed nurse as a valuable asset gained in her father's case. Furthermore, Sarah was disturbed when the following week she learned that her sister Bet 'behaves very ill to one of the nurses' – presumably more than one paid carer was now with her father – a regret reflecting as much credit to the nurse as it was an aspersion on the 'insolent temper' of her sister.

As with Sarah Hurst, observations about nurses are perhaps most prominent in accounts by unmarried women, of any age, who were relied upon to nurse relations, friends, and others. Historian Edward Gibbon attributed his very survival to nursing by his maternal aunt Catherine Porten during his childhood. This was not the nursery nursing of the dry or wet nurse, but the sick-nursing required by the youthful historian's apparent disability, constitutional frailty, and susceptibility to epidemic disease. Gibbon's brief but emotional tribute to his aunt alluded to both the physical and affective trials of nursing a beloved child: 'Many wakeful nights did she sit by my bedside in trembling expectation that each hour would be my last' in succession to 'anxious and solitary days ... in the patient trial of every mode of relief and amusement'.[96] Porten left no separate account of her experiences: other women were more forthcoming.

The spinster as nurse: Ellen Weeton, Elizabeth Ham, and Mary Lamb[97]

The narratives of three unmarried women, born between 1764 and 1783, offer detail about episodes when they nursed others. In each case they were available to nurse (being either on the spot at the time of injury or in the neighbourhood), but not specifically paid to be a sick-nurse (although they might have been employed in another capacity at the time). Each of the women developed a track record of writing, and two went into print during their own lifetimes. They exhibit the valuable combination of acting as nurses and having the scope to write about nursing, either in specific or abstract ways. In particular they offer insight into the emotional labour of nursing and its perils.[98]

Ellen Weeton, known as Nelly, could probably be identified as the female writer of lowest social status among the examples used here. Her father was a slave ship captain who died when she was young, and Nelly seemingly experienced severe material poverty in her youth (an experience not shared by her brother who was away from home training to become a lawyer). After her mother's death, various attempts to make ends meet as either a landlady (renting out her former family home in Lancashire) or as a governess/companion preceded her eventual marriage in 1814 when she was in her late thirties. Her written legacy survives in the form of a memoir, and copies of her outgoing letters which she conscientiously made before posting the originals.

Her experience of nursing came in 1810 when the child she had been employed to teach was badly injured (an accident described in a letter to her brother ten days later).[99] Nelly had been recruited by Edward Pedder of Dove Bank in Ambleside to be a governess for his daughter. Only two months into the job the child, Mary Pedder, in a rare moment of being left alone, stood too close to the fire and her apron caught alight. The fire was extinguished by Nelly's retrieval of 'the ironing blanket' – the child was rolled in the blanket by her nursery nurse (who burned her hand in the process) and other household servants. By the time the fire was extinguished Mary's face and limbs were badly burned such that her skin hung off her 'like shreds of paper', but her torso was relatively unhurt.

The key features of the resulting nursing experience from Weeton's point of view were threefold. First, attempts to put out the fire and mitigate the burns revealed a chronic lack of household access to fluid for treating the burns: 'I could find no liquid of any kind.' No water could be had suddenly, and in the immediate aftermath of the burning the attending adults resorted to the use of 'all the milk and cream [the dairyman] could get' and a small amount of hair oil. It seems that the adults on the scene knew what they wanted to do but could not carry out their intentions for first aid (a phrase only coined later and considered further in Chapter 6). Second, care was directed to both the physical and emotional needs of the child. This included preventing her from sitting or lying down (at least in the first instance, for fear she would adhere to anyone or anything that supported her), warming her feet, which were unburned, by rubbing or hot water bottles, and reassuring her that she would not die. It also entailed holding her hands during a series of fits which came on after about an hour, to prevent her pulling at the loosened skin, a duty which Weeton found terrifying. Third, the hours after Mary was injured involved careful watching and listening around her breathing and consciousness, plus reportage on her state to her father and step-mother throughout the succeeding night.

The case did not evolve from emergency to chronic nursing because, despite vocal reassurances to the contrary designed to comfort the patient, Mary died about eighteen hours after she was injured, an outcome which Weeton attributed to her underlying epilepsy. What is most striking about the account though is the combination of practical and emotional detail clustering around a fairly brief vignette of a fatal household accident. Weeton wrote, for example: 'I listened with such intense anxiety for so many hours to every breath ... that still while I am in the room where she died, I imagine I can hear her breathe.'

Elizabeth Ham was the daughter of a farmer and brewer, with numerous aunts and uncles living across Somerset and Dorset. Her memoirs were truncated and published by an unsympathetic editor in the mid-twentieth century, who dismissively described the second half of her manuscript as 'Elizabeth Ham in Search of a Husband'.[100] Ham's experience in later life included the publication of a charmingly illustrated children's grammar book, but in her late twenties and early thirties her life consisted of living with one set of relations after another, during which she was made to feel redundant as an adult woman lacking her own household.[101] It is fairly ironic therefore (with hindsight) to observe the essential work she fulfilled in other people's homes including as a sick-nurse. Ham provides a vivid example of the modern economists' assumption 'that women are primarily (or should primarily be) engaged in unpaid housework and care work for their families', to the prejudice of women's status.[102]

Her most sustained recollections of nursing relate to an outbreak of 'typhus fever' in 1812 at the house of her aunt Mary Genge.[103] Mary Ham had married Edward Genge in 1787 and the couple had at least ten children over the next twenty years. They lived at Preston Plucknett (now a suburb of Yeovil), three or four miles away from Elizabeth's residence at the time in East Coker. Since the whole family was suffering at once and 'nurses were not to be had', Ham walked to her aunt's house every other night to help nurse her uncle and cousins: 'It was a most distressing scene, hurrying from one bedside to another, every instant of the night.' After about a week the younger children were getting better but William Genge aged about 20 fell ill, and Ham received an entreaty from her aunt to come at once, this time to stay.

William was largely speechless, but not quite insensible. Ham recalled: 'For five days and nights I never left his bedside, except for about an hour one day ... and one night when I laid down in my clothes ... whilst my aunt took my place but she called me before I got to sleep.' Ham's exhaustion was compounded by the arrival of the cousins' great aunt who audibly castigated the patient for being 'a wicked and depraved young man'. Ham confessed:

> I shall never forget that moment! The poor dying youth made a violent effort to turn towards me, with an expression of the greatest terror in his poor faded face, and grasped my hand, with the expression 'Don't run away'. The only articulate words that were heard from him during his illness.

William Genge died the following day, and therefore nearly forty years before Ham started to compose her memoirs, with a consequential lack of immediacy in her writing plus the risk of distortion over a protracted lapse of time. Even so her account of caring at night, sleeplessness, and the affective work entailed in nursing relatives with (or in spite of) other relatives has an authenticity confirmed by other writers.[104]

Mary Lamb's example by contrast is one of deeds rather than words, expressive of the risks of unpaid nursing for family members. On 22 September 1796, Mary Lamb murdered her mother with a stab wound to the heart. Mary had been caring for her mother Elizabeth Lamb for a protracted period, and newspaper reports of the inquest uniformly presumed that:

> As her carriage towards her mother was ever affectionate in the extreme, it is believed that to the increased attentiveness, which her parent's infirmities called for by day and night, is to be attributed the present insanity of this ill-fated young woman.[105]

Mary went on in later life to be an author in her own right and to share accommodation with her brother Charles Lamb (writer and acquaintance of Wordsworth, Coleridge, and Hazlitt, among other contemporary literary figures). This means that the murder has been considered somewhat in the context of literary history, but not of nursing history. Mary's experiences depict both the risk of extreme pressure on attentive unpaid nurses and the availability of protection even in extremis.

The months leading up to Elizabeth Lamb's murder provided familial permission to be considered mad. Charles spent the final weeks of 1795 and the first of 1796 at a private madhouse in Hoxton, a diagnosis considered at the time to be an expression of hereditary weakness – his father's 'senses had failed him before that time'.[106] He returned home, and the earliest surviving letters of Charles and Mary Lamb are dated from the period of his recovery. The Lamb household was also one in which tension was building in the spring and summer of 1796. Charles wrote to Samuel Taylor Coleridge in a letter dated 29 June to 1 July 1796, unwittingly referring to the preconditions for the tragedy: 'My mother is grown so entirely helpless (not having any use of her limbs) that Mary is necessarily confined from ever sleeping out, she being her bed fellow.'[107] If this description of Elizabeth Lamb's infirmity is correct, and if 'limbs' is a literal reference to all four limbs including arms and legs, it suggests that Mary had to assist her mother with washing, dressing, eating, toileting, and every physical function which might otherwise be performed for oneself. Charles glosses this as a restriction on Mary 'sleeping out', in other words visiting friends overnight. It is possible to argue that this curtailment of sociability was one of the lesser impacts of being one's patient's 'bedfellow'. Mary was quite possibly in unremitting attendance, kept in the house and at her mother's side by a combination of affection and duty. Furthermore, Mary was also engaged in remunerative work at the same time. She undertook sewing to earn money contributing to her own and her parents' support and took on an apprentice in mantua-making. She was loaded with responsibility while having no outlet for leisure or respite.

In the days before 22 September, Charles was starting to perceive his sister's struggle with her mental health. He sought the advice of physician David Pitcairn, who was unfortunately away from home. This means that when Mary became violent, there had been indications of her illness if no sufficient clues to its magnitude. When she reached breaking point, she was in the kitchen of the family's small house. She threw forks at both of her parents (wounding her father on the forehead), chased her own apprentice girl around the room, and ultimately grasped a knife and stabbed her mother.

Mary never seems to have written in explicit terms about these events, nor about her state of mind during this episode, although she ruefully referred to later bouts of madness in her letters. Instead, Charles Lamb's writing provides retrospective information about the emotional strain of unpaid caring, and clues about his sister's avoidance of punishment. Charles elaborated on the newspaper reports by attributing Mary's distress in part to their mother's attitude. Elizabeth Lamb seems not to have repaid Mary's emotional investment. Charles wrote to Coleridge on 17 October 1796 that their mother 'met her [Mary's] caresses, her protestations of filial affection, too frequently with coldness and repulse'.[108] In this case, the patient's affective response to the receipt of care contributed palpably to the nurse's distress.

After the stabbing, Mary's legal position was precarious. It is not entirely clear how she evaded prosecution for murder or lengthy incarceration in Bethlem which, prior to the opening of Broadmoor Hospital in 1863, was England's only institution for the reception of people thought to be criminally insane. Her identity as perpetrator was known locally, and while the newspapers largely avoided giving her name the *Whitehall Evening Post* explicitly attributed the crime to 'Miss Lamb'.[109] The actions of her younger brother Charles were probably critical, because he immediately removed her to a private madhouse in Islington. His own previous experience as an inpatient may well have contributed to his promptitude in this respect, as he recognised his own improved mental state after a period of hospitalisation. Therefore, when the inquest reached a verdict of 'lunacy' as the cause of Elizabeth Lamb's death, there was perhaps nothing more for the state to do, as Mary was already under household restraint. More than this, however, Charles built a narrative around his sister which was supportive, committed, and which provided lifelong protection: her mental stability might have been weak, but she was to be pitied rather than punished. In the short term, Charles Lamb wrote to Coleridge with relief: 'The good lady of the Mad house, & her daughter ... love her & are taken with her amazingly, & I know from her own mouth she loves them & longs to be with them as much.'[110] After their father's death, Charles and Mary lived together for the remainder of Charles's life. He needed no further hospitalisation, but she underwent a number of periods in private madhouses. The intense risk of negativity around Mary Lamb as a spinster, nurse, and undoubted murderer was neutralised by a combination of brotherly love and her sibling's emphasis on her affectionate, unpaid, overworked, and overwrought circumstances. By taking the initiative in this way, Charles offered Mary a combination of the 'status shield' and 'virtue script' which inhibited both stigma and prosecution.[111]

'Bad' nurses, or the risks of nursing work?

What these narratives and experiences suggest, but do not make explicit, was the types of risk involved in pursuing nursing work.[112] Each of the types of task outlined at the start of this chapter carried at least one risk of physical or emotional injury for the women who nursed. Watching and regulating, for example, required the kind of constant attentiveness prized by Agnes Porter's short story despite the risk of unregulated hours, night work, and unsatisfactory periods of rest. Concentrated, unalleviated nursing could lead to 'physical and emotional exhaustion'.[113] Literary unpaid spinster nurses knew this: Mary Lamb apologised for writing to Dorothy Wordsworth when she supposed the latter was tired from nursing her nieces and nephews, and Ellen Weeton had no difficulty believing that her sister-in-law fell into 'a Pleurisy' as a result of exhaustion (having nursed her own three children through illness).[114] Gertrude Savile's final diary entry remarked on the death of Princess Caroline in 1757 as the result of a neglected rheumatism, having attended the Queen at night time 'a great deal too much for her health and strength'.[115] Other observers, and particularly male medical observers of female nurses, did not appreciate the penalties of nursing in quite the same way. Therefore, it is not necessary to impose anachronistic concepts like 'burnout' on the pre-professional nurse: instead we can acknowledge that a parallel experience of exhaustion was possible between 1660 and 1820.[116]

The most dangerous aspect of the workload falling to nurses, according to contemporary apprehensions about self-care, should have been that of nightwatching. Remaining awake overnight might be asked of nurses for a variety of reasons including continuation of treatment, observation of a patient's condition, or companionship for the dying, labelled 'the necessary fatigue of her undertaking'.[117] Unfortunately, the very act of being out of bed and awake throughout the night was typically considered perilous. Buchan's *Domestic Medicine* frequently cites nightwatching as a precursor to poor health, and while this was compounded when combined with anxiety it was clear that the physical act of wakefulness was risky on its own.[118] Furthermore Buchan was repeating a shibboleth of long-standing medical advice and alleged danger.[119] Long periods awake including at night, and 'night Workings' were cautioned against during the whole period covered by this book and physicians tried to protect themselves against severe lack of sleep.[120] It was not unknown for practitioners to dose their patients with opiates so that they (the practitioners) 'might procure sleep after many nights watching'.[121]

Yet there was a blind spot among commentators about the watchfulness required of nurses at night. Lapses of attention or concentration should have been forgivable among a group of people who routinely missed their night's sleep (and who were not obviously given the chance to catch up on their sleep during the day), but instead the women who nursed at night were permitted no leeway on these grounds. Their attention to the patient was required to be constant. A failure of attention was not apparently mitigated by multiple nights of duty, let alone a single night. One of the only people to admit this was the fictional Clarissa Harlow:

> Hers is a careful and (to persons of such humanity and tenderness) a melancholy employment, attended in the latter part of life with great watching and fatigue, which is hardly ever enough considered.[122]

As implied above, watchfulness held a specific meaning for Buchan and others in the late eighteenth and early nineteenth centuries. Insomnia might be a decent synonym for the then combination of being awake at night, being worried, and allowing one's worries to assume undue magnitude during the hours of darkness. Contemporaries might therefore have dismissed the risks of watching to nurses on the grounds that they were not inevitably prey to the same wearing experiences as those who were involuntarily wakeful. Against this, we might now set the anxieties of the sick room. These were different for people who loved their patient, compared with those whose only commitment was contractual, but as the evidence above suggests there was not necessarily a clear-cut line between the unpaid and paid nurse in this respect. There was perhaps a spectrum of emotional investment in care for the patient, which might see even the detachment of a well-paid night nurse become liable to unease in the presence of suffering or impending death (not wholly or necessarily dictated by fears for her contract ending).

Instead of admitting their weariness, nurses were effectually encouraged to make light of the risks of night nursing. Melesina Trench, for example, reproached a correspondent in 1822: 'Why did you not write for me? Perhaps you know not that as a nurse I have perfect self-command, and that the care of those I love never injured my health; nay, that the privation of sleep, and the watchfulness it induces, seems to do me good.'[123] This sentiment chimes with the claims of Mary Hays's fictional character Emma Courtney, who when nursing the man she loves experiences 'neither fatigue nor languor – my strength seemed preserved as by a miracle, so omnipotent is the operation of moral causes!'[124] Powerful love can overcome otherwise commonplace tiredness. Real women through the period (as opposed to fictional ones) marked their nursing service in terms of successive sleepless nights, as when widow Ursula Venner looked after her father Edward Clarke in 1695 and reported 'I have not been in my bed this sennight', or when Elizabeth Freke sat up for the same period of time with her dying husband in 1706.[125] Perhaps this level of endurance was a badge of pride, a mark of women's commitment. Such a point of honour might help to explain Lady East's confusion when on one occasion, in 1791, her sister Harriet and her servant Kitty both sat up at night with her husband during his well-documented episode of gout.[126] Rather than avoid night-time duty, women were sometimes competing to fulfil it. For the fictional paid nurse, the capacity to work continuously without tiring was made the basis for their existence in an essay of 1806 titled 'Usefulness of an Old Woman', reinforcing the choices of the women in Lady East's household. The focus of the article, a 'Mrs Thompson', stressed the meticulous attention of old women in contrast to the self-centred behaviour of the young: 'An old woman is never tired of anything. I am old, Sir, and I know my value in society', she piously concludes.[127] Under these circumstances it was entirely congruent that fitness for sitting up might have been the threshold which determined women's capacity to nurse at all, at least by the fictional exemplar. Trimmer's nurse Wilden gives up nursing altogether when she finds nightwatching too strenuous (coincidentally suggesting that not all older women were utterly impervious to weariness).[128]

The recognition of physical risk around night nursing, and its active repudiation by a handful of real and fictional women, raises questions about other less tangible risks such as embarrassment, revulsion, fear, or guilt. Opportunities for embarrassment are met in the literature very slightly and concentrate on the patient. Johnson's *Friendly Cautions* discussed the administration of 'clysters' or enemas as being 'commonly now resigned to the Nurse' and urged that she be expert for fear of either disgusting or injuring her patient.[129] The book does not admit that the nurse too might be disgusted, but does give detailed instructions of how to insert the clyster pipe into the anus, the nurse using her left forefinger as a guide. The consequential penalties of the sick

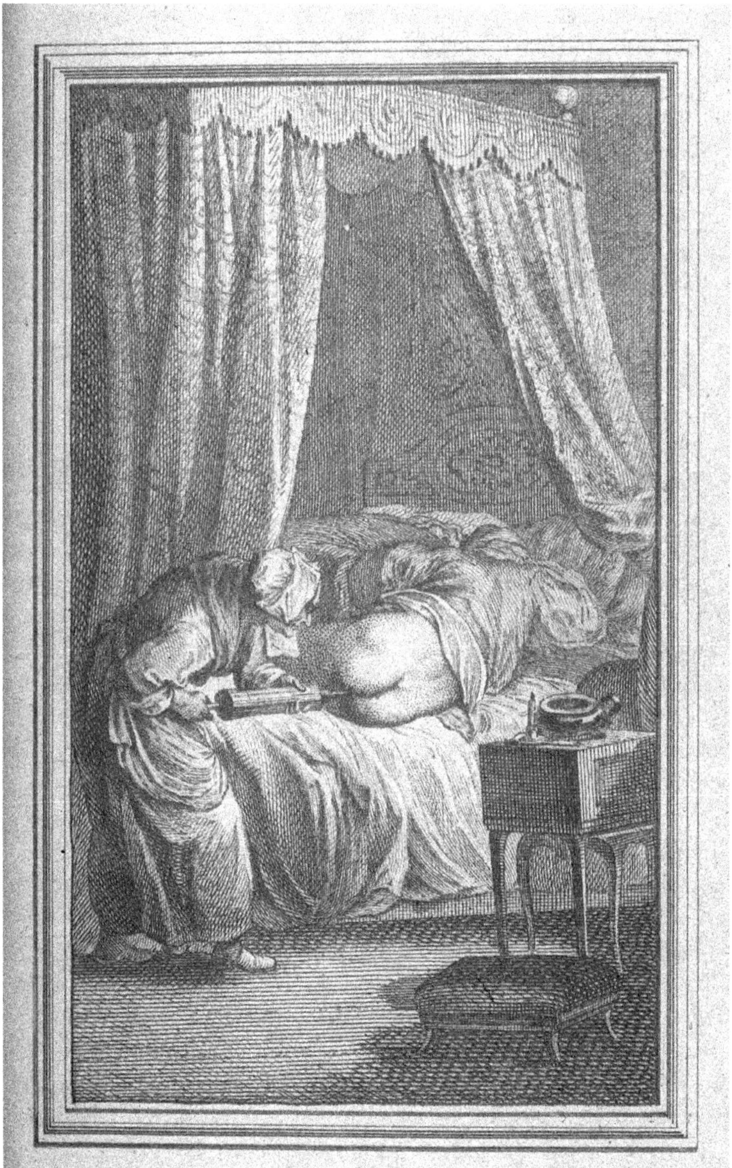

Figure 1.2 C. Eisen, A nurse gives a man an enema [1762]: engraving courtesy of the Wellcome Trust

room, identified by synonyms for anxiety and depression, beset nurses too, particularly when they had to deal with distressing physical symptoms, and expressions of pain, or patients' shattered spirits. The fact that nurses' own spirits were in jeopardy was only acknowledged by the women who knew the risks from personal experience. Dorothy Wordsworth, for example, in caring for one of her nieces in a convulsive illness of 1810, reflects on the emotional state of her brother and sister-in-law, adding 'I have had hard work to keep *my* spirits up'.[130] On a visit to Clifton near Bristol and the restorative Hot Wells, Abigail Gawthern admitted 'the appearance of so many invalids is truly distressing'.[131] Medical realisation of nurses' sufferings in similar respects was likely to be reconstrued negatively, such as in the observation that female attendants may be subject to hysteria.[132]

The risk of revulsion extended to fear of the dead body, which was admissible in unpaid nurses but apparently not considered for their paid equivalents. Gertrude Savile, for example, recounts watching the death of her friend Hannah D'Enly then immediately regarding the corpse with horror, but was this emotional freedom open to the woman who sat up with the body of John Collier, noticed above?[133] Confrontation of feeling about dead bodies was exacerbated where nurses' exposure was unanticipated, such as where they discovered the bodies of their patients or following suicides.[134]

Nurses might reasonably have feared contracting their patients' illnesses. Buchan was unusually attentive to this sort of physical jeopardy. He retailed an anecdote of a nurse who shared a bed with a child experiencing the 'bad' kind of smallpox: the nurse went on to suffer a severe case herself from which 'she narrowly escaped with her life'.[135] Similarly in considering venereal disease, Buchan feared the transmission to 'the innocent nurse' of an infected child (presumably in this case a wet nurse rather than a sick-nurse) and recommended that, rather than parents checking nurses for their freedom from infection, nurses should have children certified as 'clean'.[136] This was a rare acknowledgement of nursing risk from the medical faculty because while the danger of nursing contagious disease was well-known, concrete evidence is scattered. Daniel Gurney's nurse caught scarlet fever from her patient and died in 1809: Daniel recovered.[137] William Holland, noted above for his perception of nursing, observed in 1803 that the carer for a shepherd and his wife (both of whom had died) was now herself very ill, and in 1814 that the Wilkins family had caught an infection from the Rich family as a result of nursing.[138]

Guilt was a further risk: the need to be alert was constant, even during a patient's apparent sleep or insensibility, and a single slip of focus could prove fatal. In 1762, for example, Lady Tyrconnel's nurse was caring for her during a 'dreadful Fever'. The nurse left the patient alone presuming her to be sleeping, only to be summoned by passers-by in the street: Lady Tyrconnel was climbing out of the window, imagining she was escaping from an angry husband.[139] Edmund Burke allegedly received the dying confession of a nurse who had incautiously left her patient (a friend of Burke's) alone at the crisis of his illness when she should have given herself wholly to 'incessant watching', and ever afterwards blamed herself for his death.[140]

No type of nurse had a monopoly on any of the risks associated with their work. Paid nurses would have been no less tired than their unpaid equivalents after a sleepless night because cash income was not a protector against weariness. Unpaid nurses would have been no less susceptible to embarrassment, and may have been more so, if required (for instance) to deliver an enema to a relative. The stereotypes of ideal/voluntary and vilified/remunerated nurses are dismantled when the tasks of nursing are considered through a consideration of the nurse's (instead of the patient's) vulnerability.

Conclusion

Nurse Rooke may have been worth hearing, but she has rarely or never been heard outside the pages of *Persuasion*. Instead, her voice has been displaced by generalities about women who nursed, and about the supposedly corrupting effects of payment on tenderness. The delivery of care was largely congruent with women's broader identities throughout the period, meaning that any failure to care could constitute an indictment of individual women on the grounds of divergence from normative femininity. Consequently, historians' reliance on narratives by the observers of paid nurses has generated a one-dimensional view of their shortcomings. Paid nurses were thought inadequate on the grounds that they were likely to be emotionally inattentive, but it was easier to satirise them for being materially negligent (or only attentive to their own material needs). Emotional investment was less obvious in hired nurses, but that does not mean that they were immune to the pain or unhappiness of their patients or that they were absolved from emotion work. A patient may have thought a nurse hard-hearted at the same time that the female nurse struggled to manage her own emotions.

This survey of evidence for women's domestic nursing, from ideals, critiques, and accounts of nursing by real women, unfolds multiple alternative perspectives. Most detailed are the examples of Ellen Weeton, Elizabeth Ham, and Mary Lamb for their context and consequences of their nursing work. None of these women were paid specifically to nurse, and all demonstrate the emotional burdens of nursing. Mary Lamb was not the only domestic anti-nurse: she was the only nurse (domestic or institutional, female or male) discussed in this book who unequivocally murdered her patient. Clearly murder was a rare and extreme occurrence among nurses yet it illustrates the scope for mental disturbance arising from their work, and points to an unknown group of women whose distress manifested in other ways short of fatal violence.

The next chapter deals with the constraints of institutional working, from sources that offer less insight into women's emotions and more focus on their life-chances in social and economic terms.

Notes

1 J. Austen, *Persuasion* (London: Pan, 1971), p. 140.
2 R. Dingwall, A.M. Rafferty and C. Webster, *An Introduction to the Social History of Nursing* (London: Routledge, 1988), pp. 14–15.
3 Austen, *Persuasion*, pp. 97, 109, 113.
4 For a similar list of tasks, see A. Stobart, *Household Medicine in Seventeenth-Century England* (London: Bloomsbury, 2016), p. 20.

5 See for example P. Williams, 'Religion, respectability and the origins of the modern nurse', R. French and A. Wear (eds), *British Medicine in an Age of Reform* (London: Routledge, 1991), p. 233.
6 M. Pelling, *The Common Lot: Sickness, Medical Occupations, and the Urban Poor in Early Modern England* (London: Longman, 1998), pp. 191–2.
7 See, among many, *Rules and Orders for the Government of St Bartholomew's Hospital* (London: [no details], 1814), pp. 77–8, 85–6.
8 For the early years of the period, see T. Coxe, *A Discourse wherein the Interest of the Patient in reference to Physick and Physicians is soberly Debated* (London: C.R., 1669), p. 67. In 1761, parish nurse Mary Dew described applying a poultice and plaisters to her patient as a matter of course: www.oldbaileyonline.org (accessed 1 February 2023).
9 T. Fuller, *Exanthematologia: Or, an attempt to give a rational account of eruptive fevers* (London: Charles Rivington and Stephen Austen, 1730); for usage by historians, see for example V.L. Bullough and B. Bullough, *The Care of the Sick: The Emergence of Modern Nursing* (New York: Prodist, 1978), p. 57.
10 T. Langtree, 'Notes on pre-Nightingale nursing: What it was and what it was not' (Phd thesis, James Cook University, 2020).
11 T. Tanner, *A Practical Treatise on the Small-Pox and Measles* (Worcester: S. Bryan, 1745); R.W. Johnson, *Some Friendly Cautions to the Heads of Families* (London: David Wilson, 1767).
12 W. Grant, *An Essay on the Pestilential Fever of Sydenham, commonly called the gaol, hospital, ship, and camp-fever* (London: T. Cadell, [1775]), p. 141.
13 C.J. Lawrence, 'William Buchan: Medicine laid open', *Medical History* 19: 1 (1975), 20–35, on p. 20. The closest rival to *Domestic Medicine* was John Wesley's *Primitive Physic*, first published in 1747, which made virtually no mention of nursing.
14 C.E. Rosenberg, 'Medical text and social context: Explaining William Buchan's *Domestic Medicine*', *Bulletin of the History of Medicine* 57: 1 (1983), 22–42, on pp. 27–8.
15 W. Buchan, *Observations Concerning the Prevention and Cure of the Venereal Disease* (Edinburgh: Mudie and Sons, 1796), p. xx.
16 T. Dimsdale, W. Buchan and G. Swieten, *The Present Method of Inoculating of the Small-pox* (Dublin: John Exshaw, 1774), pp. 74–5.
17 S. Nicklin, *Address to a Young Lady on her entrance into the world* (London: Hookham and Carpenter, 1796), pp. 171–2.

18 A. Withey, *Physick and the Family: Health, Medicine and Care in Wales, 1600–1750* (Manchester: Manchester University Press, 2011), p. 178.
19 P. Wallis and T. Pirohakul, 'Medical revolutions? The growth of medicine in England, 1660–1800', *Journal of Social History* 49: 3 (2016), 510–31, on p. 517.
20 J. Alleine, T. Alleine, et al., *Life and Death of the Rev Joseph Alleine* (New York: Robert Carter, 1840), p. 91.
21 E. Hobby, *Virtue of Necessity: English Women's Writing 1649–1688* (London: Virago, 1988), pp. 80–1 for Theodosia's room for manoeuvre as the wife of a 'great man'.
22 One of the most positive treatments of a former nursery nurse turned sick-nurse is given in S. Morgan, *The Wild Irish Girl; a National Tale* (London: Richard Phillips, 1807) but where the nurse's Irish Catholic identity is critical to her character.
23 S. Richardson, *Clarissa: or, the History of a Young Lady* (London: the author, 1748), letter 5.
24 Richardson, *Clarissa*, letter 362.
25 Richardson, Clarissa, letters 426 and 481.
26 S. Trimmer, 'On nursing', *The Family Magazine* (London: J. Marshall and Co, 1788), pp. 318–23.
27 S. Trimmer, 'The good nurse', *The Family Magazine* (London: J. Marshall and Co., 1789), pp. 173–93.
28 Kitchen physick was a familiar epithet throughout the period covered here: see, for example, T. Cock, *Kitchin-Physick, or, Advice to the Poor* (London: Dorman Newman, 1676).
29 NB Florence Nightingale read some of Sarah Trimmer's output, specifically S. Trimmer, *New and Comprehensive Lessons* (London: J. Harris & J. Hatchard, 1818), although this work does not mention nursing; UK Reading Experience database: https://www.open.ac.uk/Arts/reading/UK/record_details.php?id=5374 (accessed 13 June 2023).
30 J. Martin (ed.), *The Journals and Letters of Agnes Porter* (London: Hambledon, 1998), p. 83.
31 [A. Porter], *The Triumphs of Reason* (London: the author, 1791).
32 R.C. Trench (ed.), *The Remains of the Late Mrs Richard Trench* (London: Parker, Son, and Bourn, 1862), p. 329.
33 G. Kelly, 'Opie [nee Alderson], Amelia', *Oxford Dictionary of National Biography*, https://doi.org/10.1093/ref:odnb/20799 (accessed 3 October 2022).
34 A. Opie, *Adeline Mowbray* (London: Longman, Hurst, Rees and Orme, 1805), volume III, p. 286.

35 Opie, *Adeline Mowbray*, volume II, p. 204.
36 Opie, *Adeline Mowbray*, volume III, p. 100.
37 L. Hart, 'A ward of my own: Social organisation and identity among hospital domestics', P. Holden and J. Littlewood (eds), *Anthropology and Nursing* (London: Routledge, 1991), p. 104.
38 Nicklin, *Address*, p. 170.
39 Nicklin, *Address*, p. 172.
40 P. Smith, *The Emotional Labour of Nursing* (Basingstoke: Macmillan, 1992), p. 103; Hart, 'A ward of my own', p. 102.
41 E.W. Marrs (ed.), *The Letters of Charles and Mary Anne Lamb, Volume II 1801–1809* (Ithaca, NY: Cornell University Press, 1975), p. 185.
42 M. Carpenter, 'The subordination of nurses in health care: Towards a social divisions approach', E. Riska and K. Wegar (eds), *Gender, Work and Medicine: Women and the Medical Division of Labour* (London: Sage, 1993), p. 101.
43 'Stanzas to a Sick Friend', *Ladies Monthly Magazine*, 1 August 1801, p. 137.
44 Williams, 'Religion, respectability', pp. 235, 248–9.
45 Nursing is not indexed in L. Davidoff and C. Hall, *Family Fortunes: men and women of the English middle class, 1780–1850* (London: Hutchinson, 1987), but nursing by male family members is referenced at pp. 330, 345–6.
46 W. Harris, *A Rational Discourse of Remedies* (London: Richard Chiswell, 1683), p. 170.
47 J.E. Ward and J. Yell (eds), *The Medical Casebook of William Brownrigg MD, FRS (1712–1800) of the town of Whitehaven in Cumberland*, Medical History supplement 13 (London: Wellcome Institute for the History of Medicine, 1993), pp. 19, 93.
48 Ward and Yell, *Medical Casebook*, p. 44.
49 M. Fissell and R. Cooter, 'Exploring natural knowledge', R. Porter (ed.), *The Cambridge History of Science, Volume IV: Eighteenth-Century Science* (Cambridge: Cambridge University Press, 2003), p. 149.
50 Trimmer, 'Good nurse', p. 190.
51 Carpenter, 'Subordination of nurses', p. 100.
52 This drawing of boundaries was not necessarily confined to practitioners: an essay about smallpox from 'a plain man' of 1752 found 'A nurse is as necessary in her place in this distemper as a physician'; *Gentleman's Magazine*, 22 (1752), 403–5.
53 P. Woodman, *Medicus Novissimus; or, the Modern Physician* (London: J.H. for C. Coningsby, 1712), p. 224.

54 T. Lobb, *A Treatise of the Smallpox* (London: T. Woodward and C. Davis, 1731), p. 439.
55 The death of Henry Jessard in late October 1805 from a fatal dose of laudanum given by an unnamed nurse was cited as a consequence of 'unlettered ignorance' rather than, for example, domestic dosing with potentially fatal substances: *York Herald*, 2 November 1805.
56 H. Woolley, *The Gentlewoman's Companion* (London: A. Maxwell for Dorman Newman, 1673), pp. 165–7.
57 'The Death and Adventures of Timothy Finch', *The Schemer, or Universal Satirist* (London: J. Wilkie, 1761), p. 163.
58 Trimmer, 'Good nurse', p. 188.
59 S. Bamford, *The Autobiography of Samuel Bamford, Volume I: Early Days* (London: Frank Cass, 1967), pp. 62–4.
60 *An Epistle to the Fair Sex, on the subject of drinking* (London: T. Gardner, [1744]), p. 45.
61 Trimmer, 'Good nurse', p. 175.
62 J.C. Pilkington, *Memoirs of Mrs Laetitia Pilkington*, volume III (London: R. Griffiths, 1754), p. 233.
63 E. Maynwaringe, *Tutela Sanitatis: The Protection of Long Life, and Detection of its Brevity* (London: Peter Lillicrap, 1664), p. 8.
64 J. Hargreaves, 'In the nursing homes, nurses really nurse: Nursing in private nursing homes in 1930s Britain', *Association for the History of Nursing Bulletin* (2022).
65 For the explicit contemporary supposition that nurses' withholding of prescribed medicines 'nearly approaches towards murder' see *Gentleman's Magazine* 22 (1752), p. 405.
66 Treated at length in Chapter 6. In fictional literature, Mary Wollstonecraft's character Jemima writes with horror about 'the virago of a nurse' without specifying particular harms, and in an institutional rather than a domestic context: see M. Wollstonecraft, *Maria or the Wrongs of Woman* (Oxford: Oxford University Press, 1987), p. 117.
67 For a French nurse confessing to multiple murders of ladies, see *Gentleman's Magazine* 6 (1736), p. 55.
68 'Vulgar prejudice', *Oracle and Public Advertiser*, 7 July 1796.
69 In addition to this case the occurrence of murder, coincidentally of foundling infants rather than sick adults, was investigated in Dublin in 1738; *London Evening Post*, 11–14 March 1738; M.B. Roe, *The Least of These: The Tragic Story of Dublin's Foundling Hospital* (Cheltenham: History Press, 2022), chapter 6. London's baby farms, and campaigning by Jonas Hanway in the mid-eighteenth century to reduce infant mortality, did not result in any firm allegations of murder

against specific women; J.S. Taylor, *Jonas Hanway, Founder of the Marine Society: Charity and Policy in Eighteenth-Century Britain* (London: Scolar Press, 1985), p. 115 for alleged 'killing nurses' in this context.
70 See for example E. Hall (ed.), *Miss Weeton: Journal of a Governess 1807–1811* (London: Humphrey Milford and Oxford University Press, 1936), p. 241, where the family was attended by two unmarried aunts, two paid nurses, and two servants. See also B. Hurst and S.C. Djabri (eds), *The Diaries of Sarah Hurst 1759–1762: Life and Love in Eighteenth-Century Horsham* (Cirencester: Amberley, 2009), p. 171 when a sister and a paid nurse were both in attendance on the diarist's father. Surrey History Centre, Z/588/1 Diary of Elizabeth Davis 6 October 1793 depicts the diarist nursing her sister-in-law during the day but a paid nurse being recruited to relieve her at night.
71 Berkshire Record Office, D/EX1306/1 diary of Lady East 1791–92.
72 R.M. James, 'Health care in the Georgian household of Sir William and Lady Hannah East', *Historical Research* 82: 218 (2009), 694–714, on p. 706; J.I. Wand-Tetley, 'Historical methods of counter-irritation', *Annals of Physical Medicine* 3: 3 (1956), 90–8 with particular reference to gout on pp. 96–8.
73 James, 'Georgian household', p. 710.
74 James, 'Georgian household', pp. 711–12. For a similar experience of nursing by a wife a little lower down the social scale, albeit in less detail, see Agnes Witt: A. Sutton (ed.), *An Edinburgh Diary 1793–1798* (Stroud: Sutton, 2016), pp. 78, 85, 104–5, 107–8, 117–18, 144, 165, 415–17. For brief reference to nursing by a mistress rather than a wife, see B. Cozens-Hardy (ed.), *The Diary of Sylas Neville, 1767–1788* (Oxford: Oxford University Press, 1950), p. 266.
75 Martin, *Agnes Porter*, p. 126.
76 A. Henstock (ed.), *The Diary of Abigail Gawthern of Nottingham 1751–1810* (Nottingham: Thoroton Society, 1980), p. 59.
77 M. Bevan, 'Dalrymple, William (1772–1847)', *Oxford Dictionary of National Biography*: https://doi.org/10.1093/ref:odnb/7060 (accessed 19 January 2023) for Devaynes and Hingeston as court apothecaries towards the end of the eighteenth century.
78 All references to the experiences of the Collier family may be found in R. Saville (ed.), *The Letters of John Collier of Hastings 1731–1746* (Lewes: Sussex Record Society, 2016), pp. 20–35.
79 John died on 31 December 1732, and was buried (in Westminster Abbey) on 15 January 1733. James had fallen ill by 9 January 1733

at the latest, which means that there was a period of at least six days when James was sick but John remained unburied.
80 This accords with the interim findings of the Social Bodies project funded by the Leverhulme Trust, where data from personal letters between 1680 and 1820 revealed very few references to nurses in letters authored by men; S. Fox, K. Harvey and E. Vine, 'Material identities, social bodies: Embodiment in British letters c.1680–1820', seminar paper for the British History in the Long 18th Century seminar held at the Institute of Historical Research in London and online, 5 October 2022.
81 J. Ayres (ed.), *Paupers and Pig-Killers: the diary of William Holland, a Somerset parson, 1799–1818* (Stroud: Sutton, 2000), pp. 130, 171–2, 238, 266.
82 Ayres, *William Holland*, pp. 103–5, 126, 134–5. Sarah Styling later became a murder victim, although not notably as a result of her nursing activity: pp. 183–4.
83 This meant she was not herself a natural nurse: on at least one occasion, her own mother grew weary of her attendance; see A. Savile (ed.), *Secret Comment: The Diaries of Gertrude Savile, 1721–1757* (Nottingham: Thoroton Society, 1997), p. 147.
84 Savile, *Gertrude Savile*, p. 322.
85 Savile, *Gertrude Savile*, pp. 328–9.
86 Savile, *Gertrude Savile*, pp. 70, 72. Stobart, *Household Medicine*, p. 157 gives Bridget Fortescue taking two different servants with her to London when seeking medical advice, because one of them was adept at dressing her while the other tended her ailments (and neither was deemed suitable to do the other's job).
87 Savile, *Gertrude Savile*, pp. 190, 229.
88 Sutton, *Edinburgh Diary*, p. 119.
89 E.W. Marrs (ed.), *The Letters of Charles and Mary Anne Lamb, Volume III 1809–1817* (Ithaca, NY: Cornell University Press, 1975), p. 65.
90 R.A. Anselment (ed.), *The Remembrances of Elizabeth Freke 1671–1714*, Camden fifth series, volume 18 (Cambridge: Royal Historical Society, 2001), p. 287; A. Ingram, S. Sim, C. Lawlor, R. Terry, J. Baker and L. Wetherall-Dickson, *Melancholy Experience in Literature of the Long Eighteenth Century: Before Depression, 1660–1800* (Basingstoke: Palgrave Macmillan, 2011), pp. 157–64.
91 Ayres, *William Holland*, p. 124. See also A.C. Edwards (ed.), *The Account Books of Benjamin Mildmay, Earl Fitzwalter* (London: Regency Press, 1977), p. 148 for an aristocratic employer paying for lodgings and a nurse for a coachman with smallpox.

92 Henstock, *Abigail Gawthern*, p. 83.
93 J. Swan, *The Entire Works of Dr Thomas Sydenham* (London: Edward Cave, 1742), p. 122.
94 M. Dresser, *The Diary of Sarah Fox née Champion: Bristol 1745–1802* (Bristol: Bristol Record Society, 2003), p. 14.
95 Hurst and Djabri, *Sarah Hurst*, pp. 170–1.
96 E. Gibbon, *Memoirs of My Life* (London: Penguin, 1990), p. 61.
97 Paragraphs about Ellen Weeton and Elizabeth Ham have previously been published in a short work-in-progress article as A. Tomkins, '"I helped to nurse": Unpaid care work by Georgian spinsters 1780–1820', *UK Association for the History of Nursing Bulletin* 10 (2022). I am grateful to the editor for permission to reproduce them here.
98 Smith, *Emotional Labour of Nursing*, and P. Smith and H. Cowie, 'Perspectives on emotional labour and bullying: Reviewing the role of emotions in nursing and healthcare', *International Journal of Work Organisation and Emotion* 3: 3 (2010), 227–36.
99 Hall, *Miss Weeton*, pp. 231–9, containing all references to this incident.
100 E. Gillett (ed.), *Elizabeth Ham by Herself 1782–1820* (London: Faber and Faber, 1945), pp. 7, 180–1.
101 B. Jones, 'Ham, Elizabeth (1783–1859)', *Oxford Dictionary of National Biography*, https://doi.org/10.1093/ref:odnb/45850 (accessed 12 July 2023); E. Ham, *The Infant's Grammar, or a Picnic Party of the Parts of Speech* (London: Harris and Son, 1824); Gillett, *Elizabeth Ham*, giving multiple small indications of feeling marginal, particularly from chapter 40 onwards.
102 J. Whittle, 'A critique of approaches to "domestic work": Women, work and the pre-industrial economy', *Past and Present* 243: 1 (2019), 35–70, on pp. 54–6. The risk of this prejudice was recognised in the eighteenth century; T. Gisborne, *An Enquiry into the Duties of the Female Sex* (London: T. Cadell Jun. and W. Davies, 1797), pp. 275–7, which cautioned families against treating unmarried women as unpaid drudges.
103 For references to this period of Ham's life see Gillett, *Elizabeth Ham*, p. 180.
104 At each end of the period see (for example) the Hervey letter books cited by H. Newton, *Misery to Mirth: Recovery from Illness in Early Modern England* (Oxford: Oxford University Press, 2018), p. 125 and M. De Lancey, *A Week at Waterloo* (London: Reportage Press, 2008).
105 *Morning Chronicle*, 26 September 1796.

106 E.W. Marrs, *The Letters of Charles and Mary Anne Lamb, Volume I 1796–1801* (Ithaca, NY: Cornell University Press, 1975), p. 4, letter to Coleridge of 27 May 1796 suggesting that Charles was a patient at Hoxton from mid-November 1795 to mid-February 1796; see also the letter of Robert Southey to Edward Moxon, 2 February 1836, recalling his introduction to the Lambs in 1794–95; extracted from A. Roberts et al., *Mary and Charles Lamb – Their Web Biographies*, http://studymore.org.uk/ylamb.htm (accessed 13 July 2022).
107 Marrs, *Letters of Charles and Mary Anne Lamb, Volume I*, p. 34.
108 Marrs, *Letters of Charles and Mary Anne Lamb, Volume I*, p. 52. This combination of demanding patient and emotional frigidity is reminiscent of Adela Cleveland's experience in the novel by S.H. Burney, *Traits of Nature* (London: Henry Colburn, 1812), volume V.
109 *Whitehall Evening Post*, 24–7 September 1796. This was the only report discovered (out of at least twelve between 23 and 28 September) which gave her name among the titles featured in the digitised Seventeenth and Eighteenth Century Burney Newspapers Collection: www.gale.com (accessed 19 January 2023).
110 Marrs, *Letters of Charles and Mary Anne Lamb, Volume I*, p. 48. This hospitable lady was Ann Holmes; L. Smith, *Private Madhouses in England, 1640–1815: Commercialised Care for the Insane* (London: Palgrave Macmillan, 2020), p. 95.
111 M.D. Cottingham, R.J. Erickson and J.M. Diefendorff, 'Examining men's status shield and status bonus: How gender frames the emotional labour and job satisfaction of nurses', *Sex Roles* 72: 7–8 (2015), 377–89; M. McAllister and D.L. Brien, 'Narratives of the "not-so-good nurse": Rewriting nursing's virtue script', *Hecate* 41: 1–2 (2016), 79–97.
112 Considered briefly in M. Stolberg, *Experiencing Illness and the Sick Body in Early-Modern Europe* (Basingstoke: Palgrave Macmillan, 2011), p. 57.
113 H. Newton, *The Sick Child in Early Modern England, 1580–1720* (Oxford: Oxford University Press, 2012), chapter 3, 'The family's experience of care'.
114 Marrs, *Letters of Charles and Mary Anne Lamb, Volume II*, p. 239; Hall, *Miss Weeton*, p. 241.
115 Savile, *Gertrude Savile*, p. 338.
116 For a brief survey of causes and consequences of burnout in the modern nursing profession, see among others J.S. Felton, 'Burnout as a clinical entity', *Occupational Medicine* 48: 4 (1998), 237–50, on p. 241.
117 Fuller, *Exanthematologia*, pp. 208–9.

118 See for example W. Buchan, *Domestic Medicine*, [16th edition] (London: A. Strahan, T. Cadell jun., and W. Davies, 1798), p. 88.
119 E. Maynwaringe, *Tutela Sanitatis: The Protection of Long Life, and Detection of its Brevity* (London: Peter Lillicrap, 1664), p. 37. See W. Walwyn, *Physick for Families* (London: J. Winter, 1669), p. 93 for an account of a nurse made ill having 'tyred her self with care and watching'.
120 Ward and Yell, *Medical Casebook*, p. 153.
121 N. Cotton, *Observations on a particular kind of scarlet fever* (London: R. Manby and H.S. Cox, 1749), p. 16.
122 Richardson, *Clarissa*, letter 507. The concern for nurses' risk of exhaustion was also periodically absent in the twentieth century: K. Roberts, 'An ambiguous presence: Wartime constructions of the body of the nurse', *UK Association for the History of Nursing Bulletin* 10: 1 (2022), www.bulletin.ukahn.org (accessed 12 June 2024).
123 Trench, *Mrs Richard Trench*, p. 478.
124 M. Hays, *Memoirs of Emma Courtney* (Oxford: Oxford University Press, 2009), p. 176.
125 Venner is quoted in Stobart, *Household Medicine*, p. 20; Anselment, *Remembrances*, p. 289.
126 James, 'Georgian household', p. 712.
127 'Usefulness of an old woman', *La Belle Assemblée* 1: 1 (1806), 12–13.
128 Trimmer, 'Good nurse', p. 190.
129 Johnson, *Friendly Cautions*, p. 108 [of 1767 edition]. *Gentleman's Magazine*, January 1813, p. 50 for a review of a book which mocks apprentices to medicine for the supposition of their being 'too fine a gentleman to think of contaminating your fingers by administering a clyster to a poor man, or a rich man, or a child dangerously ill, when no nurse can be found'. See I. Eyers and T. Adams, 'Dementia care nursing, emotional labour and clinical supervision', T. Adams (ed.), *Dementia Care Nursing: Promoting Well-being in People with Dementia and their Families* (Basingstoke: Palgrave Macmillan, 2007) for revulsion in the twenty-first century.
130 E.D. Selincourt (ed.), *The Letters of William and Dorothy Wordsworth, Volume II: The Middle Years 1806–1811* (Oxford: Clarendon, 1969), p. 396.
131 Henstock, *Abigail Gawthern*, p. 115.
132 W. Rowley, *The Rational Practice of Physic*, volume I (London: the author, 1793), p. 303.
133 Savile, *Gertrude Savile*, p. 84.

134 *True Briton*, 31 October 1797 report of an inquest on the suicide of Mr Bruister, when a nurse found the body.
135 Dimsdale et al., *Small-pox*, p. 98.
136 Buchan, *Venereal Disease*, pp. 153–4. Earlier medical authors had also noted this sort of risk to wet nurses; see E. Maynwaringe, *The History and Mystery of the Venereal Lues* (London: J.M., 1673) p. 84, suggesting that the nurse of a poxy child 'earns her wages very dearly'.
137 Birmingham Archives, MS 30101/C/D/10/6/44 Galton papers correspondence, letter to John Howard Galton from L.A. Patterson 8 October 1809.
138 Ayres, *William Holland*, pp. 76, 262.
139 J. Greig (ed.), *The Diaries of a Duchess* (London: Hodder and Stoughton, 1926), pp. 45–6. [untitled], *Sun*, 4 July 1793 for a fatality during a domestic nurse's brief absence.
140 A. Hayward (ed.), *Diaries of a Lady of Quality from 1797–1844* (London: Longman, 1864), pp. 16–17. Feelings of guilt have rarely been acknowledged in the modern medical workplace, let alone the historical one; F.M. Gazoni, M.E. Durieux and L. Wells, 'Life after death: The aftermath of perioperative catastrophes', *Anaesthesia and Analgesia* 107: 2 (2008), 591–600.

2

Nursing the metropolis: the ancient London hospitals of St Thomas's and St Bartholomew's

> At St. Bartholomew's, part of the charge to the Sisters when chosen, is, 'Also ye shall use unto them (the patients) good and honest talk, such as may comfort and amend them'. I doubt this is not often done by these Sisters, who are, too many of them, fine dressy ladies.[1]

This judgement by radical novelist Mary Hays about the Sisters at St Bartholomew's Hospital is unexpected: it points in the opposite direction to most criticisms of paid nurses, specifically that they were of lower social status and demeanour than was required by their employer, and instead finds them too elevated to engage with patients.[2] This perception of a snub arose, perhaps, because the Barts Sisters were unusually successful in asserting their authority in the ward over both patients and their visitors.

The women who Hays encountered may have been standoffish if they had imbibed any of the governors' pride in their hospital's history. St Bartholomew's and St Thomas's hospitals, refounded in 1546 and 1551 respectively as part of the Protestant Reformation in England, were (until the eighteenth century) the nation's only hospitals which were dedicated to patients who were physically sick.[3] Both were general hospitals, accepting surgical and medical cases, and responsive to moments of national crisis such as the civil wars of the 1640s and the final epidemics of plague.[4] They catered only to the curable poor. Prosperous patients would always choose to be treated in their own homes, and the incurable were inadmissible. Both foundations were rebuilt in the period 1660 to 1820, each exchanging their medieval accommodations for a more coherent architectural presence, expanding their patient capacity as a result.

Following redevelopment, they could both hold between 400 and 460 patients.[5]

The historiography of these hospitals has traditionally comprised proud institutional histories by former medical staff which occasionally noticed differences between the two institutions, such as on political grounds.[6] More recently Barts, at least, has provided a focus for the history of medical education in London, and the leadership of men at Barts in offering lectures.[7] Nursing activity is recognised by these authors in predictable ways: women before the 1850s are noticed as either picaresque or squalid, their working lives serving as a suitable backdrop to their well-trained successors after nursing reform. The 1995 book about nursing at Barts, written by a hospital archivist, even invokes the Dickensian image of Betsy Prig: the nurses' misbehaviour and dismissals from post 'reflect something of the restricted lives' of the hospital's female employees 'from which drink offered an easy if temporary escape'.[8] This history was, thus, entirely unqualified by the wider historiography of the early modern period or by histories of women as workers.

The institutional archives which survive for these two hospitals, at the London Metropolitan Archives and the Barts Heath Archives respectively, do not feature any collections of personal papers for nurses before 1820. Instead, they contain multiple fragments of evidence about hundreds of women who were appointed to nursing posts and who were only noticed again by hospital managers if they were party to routinely collected data or if their service was noteworthy in positive or negative ways. The St Thomas's nurses can be captured for decades at the beginning and end of the eighteenth century, where they can be combed out from the hospital's records incorporated into the London Lives dataset, to enable some occasional remarks about female staff. The St Bartholomew's archive exists solely in manuscript at the time of writing but yields information about female employees over the full period 1660–1820 (albeit with interruptions) around dates of appointment, reasons for dismissal, and conditions of service. Therefore, this chapter will consider the nursing experience at both hospitals, giving prominence to the women identifiable as working at St Bartholomew's, but extending the analysis by sporadic reference to St Thomas's nurses.

It will address, briefly, the standard charges of nurses' drunkenness, and the opposing characterisation of them in the introductory quote for this chapter as fine and dressy. Most attention will be given, though, to the more detailed and interesting evidence for nurse experiences and life-chances in terms of recruitment, tenure, and ward culture.[9] The significance of their clothing, *vice* Hays, features briefly.

Nurse careers in London played out in a rapidly evolving context. The metropolitan landscape of institutional care changed dramatically over the period as a result of the rising provision of workhouse infirmaries. There were few or no such spaces in 1700, but workhouse foundations proceeded briskly in the early eighteenth century and capacity dedicated to the sick or injured developed apace. Marylebone, for example, acquired its first workhouse in the mid-eighteenth century, and from 1775 used this 'old' workhouse exclusively as an infirmary. A new infirmary with three hundred beds was used from 1792.[10] The provision of workhouse infirmary spaces exceeded London's hospital beds in number at some point in the second half of the eighteenth century, and made a profound difference to the chances of poor patients being sent to the latter.[11] The presence of workhouse care, for all that the phrase might seem at first sight like a misnomer, is well established in studies of provincial England as well as in London.[12] Furthermore the tacit public health function filled by the expansion of workhouse facilities even had particular purchase for specific types of patient, such as those with venereal disease, in addition to the chronically ill and incurable who were inadmissible to hospitals.[13]

Unfortunately, there is little consistent empirical evidence about the identity of workhouse nurses, or detail about the nature of their institutional labour. Nursing was undertaken by fellow paupers as a part of the workhouse's central aim to set the poor to work, and in line with other forms of toil nursing could be rewarded with small cash sums rather than fully remunerated.[14] In Forehoe Hundred Workhouse in Norfolk during the early 1780s, for example, nurses of the sick poor were given two shillings and six pence per quarter (two pence less than was given to nurses of children).[15] The women (and possibly men) who undertook the work might be competent or even deserving of praise: patients in the workhouse of St Margaret's parish Westminster were judged 'well nursed' in 1732.[16] Yet detailed evidence about workhouse nurses is fragmentary. This is a shame because their opinions could be taken very seriously as people with experience of caring for the sick poor. In 1817, for example, the death of a pauper at the St Martin in the Fields Workhouse resulted in an inquest, where the workhouse nurse Catherine Ann Pigott and her assistant Mary Brown both gave evidence. Pigott in particular confirmed that the dead man's 'stomach rejected some barley-water which she gave him' and that this was evidence of his dying from want.[17] The problem lies in identifying workhouse nurses beyond exceptional cases.

The nurses of St Bartholomew's Hospital

The refounding of St Bartholomew's Hospital by Henry VIII in 1546 saw the continuation of an old tradition, the presence of female attendants or Sisters.[18] There were fifteen Sisters by the middle of the seventeenth century, and these women were joined incrementally by helpers or nurses to whom the Sisters could deputise. By around 1660 there was apparently an intention to appoint one Sister to each ward, plus one nurse/helper to selected wards, and a short time later on 21 January 1678 it was decided to give preference to helpers for any vacancies among the Sisters. The title 'nurse' gradually superseded the older label 'helper', and the two classes of worker – Sisters and nurses – were joined by a third from the mid-eighteenth century, when watchers or night nurses were recruited to each ward.[19] These latter women lived outside the hospital, unlike the Sisters and nurses who were accommodated in house, and were not generally named in the hospital records (and so are not a focus for this chapter).[20] By the end of the eighteenth century there were ninety-nine women superintended by the matron: one Sister, one nurse, and one watcher for each of the thirty-three wards.

On appointment and at intervals thereafter the Sister and nurses were read their 'charge', as confirmed in the quote at the start of this chapter. This comprised a set of behavioural rules rather than a job description. In the earliest printed version, in addition to obedience to the matron, and serving the patients, Sisters were enjoined to avoid foolishness 'and above all thynges see that ye avoyde, abhore and detest skoldying, and dronknennesse, as moste pestilent and filthie vices'.[21] In time these injunctions became composites of recommendation for comportment. By 11 June 1795, for example, the Sister was 'answerable for the conduct of the patients in her ward' which happened to include an embargo on the use of alcohol not specifically dispensed by the hospital. The terms of the 'charge' remained prominent, as it became usual towards the end of the 1810s to gather the female ward staff together and read the charge to them all on an annual basis.[22] The core tasks of the nursing staff throughout the period were to keep the wards and patients clean, deliver food or drink, and ensure that physicians' orders were followed for patients taking medicine.[23]

The rules were tightened, however, at the start of the nineteenth century by a governors' minute of 21 May 1803 covering the duties of the Sisters, and by a subsequent published edition of 1814.[24] The women had to remain in their wards after seven or eight at night (depending on the season), 'except for some great and especial cause' including risk of death and 'needful succour'. Sisters were required to attend church with patients on Sunday morning, while nurses followed them on Sunday evening. A critical addition to the explicit conditions of service was that ward staff were not to absent themselves to nurse any sick people outside of the hospital. This suggests that both the governors and the hospital's female servants were by then aware that institutional employment constituted a form of training with a commercial value that the hospital was keen to monopolise.

Early historians of nursing at St Bartholomew's Hospital identified the laundry or 'buck' as a key element of the nursing role.[25] The bedding of each ward was washed in a large tub or buck, and the Sisters took turns at this laborious and dirty work.[26] Collectively they received additional payment for doing the laundry, supplemented as either the number of wards went up or as the cost of fuel, ash, or soap increased.[27] The amounts of money involved were substantial, and the women would have argued that they should have been even higher. In 1698 the Sisters petitioned that the buck cost them thirty-five shillings to complete, when they were only allowed thirteen in recompense; the allowance was raised to eighteen shillings for every buck.[28] The women's responsibility for laundry continued until 1754, when the hospital governors realised that Sisters had long been in the habit of taking the money and promptly paying someone else to do the work. This other person, Elizabeth Johnson, who was not otherwise known to be a hospital employee, was receiving three pounds for the buck every three weeks from the hands of the Sisters.[29] On making this discovery, the governors assumed responsibility for paying Johnson and her successors as laundrywomen, and the female ward staff were only supposed to undertake small-scale washing thereafter of a type which did not require such a large tub or 'buck'.

Laundry was a well-known adjunct to the work of nursing more broadly and gave rise to some debates in provincial infirmaries as to when or whether nurses *should* wash textiles in addition to washing patients.[30] What is distinctive about the trajectory of laundering responsibilities at St Bartholomew's Hospital was the palpable reluctance of Sisters to undertake the laundry work, and their independent decision to deputise (at high cost) without reference to governors' permission. This suggests that Sisters' complaints about expense were acting as a vehicle for their desire to distance themselves from work which was laborious and dirty because it involved protracted contact with soiled patient linens. Sister Elizabeth Ladley was very probably demoted rather than promoted when she became the hospital washerwoman on 13 December 1770.[31]

Beyond laundry, it is important to acknowledge that the sick-nursing workload of the women was determined somewhat by the number of patients under their care, and further by the nature of patients and their ailments. There were between ten and fifteen beds in each ward of the main hospital throughout this period, meaning that nursing at Barts broadly conforms to the one-to-many pattern identified in Table 0.2.[32] In the late seventeenth century demand for places could be modest, not least owing to the requirement that patients pay admissions fees (on which, see more below): three wards were empty on 23 November 1689. The expansion of facilities arising from eighteenth-century rebuilding increased the hospital's capacity but not necessarily the typical workload for female ward staff since the number of beds per ward remained constant. Venereal patients were initially treated in the Lock and

Kingsland branch hospitals but were taken into dedicated venereal wards for men and women respectively within the main hospital after 1760. Patients in the surgical or 'cutting' wards, and subsequently those with venereal disease, were judged to create heavier work for nursing staff, with an impact on their wages. Beyond these venereal and surgical designations, information about patient illnesses or injuries is piecemeal.[33] Finally, the patient population per se was separating from – but not wholly divided from – London's pauper population.[34] The provision of workhouse infirmary beds meant that, across the eighteenth century, a declining proportion of patients was coming from among the parish poor.[35]

The salaries given to Sisters and helpers/nurses at St Bartholomew's Hospital were modest and were complicated in the seventeenth century by their consisting of two separate components. There was a fixed annual stipend, set at fifty shillings in 1621, augmented by weekly 'board wages' to cover the fact that female ward staff were not given their diet by the hospital: they were supposed to buy and prepare their own food. This weekly element stood at three shillings and six pence per week at the start of the period, giving the Sisters an annual income of £11 12s. This remuneration increased little or not at all until 1782 but received a decided boost in the early nineteenth century. In 1802, Sisters were given a basic income of £32 6s 10d rising to a maximum of £52 16s 7d for the Sister of the men's venereal ward, while nurses received at least £17 16s 10d rising to £24 16s 9d, also for working in the men's venereal ward. In this context, however, both Sisters and nurses could demand fee income from patients on admission.[36] For comparison, the Sisters at St Thomas's Hospital were possibly in a better position from 1731 onwards when their wages were raised to reflect the fact that the hospital no longer permitted patients to be charged fees by ward staff. This meant that Sisters at St Thomas's received a reliable annual income of between £25 and £40, where nurses received £16 to £20.[37] Fees were not abolished at Barts until 1821.[38]

In addition to remuneration in cash, Sisters and nurses lived in the hospital where they had a bed but not, seemingly, their diet. They were accommodated collectively in a Sister's dormitory until the hospital was rebuilt between 1730 and 1768, which may have contributed to collegiality in the first half of the period.[39]

Allegiance to wards rather than to other women was perhaps accentuated after the rebuild, when Sisters were given a separate room next to 'their' ward.[40]

Notwithstanding these benefits of employment, Sisters and helpers/nurses were differentiated from other female staff in the hospital, being of decidedly lower status. The matron and cook, plus in the seventeenth century the woman designated as the curer of scald heads, were 'officers' of the hospital whereas the Sisters, nurses, and helpers were denoted 'servants'.[41] This created a boundary between the female employees which might be crossed in friendship but was only crossed occasionally in person.[42] Similarly Sisters might deputise for the matron but were never regarded as suitable to replace her, and the (anomalous) formal appointment of a matron's assistant in 1690 was not apparently made by drawing on the existing ward staff.[43]

Coincidentally, joining the women on the wards, a midwife was appointed by the hospital in an ad hoc fashion, more visible in the Old Bailey records than in the journal minutes.[44] She was retained at a payment of twenty shillings per quarter in 1703, which constitutes a significant sum for a woman in a hospital where female patients were not admitted in order to give birth; the hospital governors presumably apprehended that midwifery services would be needed either for concealed pregnancies or for women where the pregnancy was evident but tangential to their reason for admission. Finally, women from beyond the existing staff could be appointed for specific nursing purposes that were not related to ward attendance: in 1677, Jane Adams was to make 'straite stockins' for the poor patients.[45]

Female ward staff may have been regarded as below officer status in terms of the hospital's internal affairs, but they could still be seen as important and visible representatives of the charity. Perhaps with this in mind, from the outset the Sisters were required to wear blue uniforms during the day, and from 1687 were supplied with white night 'rails' or bedgowns.[46] At some point it became their own responsibility to supply the white gowns.[47] The latter were even supposed to be worn ceremonially in procession when Sisters made their way to divine service, meaning these must have been quite robust or thick nightgowns.[48] Therefore, if they seemed 'fine' and 'dressy' to hospital visitors in 1804, their appearance as such was somewhat dictated by hospital policy and the women's involuntary consumption of clothing.[49] Attire may have contributed, though, to the ability of female ward staff to exhibit a haughty demeanour, as seen at St Thomas's hospital in 1709 with a complaint about a Sister's 'high carriage' and reported at Barts in 1786 as a Sister's 'imperious elevation of voice'.[50] Such an attitude may have seemed lacking in tenderness, or even inhumane, but still have comprised an important element of the nurses' ability to fulfil their role. The markers of authority that nurses devised to differentiate themselves from patients at the point of patient admissions are discussed further in Chapter 3.

The identities of new nursing appointments at Barts were not recorded in the hospital journals with scrupulous consistency. There is a notable gap in recording between 1800 and 1814, for example, when a separate book was supposedly kept to record all nurse appointments (which is now lost). The journals are indexed, but the index is imperfect, particularly for women at first appointment as nurses: by the final third of the eighteenth century, notes about promotions were more likely to be indexed. Nonetheless, 611 women were named in the journals of 1660 to 1820 as helpers/ nurses or Sisters, either at first appointment, promotion, departure or death. It is impossible to know what coverage this represents of all women employed in the 160-year period, because turnover of staff who were not named (for whatever reason) may have differed from those who we can trace throughout their careers. Estimates of female staff totals based on the number of open wards is also problematic, since the number of wards in operation at any one time could fluctuate. Burial records offer one way of estimating the scale of underreporting in journals: thirty-two women were buried at St Bartholomew the Less between 1662 and 1812, with an occupational designation of being in life the Sister of a specific ward (having died in service) who had not otherwise been found named in the journals. This number can be compared with eighty-five women buried in the hospital's parish between 1665 and 1820 who can be traced in the journals. If the propensity for Sisters to be buried and remarked on in the burial registers remained constant throughout the period, then perhaps 27 per cent of sisters were not cited in journals.[51] There is no similar test for underrecording nurses. These data combined with a rough calculation of female staff coverage of the different wards by women named as ward personnel suggest either that the journal evidence fails to credit some women with protracted tenures in post, or there is a modest undercounting of Sisters and a serious one for nurses. This unknown absence notwithstanding, the journals provide valuable, not to say unique, data for considering the lives of women inside and outside the hospital, who have otherwise been subject to generalisations at best.

Recruitment

It is not clear who made selections of women to appoint as nurses and sisters. At Barts, the matron's word seems to have counted for a good deal, and the governors saw each woman before or at the meeting which formally appointed them. In one or two cases a woman had a named sponsor. Yeo argues that the hospital employed women on the basis of their physical strength, but this seems inadequate when we consider that women could be moved between wards to match heavy duty with physical capacity and vice versa, as women might became infirm in post.[52] The rules made allowances for Sisters too weak to carry bread, beer, and meat from the kitchen to the wards.[53] The matron in 1771 claimed to be interested in women's character and disposition, and in aligning their capacities with the demands imposed by the duties of different wards.[54] Just occasionally female patients were appointed to the nursing staff, presumably where they had already demonstrated some competency.[55]

At St Thomas's women were said to have been 'recommended to the committee', although not by whom, and to be selected on the basis of their age and good health; it became a rule not to appoint women over the age of 40 (later extended to 50).[56] Even so the hospitals were possibly adopting slightly different employment regimes. In the years 1705 to 1710 St Thomas's had a policy of periodic review of nursing staff, and of systematically discharging those thought to be incapable of their service, in a way that was not obviously mirrored during any period at Barts.[57]

There is additional information about the admission of women as nurses or helpers at Barts in the 1710s, when the hospital recorded not only the names of appointees but also those of their rivals. Between 1709 and 1717 there were twenty-four occasions when multiple women sought employment at Barts, and these are expressive of hot competition for places. There was an average of five candidates for each vacancy, but some women presented themselves repeatedly to try to get in. Widow Elizabeth Woodrolfe tried six times to be chosen between 1713 and 1714, before finally being selected as a helper in June 1715.

Hospital governors at Barts may have made estimations of women's physical capacity and/or worth, but the chief of their concerns which is visible relates to women's financial vulnerability to poverty, because from the late seventeenth century the governors took an interest in where the nurses and Sisters were legally settled. As early as 1684, a Sister who had been recommended to a post by the wealthy grocer Sir John Cutler was still asked to provide security to serve the hospital and parish 'harmless' of her child.[58] A minute of 8 December 1707 required all new helpers/nurses or Sisters to offer security against their future 'infirmity'. It is not clear whether this was ever enforced strictly, but the implications of the laws of settlement (whereby employment at Barts for more than one full year would confer a settlement in the parish of St Bartholomew the Less) had made an impression.[59] Senior members of medical staff continued to underwrite Sisters' employment on occasion.[60] In the years 1770–1800 the question of a woman's settlement was regularly noted in the journals at the time of her appointment, and for the final years of the eighteenth century the weekly component of the women's wages was calibrated according to their being 'settled' or 'unsettled': higher payments went to women who could prove their settlement in another parish, a phenomenon which hospital historian Norman Moore judges meant the retention of 'better' women (Moore presumably inferring that settlement could be used as a guarantee for women's prosperity and respectability at some point prior to their hospital appointment).[61]

Reflecting these priorities, the hospital sought settlement certificates to ensure that women recruited from other parishes did not necessarily gain a new settlement in St Bartholomew the Less.

The institution's urgency to protect its home parish was conveyed to female staff via the threat of dismissal, encouraging them to secure evidence even from a distance. Illiterate Mary Stanny had a letter written on her behalf to the parish of St Michael in Bedwardine, in the city of Worcester, to secure proof of her deceased husband's settlement 'without which she will be discharged'.[62] This suggests the governors remained aware of the potential proximity of women to parish relief throughout the period, particularly if nurses and Sisters did not die in service but fell into need after their work for Barts had ended. The hospital's duties in this regard were perhaps observed the more punctiliously after a ruling from the King's Bench, which stated that the hospital itself could not be rated for poor relief (despite having pulled down dwelling houses during the rebuilding programme, and so narrowed the parish's rate base).[63] These measures made a decisive difference to the women concerned, because at least one former Sister died in a workhouse.[64] If the Barts nursing staff were not poor women at the time of appointment, both they and their employer recognised their risk of becoming so.

Tenure and promotion

The average tenure of women as hospital employees (whether as nurses alone, or as nurses and then Sisters) also belies the idea that the work was excessively or punitively arduous, or that women were all appointed in hope and quickly dismissed on discovery of their physical or behavioural frailties. Minimum and maximum tenures can be calculated wherever careers within the hospital can be charted from the time of their first mention in the journals (for the former) or where their occupation as nurses and then Sisters can be known with some certainty from first appointment to departure (for the latter). The minimum tenure for 148 women was four years, with the bulk of evidence deriving from the first half of the period. The maximum tenure for 108 women was seven and a half years, comparing favourably with the average for women at provincial infirmaries given in the next chapter and with the nurses of the Royal Infirmary in Edinburgh.[65] The longest-standing female employee was Lettice Dyne (or Ginn, or Pyne, but certainly the same woman), serving at least thirty-three years. She has been immortalised in the hospital's historiography as the Sister famously discharged in 1721 for repeatedly setting the bed curtains on fire.[66] She was also, coincidentally, the only woman employed at Barts whose ethnic origin was identified as Irish. Shorter tenures among other nurses might have arisen from an early sacking, but could also be the result of death, resignation to coincide with marriage, or another no-fault cause.

The Sisters at Barts were routinely appointed from the ranks of the helpers or nurses, and therefore we can assume that the hospital did at least approve those women who received promotion as 'well behaved'.[67] The hospital noticed occasions when women were appointed as Sisters having reached the place of 'senior' helper (meaning in this case, the helper longest in post rather than the woman who was oldest). The practice was modified on 27 March 1771, when the matron reported that the longest-standing nurse was not necessarily the most appropriate person for the post of Sister. Thereafter the hospital governors approved the promotion of the person 'most fit and proper', a judgement which we must assume was based on a combination of capacity and demeanour. A similar practice is visible at St Thomas's Hospital in the late seventeenth century, offering shreds of additional evidence that women who were promoted had received a generalised endorsement of their work. In 1694, Jane Wade was chosen Sister of Susannah's ward at St Thomas's, having worked as an assistant for some years 'and of good report', and on the same day Elizabeth Wilmshurst was made Sister in Tobias ward having 'behaved herself orderly'.[68] Mary Adams, promoted in 1700, had 'behaved herself very well' before becoming Sister of Queen's ward.[69]

At Barts there was a shortening interval between first appointment and promotion to Sister over the whole period from 1660 to 1820. From 1660 to 1740 the waiting time was typically two years and ten months, whereas between 1740 and 1820 the time spent as a mere helper or nurse fell to nearer one year and five months. This suggests either that staff turnover at Barts became more rapid in the second half of the eighteenth century, or that the increasing number of wards (from twenty to thirty-three) shortened the wait time for the more prestigious job of Sister.

Perhaps as a result the hospital had to become less picky about the women it promoted.

The data gathered here for different wards permit an even finer-grained analysis of women's movement within the hospital. On 20 January 1705 the matron reported that it was customary, on the death of any Sister, to allow the eldest Sister to take the place in the dead woman's ward 'if they desired to remove'. Ward transfers were not reliably reported, but we can see the results of the accumulation of transfers (whether owing to the matron's discretion or sisters' choice) in the turnover of female staff on Diet ward. This was a men's ward up to at least 1740, becoming a female ward by 1762. The sister of Diet had no obvious helper or nurse before the 1750s. Between 1662 and 1775 there were at least twenty-seven women who held the post of Sister in Diet ward, and there are three gaps in the known succession of Sisters meaning that we can infer the presence of at least three more women in post (where, for example, Jane Watkins died in 1674, but the next recorded Sister of Diet Elizabeth Green took up the work in 1682). The gaps may of course have been more numerous in reality, and more than one sister might have filled each known gap. This means that the maximum average tenure for sisters in Diet ward stood at 3.8 years. From this disparity between the tenure as Sister of any ward, seven and a half years, and the literal tenure of Diet ward alone, there was comparatively brisk movement of Sisters between wards according to their capabilities and preferences.[70]

Ward culture, misbehaviour, and dismissal

It is an ambitious claim, to consider ward culture in a context where neither official hospital histories nor any personal narratives can be cited to access such a feature of working life. Nonetheless, the female staff data comprising variously appointments, promotions, transfers, complaints, dismissals, and deaths can give us some idea of the tenor of life on multiple wards. The addition of coincidental ward descriptions within Old Bailey trial accounts provides focused vignettes of the interactions between different grades of nurses, and between nursing staff and their patients. Interesting, though, is the realisation that none of these materials speak to the relationship between male hospital staff and nurses.

After first appointment at Barts the governors referred to women by their title and the name of their ward rather than by their first name and surname. Yeo suggests that this practice was so engrained that other staff may not even have known the women's actual names: this reads the diction of the hospital journal too literally, as will be seen, but women attached to wards could become territorial about them. In the 1670s Mary Cotton was Sister of Queen's ward, which she spontaneously decided to decorate. When the matron then suggested that she move to Soldier's ward, Cotton

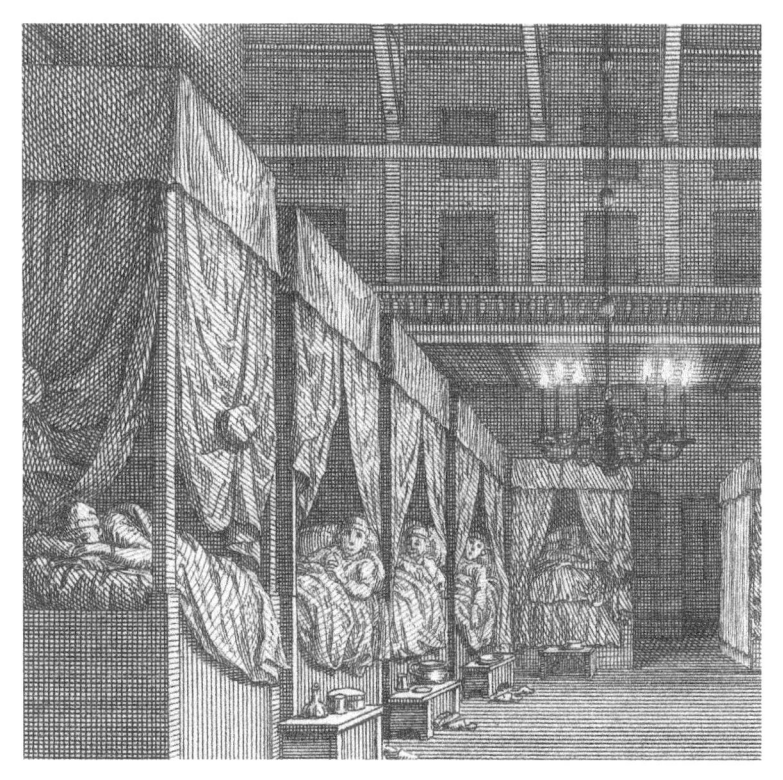

Figure 2.1 J. Folkema, detail from an etching of a hospital dormitory or ward [1702–67], showing a typical eighteenth-century arrangement of hospital beds: image courtesy of the Rijksmuseum, Amsterdam

was understandably resistant after all her 'whitening and making handsome' in Queen's. The governors reconciled her to the move by offering financial recompense for her handiwork.[71]

Wards offered variable work experiences to Sisters and nurses. Cloister ward was an ancient establishment, its name presumably having been shortened from the longer Cloister Dorter ward listed in 1571. It was a men's ward, still open in 1660 and probably closed around 1740 when the first range of the new building was opened. Ten women are known to have served as Sisters in Cloister, concentrated in the period 1681 to 1736. Of these ten, six are known to have died in post as senior female staff members, and only one complaint was ever registered for the ward. Magdalen ward had a similar profile, albeit across a longer lifespan. Magdalen was probably present in 1660 and there was still a ward bearing the name in 1800: throughout the period it was chiefly reserved for female patients. Ten out of fifteen confirmed Sisters for the ward died in post, with deaths spanning the range of years. Therefore, we can assume that these were two of the wards suited to lighter duties, where the matron might place women whose capacities were declining (either as a result of illness or old age) and where they could serve until shortly before death. Experiences of female staff in Cloister and Magdalen wards can be seen in the context of Soldier ward where no Sisters are known to have died in post, despite the ward being demonstrably open between 1672 and 1814 (and probably for the full span of years 1660 to 1820). It seems reasonable to conclude that Soldier ward was for the robust female nursing staff. Unfortunately, the mortality rates for patients in these wards cannot be known.

The presence or absence of a 'helper' in a ward, the sex of patients, and the strenuous or lighter nature of the work in a ward (specifically the Cutting or surgical ward involved heavy work) might have been expected to have some bearing on the prevalence of complaints against nursing staff by either patients or other members of staff to the hospital's governors. Instead, no pattern is visible from the available data by simple cross-referencing of these factors. Instead, a patchy but intriguing picture emerges that cuts across preconceptions about nurses and patients.

Long ward was another of the anciently named clinical spaces, among the first to be closed at the time of new building, and like Cloister was a ward for male patients. It also had a notable behaviour problem among its nursing staff in the 1680s, witnessing five complaints between 1683 and 1687 (chiefly around financial irregularity). Curtain ward, also long established, had a short-term problem, with four complaints in the three years between 1691 and 1693: was this despite the fact that Sisters were supported by helpers, or caused by the helpers' presence? Katherine ward was similarly turbulent if over a longer period, featuring eleven complaints. What underlay these patterns? The highest number of complaints (fifteen) was reported for King ward, but since a ward with this name was in continuous use between 1662 and 1820, this only gives rise to a rate of one problem reported every ten years. At the most quiescent end of the spectrum, Faith and Patience wards (both opened in the early 1750s, both for female patients throughout) reported no complaints against its female nursing staff at all. This is particularly noteworthy for Patience which was named as a venereal ward in 1760, and thereby took patients who already carried a form of problematic behavioural label, by contemporary standards, and yet who generated no problems for nurses that gave rise to a reported complaint.

Unlike the women who worked in provincial infirmaries, at Barts Sisters and helpers/nurses were permitted to exact fees from patients on admission. Hospital observers could still deprecate the manner in which fees were sought, but the fee had a function: it was conceived as repayment to the ward staff for the provision of 'earthenware and other necessaries', meaning a dedicated chamber pot. Since the fee at no stage equated to the cost of purchasing a cheap pot, and was always considerably higher, the differential was presumably intended to represent additional recompense to the ward staff for the dirty work of emptying the pots repeatedly after use. Even so, the hospital governors were keen that patient poverty did not prevent people from taking up their hospital place, confirming on 3 August 1711 that patients without the wherewithal 'shall be furnished at the charge of this hospital'. The fees were not abolished at Barts until 1821, so they remained part of the experience for nursing staff and patients alike throughout the period: the same was not the case for nurses in provincial hospitals, so the significance of fees as recompense for dirty work will be taken up in more detail in Chapter 3.

Sisters at Barts in the early eighteenth century could ask for one shilling from incoming patients, while helpers/nurses could request six pence (except for women in the venereal or surgical wards, who could ask for more).[72] In case of doubt, the rules were 'printed in a large character' and hung up in each ward to inform the patients and remind the staff about the limits of legitimate exaction of fees.[73] Wrongdoing therefore occurred where female ward staff charged more than these permitted fees, perhaps by taking 'gifts' (bribes) from patients or their friends, relations, or sponsors. In 1729, for example, Nurse Graham of the Kingsland branch venereal hospital was given half a crown by the workhouse master of St Sepulchre to persuade her to take better care of the parish's poor patients.[74] Women were reprimanded or dismissed occasionally throughout the seventeenth and eighteenth centuries on these grounds.[75] An egregious case of 1769 saw Ann Stambridge, the Sister of Watt's ward, call one of her patients 'a nasty stinking creature' and extort money in retribution for the patient's incontinence. Nonetheless complaints arising from fees or money more generally were fewer than those associated with alcohol, and both were dwarfed by other sorts of problem.

'Drunkenness and misbehaviour' were grounds for dismissal of Sisters and nurses, and this specific phrase was used prominently in the period between 1770 and 1791. Seventeen complaints of drunkenness in twenty-two years might look like a trend: but taken over the whole period, drink did not cause many Sisters to traduce their 'charge'. There were 181 instances of complaint over the 161 years, or an average of just over one problem per year reported among (by 1800) sixty-six nurses and Sisters. It is near certain that these 181 occasions were the minimum recorded complaints rather than the total of actual wrongdoing by women, but nonetheless the information about these complaints is revealing. Drink was specified in just twenty-nine entries overall. Some wards had an endemic problem, at least over a short period, as in Elizabeth ward for example where two Sisters were discharged for drunkenness within three years. Yet women were much more likely to be rebuked for miscellaneous bad conduct (which might of course have hidden various specific sins) or for very particular faults. These range from 'unwomanly carriage' in 1664 to being with child (specified 1693 and 1813). Petty embezzling was a constant low-level problem (whether of hospital property or patients' clothing) but reprimands for occasioning distress to patients fell off after 1750. Approximately 60 per cent of all complaints noticed in the journals resulted in a dismissal.

From this analysis of complaints against nurses and Sisters it is clear that intoxication was a risk but was not displayed so regularly or egregiously as might be supposed. The picture at Barts is repeated at St Thomas's in the period between 1681 and 1710, when twenty-four recorded complaints included three allegations of nurses' drinking.[76] A fair-minded historian of the Royal London hospital observed in 1962 that 'lack of moral sense and insobriety are not incompatible with kindness of heart'.[77] More importantly perhaps, the late eighteenth century was not the high point of complaints against the nursing staff at Barts: a greater concentration had arisen in the period between 1687 and 1700, when there were thirty-six complaints overall (and only one of them mentioned alcohol).[78]

A more persistent and prominent source of conflict throughout the period lay in the deployment of textiles. Female ward staff had multiple daily contacts with patients' clothing and hospital bedding, giving rise to opportunities for questionable acquisitions. The hospital rules were clear: if a patient died, their clothing was to be given to the matron, and at no time should nurses or Sisters regard hospital textiles as their own. In practice women subtracted clothes from the stock of deceased patients, pawned clothes and sheets belonging to patients or the hospital, and engaged in other behaviours with cloth which could be recognised by the matron and governors as 'embeazling'. Some women unwisely continued to make free with bedding even after it was conspicuously marked as hospital property.[79] We might now understand why the hospital's female servants regarded some perquisites of this sort as their right. Servants in private households were able to secure cast-off clothing from their employers as an additional source of benefit and, as in the hospital, there could be vigorous domestic disputes over entitlements to items variously construed as payments, gifts, loans, and thefts.[80] Nurses and Sisters could have reasoned that the cloth goods that passed through their hands were resources to be used to advantage, 'part of the moral economy of service', a supposition that was only challenged when their behaviour was noticed.[81]

These sorts of issues extended down the scale of hospital resources to the smallest of petty textiles such as tow rags and pledgets, as meagre perks or as problematic objects when out of place. The Sister of King ward was dismissed in 1770 for filching the rags otherwise allocated for patient use, while generalised reproach (or threat of dismissal) was reserved for women who chose the easiest way of disposing of used bandages and pledgets by putting them down the privy.[82] Fabric items were also the occasional cause of friction between the women (as opposed to between female employees and hospital as employer). Egregious instances were tried as felonies, as where helper Elizabeth Hawkins was prosecuted by the Sister of Long ward for multiple thefts including handkerchiefs and a muslin apron.[83]

Clearly dissatisfaction and irritation could be features of life at Barts as they are likely to be for any institution.[84] Nonetheless, nurses have been done a disservice where historians have regarded complaint as a defining feature of reactions to nurses. For example: at Barts, unfounded complaints against female staff gave rise to energetic rebuttals by the hospital board. A letter signed by J. Browne was received in 1729, accusing the Sister and nurse of the Cutting ward of 'several abuses' towards the patients. On 1 May the governors questioned the surgeons and the then cohort of patients in the ward who all contradicted the claim, crediting the female ward staff with 'great care tenderness & compassion to the patients' and reassuring the governors that the allegations were 'false and scandalous'. But internal vindication was not sufficient: an advertisement was placed in two newspapers asking 'Browne' to attend at the hospital to give further information: a marginal note in the minutes confirms that no one showed up.[85]

Complaints from outside were therefore occasions for the display of support for nurses by the hospital's governors and medical men: a track record of working at Barts arguably offered women a modest status shield. Another instance in 1749 shows that judgements could differentiate between women in otherwise identical circumstances during an internal dispute. Mary Vaughan the Sister of Sailor's ward and Sarah Field the Sister of Soldier's ward were both dismissed for using ill language and unmannerly behaviour towards the porter and steward. Sarah Field was allowed to go without protest, but the surgeons of the hospital petitioned for Mary Vaughan's reinstatement as 'a very sober person and very diligent and carefull in her ward'. She was restored to her place on promising not to give cause for complaint in future.[86]

Defence or condemnation of female ward staff was the only time that interactions between them and the male medical practitioners can be glimpsed at Barts.[87] As flagged in the Introduction, nurses only appear in the most meticulous of medical practitioners' personal papers, and even then they were rarely noticed. At St Thomas's in 1801–02, student Hampton Weekes recognised the Sisters chiefly when they undertook extramural service nursing his colleagues (rather than their routine work on the wards). William Attree was a dresser for Astley Cooper and shared the same lodgings as Hampton Weekes; when Attree became very ill, the medical men around him speculated that he might have suffered a dissection injury of a type which regularly killed or disabled medical students. Attree underwent bloodletting with leeches, fomentation, and poultices, and took a long time to recover: he also had one of the hospital Sisters sitting up with him for at least a few nights, before employing his own private nurse.[88] Similarly the hospital's physician George Fordyce had a Sister 'constantly there to nurse him' during his decline into death, an informal duty which presumably took her away from her proper attendance on a ward for long periods.[89] What is clear is that Weekes does not provide any confirmation of Sisters' poor behaviour or tendency to drink. He never noticed drunkenness; specifically, he did not deprecate the use of Sisters to nurse the medical staff on the grounds of their inattention and insobriety. The only occasion when he recorded activity which would have been deplored by hospital governors was when he delivered the child of a night nurse, who unexpectedly went into labour while working on Mary's ward.[90] On the contrary, Weekes credited one Sister with making a critical discovery in the progress of a child's surgical case.[91]

If dismissal of nursing staff was necessary and not subject to mitigation, St Bartholomew's Hospital did not dismiss women very quickly after appointment: the shortest suspected term of office was experienced by Mary Ellison, appointed in November 1772 and discharged the following March for undifferentiated 'misbehaviour', but she was not at all typical. A minimum tenure can be calculated for fifty-one of the women who were sacked, and they managed over four years on average before losing their place. We might give this information a negative or positive reading: either women held their posts for years without their chronic misconduct resulting in dismissal, or women were generally satisfactory until the stresses of their job, increasing age and tetchiness, or other deteriorating factors pushed their behaviour too far to be unremarked or condoned.

The example of Grace Porter shows how difficult it could be to balance the requirements of the job against the personalities of the women employed. She first appeared in the journal in 1735 at the time of her appointment as a nurse and was made a Sister in 1738. She was not named again until 1751. On 9 January of that year she was dismissed as the Sister of Treasurer ward for (among other faults) rudeness and unkindness to patients. Porter petitioned to get her job back, and the governors minuted on 16 January that 'she was very capable of her business [as her tenure of at least sixteen years implied] and had always been careful of her patients, but sometimes subject to a violence of temper'. She was eventually and decisively sacked in 1755 allegedly following many subsequent complaints of misbehaviour (seemingly not noted in the journals), but the hospital's dilemma was clear: Grace Porter was a decent nurse from the perspective of conducting tasks, but her personality was not necessarily suited (or became increasingly unsuited with age) to patience with patients and/or co-workers.

Similarly, the career of Mary Campbell offers a composite illustration of the limits to the responsibilities demanded of Sisters, and the failings tolerated among them. She was appointed as a helper in the Cutting ward in April 1693 and fulfilled the role sufficiently well to be promoted to Sister of Cutting in July 1698. In August of the same year she tried to test the extent of her authority by refusing to take her turn at the buck: she was ordered to undertake the laundry which fell to her lot, and similarly ordered to give up the key to the door opening into the Long Walk. Campbell's behaviour continued to be inappropriate: in October she was reprimanded for staying out of her ward late at night and keeping company with 'men'. Even so she remained as the Sister in Cutting ward until 1701, and on her replacement it was not stated that she had been dismissed for infractions. Instead she was retained, briefly, to wash the patients' linen (as opposed to the hospital linen) in her former ward. Given the potential of keys to express power in an institutional context, it is noteworthy that Campbell was the only member of nursing staff asked to surrender one. Was she unusual in gaining control of a key at all?

Most importantly, women's careers as hospital servants could end honourably without their giving rise to complaint or being dismissed. Given that only a small proportion of staff departures were marked by complaints being noted in the journals, women may have resigned for any number of reasons that did not incur displeasure. Women who left their employment to get married, for example, or who gave up their posts shortly after marriage, were noted six times within the short period 1705 to 1721, and there were certainly more such occasions that were not minuted even within this seventeen-year slot.[92] Martha Butterfield, for example, was a helper who moonlighted as a searcher of the dead for her home parish of St Sepulchre. She was appointed as a searcher until such time as she was promoted at the hospital to the place of a Sister and therefore occupied full-time in charge of a ward. Yet she never reached this threshold because in 1715 she got married; neither her appointment nor her discharge was recorded by the hospital.[93]

Therefore, ward culture need not have been dominated by complaint, and day-to-day nursing practice was occupied with an array of the tasks and responsibilities discussed in Chapter 1. Routine relationships at Barts were only recorded, though, when the events or conversations which took place on wards became of wider significance, as they occasionally did in the prosecution of criminal trials in testimony aired at the Old Bailey (serendipitously within shouting distance of the hospital).

The prosecution of Isabella Buckham – age unknown – for infanticide in December 1755 sheds valuable light on ward dynamics.[94]

Briefly, Buckham was ill in Faith's ward apparently with dropsy, and in the early hours of 20 November she visited the privy or 'vault' before complaining of wet sheets. The bed was found to be covered in blood, and the body of a male infant was found in the cess pool. When brought to trial, Buckham's defence was that she was not in her senses at the time her child was delivered in the privy, and she was acquitted. Beyond the potential infanticide, however, the trial transcript gives the sequence of events revealed in Faith's ward that night, the opinions exchanged between the nurse Ann Smith and the other patients, and the role of the ward Sister.

Firstly, Ann Smith was sitting up by the ward fire between one and two in the morning, and a number of her female patients were also awake. She responded to Buckham's evident discomfort by emptying her bedpan, supplying it a second time for her 'puking', and warming a flannel petticoat to wrap around her waist. Smith would not pin on the petticoat for fear of pricking Buckham, but otherwise she was apparently attentive and responsive to her patient. This is also an instance where the nurse's familiarity with petty textiles, in this case a petticoat, became important given the blood and other marks which were later regarded as germane at the trial. The nurse reported of the petticoat 'we saw the print of the child in it'.

Second, other patients were drawn into Buckham's story, when they allegedly heard a child cry, and then when the sheets were found to be bloody. Nurse Ann Smith took the sheets to 'Molly' Elger, also a patient in Faith's ward, and said to her 'Look here, she says she never had a child.' Mary Elger and three other patients, Margaret Bland, Ann Wing, and Mary Old, gave evidence at the trial and refused to swear that the body which had been discovered was that of Buckham's son.

Third, the ward Sister Mary Lewis was alerted to these events, and took charge. She told Buckham that she definitely had borne a child and sent for the midwife. The unnamed midwife delivered the afterbirth and nurse Smith carried it away in a basin, providing in miniature an illustration of how the power dynamic between nurses and Sisters worked. Lewis instructed the midwife, while Smith cleared up after her. Lewis was asked whether Buckham was out of her senses, to which she replied 'I can't tell, for I was almost out of mine.' This may have been a reference to her own loss of sleep, or to how unusual it was for a woman to give birth in one of the female wards, or perhaps at her distress at the bloodied state of her ward (clots fell to the floor when the sheets were taken from Buckham's bed). It could also be evidence of further female solidarity, this time of the ward Sister with the accused patient.

This is not a deeply surprising story, but it is nonetheless a revealing one. It shows the ward working in some ways we might have anticipated – the nurse did the dirty work that the sister gave her – and in ways we could not have supposed, namely the collective voice of the nurse and female patients testifying to the fact of a birth but ambivalent about decisively linking the child's body to Buckham.

Under circumstances like this, ward culture became significant as a matter of wider public concern for Londoners; we can now also accord it some weight as indicative of the value for trusted female staff. A Mrs Horton, a Sister not otherwise identified in the hospital archives, sat up for most of the night in August 1737 with her patient William Reynolds, whose death gave rise to a murder trial.[95] Horton's testimony apparently carried some weight with the jury. She talked to Reynolds in his final hours and reported that he had exonerated the defendant 'and was very uneasy when he heard he was taken up'. The alleged attacker, William Runnington, was acquitted.

Recognition and trust, benefits and pensions

As the Old Bailey data suggest, trust in nursing staff could be displayed by patients and by the outside world, as well as by the hospital governors. For example: patients needed access to goods and services, and the hospital's female servants could influence or control their spending. In 1744 the hospital forbade its servants from selling items to patients directly, and in 1746 the governors ordered that none of the Sisters or nurses 'do divert or by any ways oblige the patients to buy their necessaries at any particular shop'. The governors perhaps anticipated that female ward staff would benefit financially from shopkeepers under such exclusive arrangements. But when the shop came to the patient, the results were chaotic. In April 1754 the hospital reported frequent complaints about disorderly persons 'crying and selling all manner of commodities' about the staircases and wards, meaning that patients who were not in the mood to buy were disturbed, and hospital property was pilfered. The immediate solution was to place hatches in the doors and require the porter and beadles to regulate the commercial traffic, but while this might have limited the salespeople's access to their customers, it did not take away from the pivotal role of nurses and Sisters (who could leave the hospital and undertake purchases as the patients' intermediaries). This deputising of female ward staff in making purchases for patients continued until the end of the period.[96]

Sisters were therefore trusted by patients to carry their word and their money beyond the ward. They could also be trusted by the hospital to deputise for officers in their absence, and this is most obvious in relation to the branch hospitals. A letter of 1747 testifies to the trust placed in Sister Elizabeth Russell in the arrangement of money matters, and to her literacy given that she wrote to Edward Nicklin, one of the churchwardens of St Bartholomew the Less, in her own hand. In 1760 the men's and women's Lock hospitals for venereal patients were closed, as it was found uneconomic to maintain them. Each hospital had one Sister, both of whom looked to Barts for their future survival: one was given a pension, and the other, younger woman was taken on as a Sister at the central site. But in order to divest themselves of the two properties, the hospital required both women to remain at the former branch hospital premises 'to show the same till let'.[97]

Recognition within the hospital was reflected in a diluted way when women stood at the boundary of the hospital or went out of their ward to engage with the wider metropolitan world. In this capacity they acted as the conduits for information. The Refuge of the Destitute, for instance, was a charity which aimed to offer poor men and women a fresh start in life from the first decade of the nineteenth century. Its core clientele was found among people at risk of imprisonment, those recently discharged from prison, or young women abandoned by their sexual partners, with the aim of offering temporary accommodation and a route to respectable employment.[98] The facilities of the Refuge became known to the nurses and Sisters of St Bartholomew's because it became quite usual for beneficiaries to be admitted to the hospital first for a cure for physical ailments, and only later admitted to the Refuge for moral reform. Sisters became instrumental to the charity when they recommended patients or friends of patients to apply there for relief. Illustrating this point, in 1813 17-year-old servant Elizabeth Brill was caught in an act of petty theft from her employer. She attempted suicide by cutting her throat, was taken to St Bartholomew's, and recovered. At the time of Brill's discharge from hospital, 'Mrs Aldred', meaning the Sister of Aldred ward, took Brill to the Refuge in person to testify to her good conduct during her time in the hospital and under her care.[99]

The benefits of hospital allegiance could work in reverse, as it were, whenever Sisters or helpers/nurses ended their employment only to be admitted as patients. Margaret Rouse, 'many years a Sister' and not able to fulfil her duties by reason of age, was admitted to one of the women's wards in 1678; Hester or Esther Grimes, initially a helper in Magdalen ward, died as a patient in Martha ward in 1712.[100] It was customary (at least in the 1720s) for women to receive physic free of cost, if they fell ill in service.[101] Benefits were even extended to those Sisters whose illness coincided with misbehaviour. On 22 November 1707 Ann Jones, the erstwhile Sister of Martha ward who was discharged for disordering herself with drink, was simultaneously admitted for the cure of her sore leg. Evidence is thinner for the second half of the period, but we can infer or identify former Sisters among the patients occasionally.[102] And as we have seen, Sisters in particular were permitted to die in service, with honourable burial in St Bartholomew the Less and remission of burial fees reserved for the most highly valued staff as 'a faithful servant, carefull of the poor'.[103]

Female staff could also be pensioned. At St Thomas's an early form of superannuation emerged in 1707 when the Sisters of Abraham's and Job's wards were found incapable of further service, being lame and blind respectively, but deserving of 'provision' as worthy 'old servants'. The hospital elected to give them accommodation in the institution, a choice of the hospital diet or two shillings and six pence per week in lieu, plus twenty shillings per annum for clothes.[104] The following year the Sister of Lydia's ward was given the same allowances, demonstrating this was not merely a one-off instance of munificence, although by 1709 it was being left to the treasurer's discretion whether women would be given the allowances of 1707 or sent to their parish of settlement.[105]

At Barts women were supported more generously, particularly from the late eighteenth century onwards. A pension rewarded women for their good and lengthy service. Lettice Dyne, noticed above as employed for thirty-three years, was given a pension of £10 a year in 1721. When the Kingsland branch venereal hospital was closed around late 1760, the nurse who had been in post for eleven years petitioned on the grounds of her age and infirmity and was also given £10 a year. From 1784 onwards, some Sisters who grew frail and unsuited to working on the wards were given pensions of sixteen guineas per year for the remainder of their lives.[106] This practice became marked in the years after 1800, when at least eleven pensions were granted up to 1820. Women who had remained at the position of nurse had more difficulty in securing support in old age, but the governors could be persuaded by a compelling case. In 1815 Elizabeth Stock secured a payment of one shilling per week, initially for one year. The grant was repeatedly renewed, up to at least 1825. This obviously made her much less favoured than the superannuated Sisters (Stock was only getting £2 12s per year rather than £16 16s) but this was perhaps a sign of the hospital's growing commitment to its former employees at lower levels by the end of the period.

It is also clear that the practice of pensioning female staff did not end after 1820, at a time when complaints about nurses and calls for nursing reform were on the rise. Fortune Fryer started working at the hospital before 1820. On retirement she returned to her native Hampshire to live with her brother and reported her hospital pension as her source of income in the census of 1851.[107]

Female staff and 'family'

Unearthing family stories for the Barts nurses involves genealogical difficulties. The female ward staff of the two ancient hospitals were chiefly identified by their first names and surnames, and rarely by other details such as a specific age or a parish of origin, making it difficult to trace them with any certainty in parish registers. Women's marital status was relevant to their recruitment to Barts, as the hospital took single women and widows but did not knowingly recruit wives, and women who married while in post were discharged (if they did not 'surrender up' their place in a timely way).[108] This means that the label 'widow' might feasibly be used to authorise connections between the women listed as a member of nursing staff and those with the same names occurring in digitised parish or city sources. For the most part, regrettably, these shreds of information are insufficient to justify identification of the women beyond the hospital archive in the vast majority of cases.

Genealogical research on selected women who have the virtue of either a highly distinctive surname, or a parallel source which categorically states they were employed by Barts, suggests that it was not the newly widowed who applied for or secured jobs there.

On the basis of this (admittedly very small) sample, women obtained work at Barts five years or more after the onset of widowhood, at least in the first half of the eighteenth century. This suggests that the future nursing staff were left in increasingly straitened circumstances, able to find other ways to get by for a number of years but ultimately seeking employment that was akin to menial service yet which supplied both accommodation and community. The two exceptions to this picture for whom we have evidence

Table 2.1 Women employed as Sisters, helpers, or nurses at St Bartholomew's Hospital for whom the onset of widowhood can be dated

Name	Widowed	Recruited or first named at hospital
Martha Azire	1746	1753
Priscilla Diggons	Before 1710	1715
Ann Fawdray	c.1747	1756
Hannah Fitzar	1723	1735
Jone Mottram	1684	1701
Mary Stanny	c.1748	1758

relate to Widow Chaloner and Elizabeth Blake, each formerly the wife of one of the beadles at the hospital, and appointed to nursing positions very soon after widowhood: John Blake died in 1763 and Elizabeth was made the Sister of Treasurer ward in December 1763, apparently without having to serve an apprenticeship as a nurse and despite the fact that she had two young children.[109] The widow of Walter Chaloner was similarly appointed before her husband had been for dead one year.[110] Thus prior contact with the hospital served as a form of economic safety net for widows of staff and as an opportunity for largesse on the part of the governors.

Surrounded constantly by the sick and regularly by the dying, the Sisters and nurses were apparently called upon to witness wills, or could even be invited to act as an executrix. The governors perceived the potential for patient exploitation, and ordered on 30 June 1711 that anyone made an executrix required the ratification of a hospital official 'to know and be satisfied that it is the Patient's voluntary will' rather than a deceptive or exploitative fraud. This injunction remained in the printed edition of the hospital rules of 1814.[111]

More significantly Sisters could be testators. Details of the people whose wills or administrations were handled by the Prerogative Court of Canterbury (PCC) have been digitised, making them easy to search.[112] The PCC proved wills for testators who left property to the value of £5 or more spanning two or more dioceses and therefore granted probate for people who had significant material substance, a brief which was not (on the face of it) a good fit for women employed in nursing. Even so, wills have been found for a small minority of the Barts Sisters, i.e. twenty-two documents proved 1714 to 1820 and a further two proved after 1820 for women at work during that year. Nothing substantive can be made of these from the point of view of the women's likely wealth. They can be used to uncover family stories more decisively, as widows named their children and single women named their siblings as beneficiaries.

Jane Collier's will seems to show that she worked at the hospital alongside her biological sister or sister-in-law. She and Mary Catterall were appointed as nurses on the same day in March 1735/36, and both worked in Barts, albeit in different wards, until Mary's death in 1746. When Jane made her will in 1767 she asked to be buried in the same grave with her brother and sister, Humphrey and Mary Catterall. This shows, incidentally, that Protestant non-conformity was no barrier to appointment, since the plot in question lay at Bunhill Fields (an exclusively non-conformist burial ground), and relevant burials for Mary and later Jane can be found there for 1746 and 1767 respectively. Non-conformity might also explain why Jane Collier had to be urged to be more frequent in her attendance at church in 1756. It is not clear on what grounds Jane referred to Humphrey and Mary as her brother and sister. They may have been her brother and sister-in-law, her brother-in-law and sister, or the relatives of Jane Collier's dead husband (if Mary had been Cattrall née Collier) and therefore were both in-laws. The only thing that is clear is that Jane's identity became subsumed with theirs on her burial. Jane Collier was buried as Mrs Jane Cattrall 'from St Bartholomew Ospitle'.[113]

The real value of the wills, however, lies in their ability to provide sidelights on relationships between the female employees of Barts. Sisters named others among the female hospital employees in a majority of wills – fifteen out of twenty-four. Four mentioned other women only as witnesses, but eleven left bequests and/or appointed executrices from among female colleagues. The most enmeshed Sister on this score was Mary Pew, who wrote her will and died in 1777. She was the Sister of Lazarus ward, one of the venereal wards, in a post she had held since July 1770. Family bequests took up £80. But she also appointed Elizabeth Gray, sister of Colston's ward, as joint executrix with one Edward Parkes, of Ratcliffe Highway, both of whom received £10 for their trouble. Furthermore, she gave Ann Ashby the nurse of Lazarus ward (in life, her closest colleague) £3, a further £3 to the hospital porter, and five shillings to each of the four hospital beadles.

In noticing hospital officers and servants among their beneficiaries, Sisters were adopting the practices of their alleged betters. They were showing largesse, and even patronage. Elizabeth Caton, who died in 1721, signalled her familiarity with funereal custom when she left money to buy a pair of kid gloves for every one of the then twenty sisters and made additional gifts including to the matron (who was definitely supposed to be her social superior). A Sister at the end of the period, Mary Owen, did not die until 1848 when she left the bulk of her estate, £250, to the hospital's Samaritan Fund. Investment in the institution during life fostered parallel commitments in death.

This pattern of behaviour provides tentative grounds for reading women's substantive allegiances into their long hospital service. Residence in the hospital over a number of years, perhaps sleeping in the same Sisters' room, and close working first as junior ward staff and then as Sisters, conferred at the least a level of personal knowledge about one another. The logical opposite to friction between women, shown just occasionally as 'misbehaviour', was that they developed deep friendships, with post-mortem instructions expressive of their viewing colleagues as adoptive kin. This construction provides the most likely interpretation for testamentary actions by Jane Ayliffe and Martha Barker, both Barts hospital Sisters, who were also friends and who died within a year of each other. Ayliffe named her 'well-beloved friend' Barker as her executrix and sole beneficiary, while Barker's sole beneficiary was Jane's grandson Samuel Ayliffe. Barker chose as her own executrix one Mary Clayton, identified as Samuel Ayliffe's aunt and presumably (if not certainly) Jane Ayliffe's married daughter. Both of the will makers used a man called John Dale as one of their witnesses, a man in the same line of work as Samuel's father. These women's lives became extensively entangled, with the result that they chose one another in preference to survivors in their own natal or conjugal families.

Hospital employees could become further embedded in each other's family lives. In 1820 Lydia Weston, formerly Sister of Faith ward, was tried at the Old Bailey for theft from the hospital, found guilty, and sentenced to transportation. If taken at face value, this would look as though Weston had an exceptionally negative experience of working at Barts. The full story is more complicated. She had forged an important friendship at the hospital with Lucy Eyres, Sister of Sitwell ward, and when Eyres got married (to the evocatively named Thomas Crowne), Weston was one of the witnesses at her wedding. The couple's first child was baptised less than a year later as Lucy Lydia Crowne, strongly implying that the affection between the two women gave rise to a permanent memorial in the child's naming. Yet Weston's affiliation with the hospital went even further. While awaiting transportation she petitioned for leniency on the grounds of a diagnosis of uterine cancer, and her request was heeded: she was permitted to remain in the country if she served out the remainder of her term or of her life (whichever should prove the shorter) as a patient of St Bartholomew's hospital.[114]

These examples provide an important counterweight to any impression that the female servants of the hospitals tended to clash with one another as rivals for resources, patient affections, or other benefits. Rather this evidence indicates that fellow female employees, and the hospital itself, could act like a family, even for its most refractory members.

Conclusion

In February 1807 Barts played a bit part in a public catastrophe. The crowd which gathered to witness the executions of John Holloway and Owen Haggerty (for a murder on Hounslow Heath) was numbered in the tens of thousands. When the crush became uncontrollable, over forty people were smothered or trampled to death, and many more were 'terribly bruised'. The dead and injured alike were taken to Barts, where Elizabeth ward was given over to act as a morgue and seven other wards took emergency admissions. The *Morning Post* interviewed the three men admitted to King ward, who told tales of people flooding out from side streets and alleys toward the location of the scaffold and being trodden into insensibility. The journalist also spoke to the unnamed Sister of King ward, who was described as 'about 56, low in stature, but of a robust constitution, and perfectly collected'. She had been outside the hospital and caught up in events, being forced into the crowd at the top of Skinner Street. She emerged relatively unscathed 'and was much elated in having experienced such a wonderful escape'.[115]

This is the first known newspaper interview with a member of institutional nursing staff. Coincidentally, it provides the kind of vignette that might have been anticipated by this research on Barts nurses, of a woman in her mid-fifties in good bodily heath who, on questioning, was as focused on her own health as she was on the fates of her patients. This is not the attitude that was later expected of trained lady nurses from the mid-nineteenth century onwards, but is in line with a group of women who were not socially differentiated in the way that they were by the later 'ward' system. Sisters at Barts were recruited from among the nurses, and as such had practical experience of delivering hospital care but no higher original social standing than others of the hospital's ward staff. They were probably not drawn from among London's paupers, but the hospital was acutely aware of their risk of falling into destitution in later life, taking measures to record women's legal settlement.

Their lack of prosperity or social distinction notwithstanding, this chapter has shown that Barts Sisters, nurses, and helpers were not, for the most part, drunk and unreliable. They were instead valued employees with leverage within the hospital and in the wider London community. They may have appeared standoffish to the novelist Mary Hays, author of the introductory quote, but events of Isabella Buckham's infanticide case present a rather different picture of staff–patient relationships as somewhat hierarchical yet decidedly collaborative. The women performed well in context and were rewarded accordingly, despite their personal risk of poverty. From the perspective of 1820 and earlier, the history of nursing at Barts looks very positive.

London in the eighteenth century led the movement to build more hospitals and offer increasingly specialised medical institutions. The next chapter examines the consequences of the extension of this movement for nursing employment and experience across the counties of England and includes contextual aspects of nursing work which affected London and provincial nurses alike.

Notes

1 *Gentleman's Magazine* 74 (1804), 709–10, letter from 'Eusebia', otherwise known as the novelist Mary Hays.
2 At the date of this quote, the Sisters at Barts were recruited from the ranks of the nurses, and so were not socially superior to the other members of nursing staff.

3 H. Richardson, *English Hospitals, 1660–1948: A Survey of their Architecture and Design* (Swindon: Royal Commission on the Historical Monuments of England, 1998), p. 1.
4 N. Moore, *The History of St Bartholomew's Hospital*, volume II (London: Arthur Pearson, 1918), p. 764 for the implication that Barts admitted or treated plague sufferers in 1665.
5 *Medical Register for the Year 1783* (London: Joseph Johnson, 1783), pp. 31–2.
6 In the case of Barts see Moore, *History*, p. 797 for Tory influence over the hospital in the late seventeenth and early eighteenth centuries.
7 K. Waddington, *Medical Education at St Bartholomew's Hospital 1123–1995* (Woodbridge: Boydell Press, 2003), pp. 33–6.
8 G. Yeo, *Nursing at Barts: A History of Nursing Service and Nurse Education at St Bartholomew's Hospital, London* (Stroud: Alan Sutton, 1995), chapter 2 and specifically p. 11.
9 Unless otherwise stated, all references for this chapter derive from the St Bartholomew's Hospital volumes of minutes of the board of governors at Barts Health Archives, references SBHB/HA/1/5, 1647–65, to SBHB/HA/1/17, 1815–26, at the specific day, month, and year given in the text. Barts nurses were referenced lightly in S. Mendelson and P. Crawford, *Women in Early Modern England 1550–1720* (Oxford: Clarendon, 1998), pp. 339–41.
10 A.R. Neate, *St Marylebone Workhouse and Institution, 1730–1965* (London: St Marylebone Society Publications, 1967), pp. 5–7.
11 K. Siena, 'To the hospital or the workhouse? The provision of medical care for the poor in eighteenth century London', *London Journal* 48: 1 (2023), 47–69.
12 J. Boulton and L. Schwarz, 'The medicalisation of a parish workhouse in Georgian Westminster: St Martin in the Fields, 1725–1824', *Family and Community History* 17: 2 (2014), 122–40; A. Tomkins, 'Workhouse medical care from working-class autobiographies, 1750–1834', J. Reinarz and L. Schwarz (eds), *Medicine and the Workhouse* (Rochester, NY: Rochester University Press, 2013).
13 K. Siena, 'Contagion, exclusion, and the unique medical world of the eighteenth-century workhouse: London infirmaries in their widest relief', J. Reinarz and L. Schwarz (eds), *Medicine and the Workhouse* (Rochester, NY: University of Rochester Press, 2013).
14 *An Account of the Work-houses in Great Britain* (London: Brown, 1732), p. 42 relating to the parish of St Giles in the Fields, and p. 177 relating to Charity Hall in Kingston upon Hull.

15 Norfolk Record Office, C/GP 8/3 records of the Forehoe Poor Law Union, minute book 1780–82; I am indebted to Susannah Ottaway for this reference.
16 *Account of the Work-houses*, p. 61.
17 'Coroner's inquest', *The Times*, 30 October 1817.
18 Moore, *History*, chapter 28.
19 Yeo, *Nursing*, p. 13.
20 For use of the term 'watcher' and speculation about overlap with nursing, see I. Mortimer, *The Dying and the Doctors: The Medical Revolution in Seventeenth-Century England* (Woodbridge: Royal Historical Society, Boydell Press, 2009), pp. 146, 158, 160–2. For longer consideration of the perils of institutional night nursing, see Chapter 3 below.
21 *The Ordre of the Hospital of S. Bartholomewes in Westsmythfielde in London* (London: [no details], 1552).
22 Barts Health Archives, SBHB HA 1/17 minutes of the board of governors 1815–26, on 8 February 1817, 6 February 1818, 18 January 1819, and 14 January 1820.
23 The rules at St Thomas's Hospital were very similar: B Golding, *An Historical Account of St Thomas's Hospital Southwark* (London: Longman, Hurst, Rees, Orme, and Browne, 1819), pp. 206–12.
24 *Rules and Orders for the Government of St Bartholomew's Hospital* (London: [no details], 1814).
25 Moore, *History*, pp. 763, 768; Yeo, *Nursing*, p. 8. See also L. Falcini, 'Cleanliness and the poor in eighteenth-century London' (PhD thesis, University of Reading, 2018), p. 222 onwards for the role of nurses at St Thomas's Hospital in cleanliness including laundry.
26 For more about buck washing, see Falcini, 'Cleanliness', p. 118.
27 Barts Health Archives, SBHB HA 1/9 minutes of the board of governors 1708–19, 13 August 1715.
28 Barts Health Archives, SBHB HA 1/8 minutes of the board of governors 1689–1708, 30 June 1698, and 30 July 1698.
29 Moore, *History*, pp. 760–1; Yeo, *Nursing*, p. 8. Barts Health Archives, SBHB HA 1/12 minutes of the board of governors 1748–57, 22 and 29 March 1754.
30 S. Williams, 'Caring for the sick poor. Poor Law nurses in Bedfordshire, c.1770–1834', P. Lane, N. Raven, and K.D.M. Snell (eds), *Women, Work and Wages in England, 1600–1850* (Woodbridge: Boydell, 2004); for a further discussion of laundry see Chapter 3.
31 NB St Thomas's Hospital required washerwomen to indemnify the institution against loss of property, signifying a lack of inherent trust in these employees: Falcini, 'Cleanliness', p. 226.

32 J. Howard, *An Account of the Principle Lazarettos in Europe* (Warrington: W. Eyres, 1789), p. 132; Moore, *History*, p. 759; *Some Account of St Bartholomew's Hospital London* (London: J. Smeeton, 1800), p. 12. There were fourteen beds in Queen Ward in 1729; see Barts Health Archives, SBHB HA 1/10 minutes of the board of governors 1719–34, 6 February 1729. Lock and Kingsland hospitals were different in both their capacity and their likelihood of recruiting patients; K. Siena, *Venereal Disease, Hospitals, and the Urban Poor* (Rochester, NY: Rochester University Press, 2004), pp. 98–100.

33 Evidence of patient admissions and case notes has not survived for this period beyond some lone examples, but see J. Freke, *An Essay on the Art of Healing* (London: W. Innys, [1748]), pp. 89–91 for a case of elephantiasis with possibly repulsive consequences for the nurses of Barts.

34 Three paupers from St Martin's Workhouse over 1760–61 were sent to St Bartholomew's Hospital suffering variously with a cancerous tumour on the testicle, a sore breast, and having lost the use of their limbs: London Lives references smdswhr_391_39108, smdswhr_387_38778, and smdswhr_393_39306; www.londonlives.org (accessed 16 September 2022).

35 Boulton and Schwarz, 'Medicalisation', p. 128; Siena, 'Hospital or the workhouse'.

36 Moore, *History*, pp. 761–2, 769–71.

37 St Thomas's Hospital minutes of the court of governors 14 July 1731, London Lives reference LMTHMG553010430; www.londonlives.org (accessed 17 August 2022).

38 Yeo, *Nursing*, p. 22.

39 Yeo, *Nursing*, pp. 7, 8.

40 Yeo, *Nursing*, p. 12.

41 Barts Health Archives, SBHB/HA/1/6 minutes of the board of governors 1666–75, minute of 11 November 1669, list of officers including Katherine Ingram for scald heads.

42 Moore, *History*, p. 761 reports that Sister Susan Coake was appointed as the hospital's cook in 1664, while the governors' minutes record that on 19 June 1708 Mary Crane, Sister of Magdalen ward, was made cook.

43 Barts Health Archives, SBHB/HA/1/8 minutes of the board of governors 1689–1708, Mary Pultney, mentioned 28 June 1690, was not otherwise listed as a helper or Sister. The early nineteenth-century rules gave Sisters a role in deputising for the matron by rotation; *Government of St Bartholomew's*, p. 82.

44 Barts Health Archives, SBHB/HA/1/8 minutes of the board of governors 1689–1708, 16 January 1703; Old Bailey Online t17621208-26, www.oldbaileyonline.org (accessed 23 August 2022).
45 Barts Health Archives, SBHB/HA/1/7 minutes of the board of governors 1675–89, 23 July 1677.
46 Barts Health Archives, SBHB/HA/1/7 minutes of the board of governors 1675–89, 22 March 1687.
47 *Government of St Bartholomew's*, p. 82.
48 Yeo, *Nursing*, p. 18; Moore, *History*, p. 771 for a memory of the Sisters going to church in their white nightgowns in the first half of the nineteenth century.
49 J. Styles, 'Involuntary consumers: Servants and their clothes in eighteenth-century England', *Textile History* 33: 1 (2002), 9–21.
50 St Thomas's Hospital minute books of courts and committees 29 June 1709, see London Lives LMTHMC552030132, www.londonlives.org (accessed 24 August 2022); W. Nolan, *An Essay on Humanity: Or a View of Abuses in Hospitals* (London: J. Murray, 1786), p. 11.
51 Thirty-two represents 27 per cent of the 117 total recorded burials for Sisters.
52 Barts Health Archives, SBHB/HA/4/1 board of governors' order book 1653–1739, on 22 July 1672.
53 Barts Health Archives, SBHB/HA/4/1 board of governors' order book 1653–1739, on 21 October 1661.
54 Yeo, *Nursing*, pp. 13–14.
55 Barts Health Archives, SBHB/HA/1/ 7 minutes of the board of governors 1675–89, 19 March 1677.
56 St Thomas's Hospital minutes of the court of governors 21 June 1683, 22 August 1694, 5 May 1703, 6 December 1706; see London Lives LMTHMG553010034, LMTHMG553010102, LMTHMG553010191, LMTHMG553010235, www.londonlives.org (accessed 24 August 2022).
57 St Thomas's Hospital minute books of courts and committees 9 November 1705, 14 February 1706/7, 25 June 1707; see London Lives LMTHMC552030008, LMTHMC552030046 and LMTHMC30063, www.londonlives.org (accessed 24 August 2022).
58 Barts Health Archives, SBHB/HA/1/7 minutes of the board of governors 1675–89, 25 October 1684. There was a separate issue around the risk that the hospital would attract the depositing of abandoned children, giving rise to additional cost to the parish; Barts Health Archives, SBHB/HA/1/7 minutes of the board of governors 1675–89

Nursing the metropolis 125

30 May 1685, when a hospital beadle was punished for failing to prevent an infant being left in the cloisters.
59 For example Barts Health Archives, SBHB/HA/1/10 minutes of the board of governors 1719–34, 1 October 1730, when Margaret Collins was promoted from senior helper to Sister and she produced a certificate of her settlement in St Michael Cornhill. St Thomas's hospital governors were alive to the same risks: St Thomas's minute books of courts and committees 17 November 1710, see London Lives LMTHMC552030171, www.londonlives.org (accessed 24 August 2022).
60 Barts Health Archives, SBHB/SA/20/1 indemnity for Sarah Mansell's employment by surgeon Percival Pott, 1757.
61 Barts Health Archives, SBHB/HA/1/14 minutes of the board of governors 1770–86, 12 July 1782; Moore, *History*, p. 769.
62 Email from Barts Health Archives July 2020 with information about Mary Stanny's correspondence being supplied by personal communication from David Everett.
63 F. Const, *Decisions of the Court of King's Bench upon the Laws Relating to the Poor*, volume I (London: Whieldon and Butterworth, 1793), pp. 111–12.
64 St Martin in the Fields pauper settlement examination for Ann Fawdrey, 13 September 1756, London Lives smdsset_84_55871, www.londonlives.org (accessed 17 August 2022).
65 G.B. Risse, *Hospital Life in Enlightenment Scotland: Care and Teaching at the Royal Infirmary of Edinburgh* (Cambridge: Cambridge University Press, 1986), p. 76.
66 Yeo, *Nursing*, p. 11
67 Barts Health Archives, SBHB/HA/1/7 minutes of the board of governors 1675–89, 21 January 1678; SBHB/HA/1/9 minutes of the board of governors 1708–19, 17 April 1714.
68 St Thomas's Hospital minutes of the court of governors 17 January 1693/4, see London Lives LMTHMG553010099, www.londonlives.org (accessed 24 August 2022).
69 St Thomas's Hospital minutes of the court of governors 5 June 1700, see London Lives LMTHMG553010142, www.londonlives.org (accessed 24 August 2022).
70 There is only one known instance of a demotion: Barts Health Archives, SBHB/HA/1/7 minutes of the board of governors 1675–89: on 16 February 1684 the Sister of Naples ward was found to be deaf, so was made a helper.
71 Barts Health Archives, SBHB/HA/4/1 board of governors' order book 1653–1739, 22 July 1672.

72 Barts Health Archives, SBHB/HA/4/1 board of governors' order book 1653–1739, 26 March 1716; SBHB/HA/1/10 minutes of the board of governors 1719–34, 18 November 1731. A similar fee structure operated in St Thomas's hospital until July 1731 when fees were abolished (much earlier than they were at Barts); see St Thomas's Hospital minute books of courts and committees 7 July 1731, London Lives LMTHMC552040128, www.londonlives.org (accessed 24 August 2022).

73 Barts Health Archives, SBHB/HA/4/1 board of governors order book 1653–1739, 12 October 1723.

74 Siena, *Venereal Disease*, p. 144. NB Nurse Graham is missing from my own list of Barts' female ward staff.

75 Barts Health Archives, SBHB/HA/1/ 9 minutes of the board of governors 1708–19, 8 July 1710; SBHB/HA/1/10 minutes of the board of governors 1719–34, 2 February 1727 and 10 November 1731; SBHB/HA/1/12 minutes of the board of governors 1748–57, 7 March 1748 and 9 January 1751; SBHB/HA/1/13 minutes of the board of governors 1757–70, 11 October 1769.

76 These data have been compiled by reference to the digitised records for St Thomas's Hospital on the London Lives website, under the headings of the court and committee minute books and the minutes of the court of governors. All three instances of female ward staff drinking were recorded in 1707–08.

77 A.E. Clark-Kennedy, *The London: A Study in the Voluntary Hospital System, Volume I: The First Hundred Years 1740–1840* (London: Pitman, 1962), p. 37.

78 NB Beadles and other members of hospital staff were occasionally found guilty of drunkenness too, but beadles did not go on to become professionalised or vilified collectively for their drinking (unlike nursing staff).

79 Barts Health Archives, SBHB/HA/1/15 minutes of the board of guardians 1786–1801, 17 December 1800.

80 T. Meldrum, *Domestic Service and Gender 1660–1750: Life and Work in the London Household* (Harlow: Longman, 2000), p. 200.

81 Meldrum, *Domestic Service*, p. 203.

82 Barts Health Archives, SBHB/HA/1/13 minutes of the board of Guardians 1757–70, 20 February 1770, SBHB/HA/1/14 minutes of the board of guardians 1770–86, 30 May 1771, and SBHB/HA/1/15 minutes of the board of guardians 1786–1801, 21 May 1788; see also Sisters reproved for suffering dressings to stop the water spouts: SBHB/HA/1/12 minutes of the board of guardians 1748–57, 20 September 1749.

83 Old Bailey t17311208-6, www.oldbaileyonline.org (accessed 24 August 2022).
84 E.g. in 1692 Katherine Barnes, Sister of King's ward, was dismissed for raising scandalous reports about Elizabeth Rowley, Sister of Curtain ward. Rowley was, admittedly, required to prove she had not left Lichfield under a cloud, for living with a man not her husband, but she seems to have kept her place until she died seven years later. For friction between women see also Barts Health Archives, SBHB/HA/1/9 minutes of the board of governors 1708–19, 24 February 1711 and SBHB/HA/1/14 minutes of the board of governors 1770–86, 20 June 1781. NB quarrelling and worse was not confined to female servants; SBHB/HA/1/10 minutes of the board of guardians 1719–34, 28 March 1728, for fighting between the male box-carriers.
85 The text of the advertisement has not been found by reference to the digitised Burney collection of newspapers.
86 Barts Health Archives, SBHB/HA/1/12 minutes of the board of guardians 1748–57, 16 March and 13 April 1749.
87 For other examples of a dismissal among nursing staff being reversed on the intercession of medical men, see Barts Health Archives, SBHB/HA/1/10 minutes of the board of guardians 1719–34, 25 November 1731 and SBHB/HA/1/15 minutes of the board of guardians 1786–1801, 6 March 1800.
88 J.M.T. Ford (ed.), *A medical student at St Thomas's Hospital, 1801–1802: The Weekes family letters* (London: Wellcome Institute for the History of Medicine, 1987), pp. 80, 115.
89 Ford, *Weekes*, pp. 166–7.
90 Ford, *Weekes*, p. 186.
91 Ford, *Weekes*, p. 207.
92 Regrettably, none of the ceremonies can be traced reliably among London's digitised marriage registers.
93 K. Siena, 'Searchers of the dead in long eighteenth-century London', K. Kippen and L. Woods (eds), *Worth and Repute: Valuing Gender in Late Medieval and Early Modern Europe: Essays in honour of Barbara Todd* (Toronto: Centre for Reformation and Renaissance Studies, 2011), p. 131; marriage of 1715 at St Sepulchre of Martha Butterfield to James Weight identified using www.findmypast.co.uk (accessed 24 August 2022).
94 Old Bailey t17551204-27, www.oldbaileyonline.org (accessed 1 October 2019).
95 Old Bailey t17370907-43, www.oldbaileyonline.org (accessed 17 August 2022).

96 'Old Bailey', *Morning Chronicle*, 16 September 1819.
97 Barts Health Archives, SBHB/HA/1/13 minutes of the board of governors 1757–70, 12 December 1760. At St Thomas's, the testimony of the Sister in Abraham's ward even contributed to the suspension of the steward: St Thomas's Hospital minute books of courts and committees 17 June 1703, see London Lives LMTHMC552020116, www.londonlives.org (accessed 17 August 2022).
98 P. King (ed.), *Narratives of the Poor in Eighteenth-Century Britain, Volume IV: Institutional Responses: The Refuge for the Destitute* (London: Pickering and Chatto, 2006), 'Introduction'.
99 King, *Narratives*, p. 174; see also p. 198 for a nurse recommending the Refuge to the fellow servant of a patient.
100 St Bartholomew the Less, burial of 21 October 1712, www.findmypast.co.uk (accessed 17 August 2022).
101 Barts Health Archives, SBHB/HA/1/10 minutes of the board of governors 1719–34, 14 May 1720. See also truss made for former nurse Alice Wooley, SBHB/HA/1/7 minutes of the board of governors 1675–89, 5 February 1677.
102 Hannah Polley, for example, was admitted as a Sister in 1790 but was buried from the hospital as simply a spinster in 1800, suggesting she moved from staff member to patient. See also Lydia Weston discussed at the end of this chapter.
103 For example, see Barts Health Archives, SBHB/HA/1/10 minutes of the board of governors 1719–34, 5 May 1731.
104 St Thomas's Hospital minute books of courts and committees 25 June 1707, see London Lives LMTHMC552030064, www.londonlives.org (accessed 24 August 2022).
105 St Thomas's Hospital minute books of courts and committees 1 June 1708 and 2 December 1709, see London Lives LMTHMC552030104 and LMTHMC552030152, www.londonlives.org (accessed 24 August 2022).
106 Barts Health Archives, SBHB/HA/1/14 minutes of the board of governors 1770–86, 15 October 1784.
107 The National Archives (NA), HO 107, census of 1851 for Owslebury Green, Hampshire.
108 For example, Barts Health Archives, SBHB/HA/1/7 minutes of the board of guardians 1675–89, 20 August 1688; SBHB/HA/1/8 minutes of the board of guardians 1689–1708, 17 May 1690, 12 July 1690, and 2 December 1695; SBHB/HA/1/9 minutes of the board of guardians 1708–19, 14 February 1712/13 and 26 June 1714.

109 Barts Health Archives, SBHB/HA/1/13 minutes of the board of governors 1757–70, 4 October 1763 and 21 December 1763.
110 Burial of Walter Chaloner on 16 January 1722, www.findmypast.org.uk (accessed 22 August 2022); in journal minutes Widow Chaloner was appointed on 27 November 1722 as a 'nurse' at a period when most junior female ward staff were called 'helpers'. Therefore I surmise that Chaloner was appointed to a more senior position from the outset. A third beadle's widow, Faith Cracraft, was also appointed a Sister but it is not known at what date between her husband's death in 1710 and her own demise in 1720.
111 *Government of St Bartholomew's*, p. 80.
112 PCC wills and administrations can be found via the National Archives catalogue Discovery at https://discovery.nationalarchives.gov.uk/ (accessed 14 June 2024). Wills for people with property in only one diocese or with very modest estates of under £5 were proved by consistory, commissary, or peculiar church courts. The latter were much more likely to deal with the estates of the poorer women who became nurses, but the presence of nurses among their collections is more difficult to establish.
113 Burial of 10 September 1767 at Bunhill fields burial ground identified using www.findmypast.co.uk (accessed 24 August 2022).
114 NA HO 17/97.
115 'The dreadful catastrophe at the Old Bailey', *Morning Post*, 25 February 1807.

3

Nursing provincial infirmaries 1735–1820[1]

What feeling heart but swells with indignation,
To see yon Fury in a human shape
Insult poor wretches she was plac'd to cheer,
And sharpen sorrows she was bound to succour...
Her tongue kills more than the ablest doctors cure.[2]

Joseph Wilde's experiences as a patient in the Devon and Exeter Infirmary in 1809 were mixed: he applauded the charity, while finding fault with the diet and (as the quote above suggests) deploring the attitude of the female ward staff.[3] He does not make explicit complaint about their actions but chastises them for their discernible lack of proper feeling. Wilde's perception of infirmary nurses in practice diverged from the charities' hopes in theory: when the Sheffield Infirmary was projected for example, the founders anticipated that patients would be cared for by 'prudent, active, and experienced nurses', so women with pragmatic rather than sentimental qualities to the fore.[4] James Lucas, sometime surgeon at the Leeds Infirmary, stressed the importance of (and coincidentally admitted the possibility of securing) a nurse who was both clever and humane.[5] Wilde's poetic invective aligned pretty nearly, though, with the negative stereotype for paid domestic nurses discussed in Chapter 1, and historians to date have offered only piecemeal reasons to demur from his judgement in the case of pre-1820 institutional nurses. William Howie's article about cultures of complaint in the Salop Infirmary apparently confirmed apprehensions about the 'unreformed' nurse as ignorant and untrustworthy, whose relationship with other staff, employers, and patients was fraught.[6] Anne Borsay has tentatively observed (also within one institution) that complaint and dismissal was a fact of life across all classes of infirmary staff.[7] There are now reasons, however, to give wholesale reconsideration to infirmary nurses specifically in light of their experiences in post and the risks they ran.

This chapter begins with a survey of the growth in provincial infirmaries across England from 1735 to the end of the period and its implications for female staff. It goes on to analyse the experience of nurses who worked at a range of provincial infirmaries, all of which opened before 1783. It draws on hospital records to consider the explicit and tacit expectations for nurses employed by infirmaries, and to chart the tenures and work experiences of nurses in central England with a particular focus on Gloucester, Liverpool, Shrewsbury, and Stafford where hospital board minutes are detailed in respect to nurse recruitment, behaviour, and discharge. The discussion below focuses on the gap between historic conceptions of the pre-reform nurse in these new institutional forms and the reality of working relations between nurses, patients, governors, and staff. In the eighteenth century these interactions were clearly human, faulty, and occasionally tense, but were consensual or respectful most of the time. The second half of the chapter takes up some of the themes treated somewhat in Chapters 1 and 2 but emphasised in the Introduction around the risks to nurses, and specifically the penalties of dirty work in an institutional context. These perspectives, on the women who nursed and on their working environment, provide ample grounds for a positive reassessment of infirmary nurses.

The English infirmary movement

In 1660 there were only two hospitals for the sick in England, both located in London. By 1820 there were thirty-six residential institutions for the sick poor spread across most of England.[8] The majority of the new foundations were county infirmaries accepting both medical and surgical cases.[9] Infirmaries formed part of a new philanthropic movement underpinned by lifetime giving rather than testamentary bequests.[10] They also diverged from the historic character of hospital-as-almshouse, because they offered temporary accommodation to the sick, or outpatient facilities, rather than semi-permanent residences to older people.[11] Infirmaries aimed to restore curable, sick, or wounded, and chiefly adult poor to health in order to return them to productive work. Institutions' rules were framed to reinforce these priorities, because they generally excluded the incurable, the very young, the chronically sick, and morally controversial patients such as unmarried pregnant women.[12] The infirmary agenda was one of civic virtue rather than unqualified Christian benevolence, despite the prominence of Anglican clergymen and nonconformist divines among the founders, subscribers, and governors.[13]

Infirmaries tended to be founded with between two and four wards, where the primary distinction between them was based on the gender of patients and (sometimes) on suffering with a particular diagnosis. In Shrewsbury the venereal patients were housed in the garret ward, for example, while Chester developed innovative practices relating to the separation and treatment of fever patients inside the hospital.[14] Further refinements might be made when the buildings were extended or at the behest of the honorary physicians and surgeons of the establishment, most obviously by creating an operating room or separating the surgical from the medical patients.[15]

All these new hospitals required female nursing staff. It is not clear how many women had been employed across the country by 1820, although a calculation based on the women identified for this chapter suggests that a bare minimum of 1,500 women and probably in excess of 2,000 held posts as nurses in one of the provincial infirmaries between 1735 and 1820.[16]

It is possible to apprehend the approximate scale of work infirmary nurses undertook by surveying the number of beds for the sick that were offered in each place or by the number of inpatients they cared for annually. Numbers of infirmary beds can be known for specific years.[17] In addition, Chester Infirmary's governors had the foresight to make a survey of annual inpatient totals at multiple infirmaries throughout England.[18] This was undertaken to compare the costs of inpatient care at Chester with other locations for insight into more economical models of infirmary management. Information was requested by Chester from 1787–88 through to

Table 3.1 English provincial infirmaries and their capacities 1735–1820

	Founded / opened	Beds …	… in year	Inpatients …	… in year	Patients per bed per annum (approx)
Bristol	1735	140	1783	1406	1787–88	10.04
Winchester	1736	60	1737	381	1787–88	6.35
York	1740	58	1783	401	1808–09	6.91
Devon and Exeter	1741	160	1783	979	1787–88	6.12
Bath	1742	112	1751	389	1805–06	3.47
Northampton	1743	60	1783	470	1792–93	7.83
Worcester	1746	40	1771	361	1802–03	9.03
Salop in Shrewsbury	1747	70	1783	503	1789–90	7.19
Liverpool	1749	120	1783	965	1787–88	8.04
Newcastle	1751	60	1783	702	1804–05	11.70
Manchester	1752	65	1783	713	1798–99	10.97
Chester	1755	70	1783	615	1787–88	8.79
Gloucester	1755	120	1783	708	1788–89	5.90
Cambridge	1766	50	1783	308	1800–01	6.16
Salisbury	1766	75	1783	343	1787–88	4.57
Stafford	1766	80	1783	340	1804–05	4.25
Leeds	1767	40	1783	861	1806–07	21.53
Lincoln	1769	40	1783	170	1803–04	4.25
Oxford	1770	94	1783	594	1787–88	6.32
Norfolk and Norwich	1771	100	1783	534	1789–90	5.34
Leicester	1771	40	1783	457	1787–88	11.43

Table 3.1 (continued)

	Founded / opened	Beds ...	... in year	Inpatients ...	... in year	Patients per bed per annum (approx)
Hereford	1776	30	1783	203	1787–88	6.77
Birmingham	1779	40	1783	749	1787–88	18.73
Nottingham	1782	44	1782	421	1787–88	9.57
Hull	1782	20	1783	250	1800–01	12.50
Truro and Cornwall	1791	20	1799	79	1805–06	3.95
Durham	1792	Not found	N/A	66	1805–06	
Bath City	1792	18	1792	91	1808–09	5.06
Kent and Canterbury	1793	24	1792–93	109	1794 only	4.54
Sheffield	1797	Not found	N/A	395	1806–07	
Bedford	1803	6	1803	163	1805–06	27.17
Taunton and Somerset	1809	26	c.1820	Not found	N/A	
Derby	1810	80	1817	232	1811–12	2.90
Lancaster	1815	5	1815	27	1816–17	5.40
Colchester	1818	80	1820	150	1820 on	1.88
North Staffordshire	1819	20	1819	27	1819–20	1.35
Presumed minimum total by 1820		2067		15162		
Average minimum		60.79		473.81		7.79

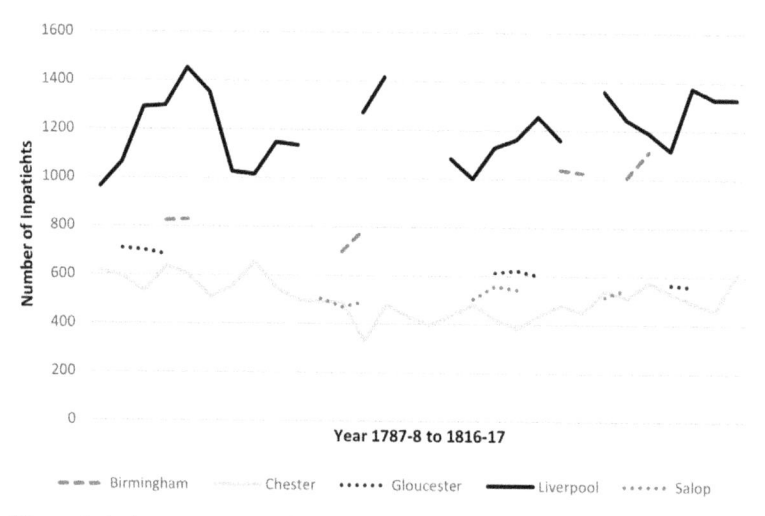

Figure 3.1 A comparison of annual inpatient numbers at the Birmingham, Chester, Gloucester, Liverpool, and Salop infirmaries 1787/88 to 1816/17

1816–17, but it is not clear what methodology each infirmary used to reach the number sent to Chester's inquiry; for example, the number of inpatients reported at Birmingham in 1787 to 1788 does not equate to an average of the numbers quoted by Reinarz for 1787 and 1788.[19] Also the infirmaries beyond Chester were either investigated sporadically, or sometimes chose to ignore the request for information, since most locations are represented by fewer than ten years of data and only Liverpool appears in as many as twenty-five years. Even so this yields an approximate picture of annual inpatient workload for nurses.

The notional number of beds is sadly problematic as a precise gauge of workload for nurses, given that infirmaries might not operate at full capacity: hospitals tended to close beds temporarily under financial stress.[20] Alternatively institutions might routinely place two patients in a bed.[21] The instability of bed numbers to patients *in situ* also renders the ratio of beds to nurses awkward, although it is notable that the numbers of nurses thought necessary to staff beds varied widely; Birmingham posited the need for five nurses to cater for forty beds, while Chester apparently employed two for a hundred beds.[22] Where details are given of the staff–patient ratio, the sparsity of nurses is confirmed: for most of the eighteenth century, the assumption in provincial infirmaries was that one nurse could feasibly cater to twenty or more patients at a time. This was the case in the newly opened Manchester Royal Infirmary, which employed one nurse for twenty-four patients, and among others of the institutions scrutinised here. This workload was only sustainable because nurses were supposed to be assisted by the ambulant patients. Rules for patients required them to act as deputies to ward nurses, apparently including most of the tasks falling otherwise to nurses around both caring and cleaning.[23] Institutions do not shed much additional light on patient workloads, or the lines of responsibility between nurses and patients, although the Manchester Royal Infirmary made a new rule in 1771 that patients should not apply poultices (presumably to themselves or each other) without a nurse being present, and Shrewsbury's minutes in 1786 refer to male patients assisting to 'foment' one another (i.e. to bathe a part of their body, often with the application of warm wet cloths).[24]

The ratio of annual inpatient numbers gives another impression of nursing workload, albeit stretched over twelve months. When divided by the bed numbers, the approximate count of inpatients per bed per annum potentially illustrates the pace of patient turnover in each location. The staff at Bristol and Liverpool infirmaries saw the highest numbers of inpatients in each year, but they were not necessarily the most heavily worked in terms of patients per bed. The number of patients per bed in Leeds is undoubtedly anomalous and can be attributed to an increase in bed numbers between 1783 and 1807, but the number in Birmingham seems likely to be more accurate. Birmingham was perhaps better at either curing its patients or discharging them promptly if it became apparent that they were securing no benefit from institutional care.

These estimations of beds, annual workload, and female staff numbers, sketchy as they are, indicate a central feature of infirmary life in this period – namely that nurses were not expected to give close attention to all patients all of the time. Wards and beds were lightly staffed, and the women designated as nurses could not perform all the nursing tasks of the infirmary. This structure left the nurses in charge of wards, rather than strictly of patient care.

It was awkward, then, that infirmary nurses did not have the benefit of a clear job description when hospitals opened. The initial rules governing institutions gave general stipulations about the cleansing of wards, obedience to the matron, and tenderness to patients.[25] All other aspects of the role had to be learned from experience since there seem to have been no arrangements for training: women learned what was required of them while already on the job. A second edition of rules, such as those printed for the Salop Infirmary in 1792 (forty-six years after the hospital's opening), demonstrated the ways that hospitals learned to be more precise in framing requirements for staff. The updated rules contained specific guidance about the disposal of deceased patients' effects, the treatment of dirty textiles, the handling of medicine containers, and the management of patient behaviour.[26]

Unlike their metropolitan counterparts at St Bartholomew's Hospital, provincial nurses were less likely to be differentiated between senior nurses or Sisters and their helpers or assistants. The rules of the York Infirmary allocated salaries to upper and under nurses from the outset, but York was unusual in several respects having not simply copied the rules of other institutions in relation to nurse employment.[27] Shrewsbury and Stafford recruited 'assistant' nurses in numbers only from the 1780s, but Liverpool and Gloucester did not differentiate between the members of permanent nursing staff during this period. This means that nurses, once accustomed to institutional duties, had no obvious way to improve their experience unless by petitioning collectively for higher wages.

There was similarly no scope for 'promotion' since the post of matron was not open to nurses, but they may have gained useful experience for the pursuit of subsequent employment in domestic nursing. One advertisement appealing for nurses to work at the Salisbury Infirmary in 1796 underlined the way that the post ensured applicants would be 'taught how to look after sick people', which suggests that the hospital managers were construing infirmary work as valuable in the labour market.[28] There were other ways for poor women to gain on-the-job experience that was valuable for fostering nursing skills in alternative public institutions. Just as the capacity of the ancient London hospitals was augmented for poor patients by the infirmary wards in metropolitan workhouses, so were provincial infirmary beds established in addition to workhouse beds for the sick. There is no reliable way to count the latter, particularly since workhouses admitted the chronic patients that were rejected by infirmaries and may have placed the sick poor in ordinary dormitories rather than in dedicated wards for illness, injury, disability, or the complaints of old age. Nonetheless, some parishes beyond London had extensive facilities for the sick, such as in the parish of St Mary's Nottingham.[29] Nurses were among the salaried staff of the Bristol Workhouse, and the fourteen nurses in the Liverpool Workhouse were distributed across the lying-in, venereal, fever, and lunatic wards.[30] Unfortunately provincial workhouse nurses remain as anonymous as their London counterparts, and their experiences or career prospects are equally unknowable from the sources that have been annexed to date. Therefore, we might posit that (at least in the eyes of infirmary trustees) a hospital nurse might have been expected to enjoy a greater social cachet than a workhouse nurse, with no sense of whether the women concerned were affected by such niceties of social differentiation. We might also notice that while the significance of the patient narrative has been characterised as in decline (for the purposes of medical diagnosis), the nurse narrative has always been missing from infirmary histories.[31]

Nurse salaries, tenures, and relationships with other staff

A sample of eight out of the thirty-six infirmaries founded in England between 1735 and 1820 was investigated for data about nursing staff. All eight were opened before 1780, ensuring a run of at least forty years of hospital records before 1820 in each case.

Infirmary weekly board minutes were frequently laid out in similar ways, not least because the secretary of a new infirmary might visit one or more existing institutions to learn the ropes. Nurse employment information was not a category of regular data in its own right, however, not least because minutes of women's resignation or dismissal took place at irregular intervals. Some hospitals developed an administrative habit of recording all appointments and discharges of nurses, but only Stafford retained this practice throughout the period. Other places named nurses coincidentally

Table 3.2 Institutional records sampled for nursing data

	Foundation year	Minutes surviving	Nurse employment recorded consistently
Birmingham	1766	1779–1820	No, but some nurses named
Chester	1755	1755–1820	No, but some nurses named
Gloucester	1755	1755–1820	No, but many nurses named
Liverpool	1745	1749–1820	1749–86
Manchester	1752	1756–1820	No, but some nurses named
Shrewsbury	1745	1745–1820	1747–1804
Stafford	1766	1766–1820	1766–1820
Worcester	1746	1745–1820	No, but some nurses named

when they listed salaries paid, while others only referred to nurses on extraordinary occasions (such as where women were dismissed for egregious fault) or in passing, in reference to a new duty. This means that while these collective minutes yield 311 named nurse appointments (somewhat fewer individual women, given the reappointments discussed below), the employment tenure is only reliably available for 223 appointments.

The criteria for recruitment were rarely given in infirmary minutes, but in Shrewsbury careful note was made of the justification for two-thirds of the nurse appointments between 1781 and 1792. The women were generally approved for being 'recommended by persons of credit' – via testimonials from former employers for their erstwhile domestic servants – or on the basis of women's sobriety and honesty. Further clues about the former identities of infirmary nurses are essentially opaque, because reliable linkage with women of the same names in marriage, burial, or other genealogical sources is highly problematic. For twenty-four of the women, even their first name is unknown. Fortunately, a good deal of their working experience can be deduced from the hospital minutes.

Infirmaries were interested in sector norms for their servants' wages. Gloucester went so far as to solicit information about payments to nurses from its nearest comparable institutions (in Bristol, Oxford, and Worcester) where interestingly the inquiries included a question about the number of patients they each had on average in a year.[32] Nonetheless, nurse salaries were relatively

Table 3.3 Comparative table of nurse wages and tenures in selected infirmaries

Infirmary	Nurse wages	Tenure
Birmingham	£4 4s + £1 1s for tea and sugar + £1 1s gratuity 1779	
Chester	£3 + £1 gratuity in 1756 only; £5 + £1 gratuity 1768–87; £6 + £1 gratuity 1787–1802; £10 or 3s 10d per week from 1804	
Gloucester	£4/£5 + gratuity raised to £5/£6 + gratuity in 1799 [NB gratuity presumed to be worth £3 3s throughout]	2 years 8 months (based on sample of 32% of 72 named nurses)
Liverpool	£3 + £1 gratuity 1749 only; £8 8s + up to £2 2s gratuity from 1814	1 year 4 months (based on 91% of 93 named nurses)
Manchester	£3 in 1752	
Shrewsbury	£3 + £1 gratuity 1747–55; £4 for women's nurse and £5 for men's nurse 1784–92; nurse in men's ward salary increased from £6 5s to £8 10s, nurse in women's ward from £6 5s to £8, nurse in venereal wards from £6 5s to £7 10s, and under nurse in men's ward from £4 to £6, all in December 1815	2 years 9 months (based on 88% of 76 named nurses)
Stafford	£3 + £1 gratuity; £4 + £1 gratuity and more for sitting up, 1788 onwards; 1796 pay for women's nurse raised to match that of the men's nurse; from 1810, men's nurse £8 8s + £1 1s in lieu of tea, £1 1s in lieu of ale, and £1 gratuity, women's nurse £7 7s but same other allowances as the men's nurse	3 years 10 months (based on 100% of 39 named nurses)
Worcester	wages increased from £4 to £6 per annum in 1774, with annual gratuity of £1 1s; increased from £7 to £7 7s in 1806; increased to £9 9s in 1808; further increased to £10 10s from 1818	

poor across England, on a par with those of the lowliest live-in servants.[33] Payments were often identical to those paid to infirmary cooks, maids, and laundresses. The equivalence of these salaries was also expressive of women's interchangeable roles, as in at least three infirmaries women moved in and out of nursing but remained in the hospital's employment as maids, cooks, or other servants (but never matrons). This level of remuneration fits with expectations for female agricultural workers and domestic servants reporting wages in settlement examinations in the 1760s.[34]

The value of an additional gratuity, though, could rise significantly in response to trustees' perception of a nurse's value or in reaction to a specific challenge well met. At Chester, Nurse Jones's gratuity was raised to the same value as her salary in 1757, giving her a total income of £6 per year.[35] Additional income could accrue from sitting up with patients at night (on which see more below), or from an acknowledgement that some dietary supplement might be justified. The nurses at Chester were allowed an extra ten shillings a year for tea from 1782.[36] Finally, there might be other sorts of benefits on offer for nurses: when John Howard surveyed the English infirmaries in the 1770s he noted that at Norwich the nurses were given urine as a perquisite. This was presumably sold by the women as an industrial raw material for extra income, although Howard thought the practice 'improper'.[37]

Given these financial prospects, infirmaries faced a perennial problem in schooling their nurses to refuse (or avoid requesting) presents and financial gratuities from patients and their families. Nurses lacked explicit access to the perquisites available to domestic servants.[38] But governors could appreciate the nurses' point of view. In December 1797, the Stafford board heard a complaint to the effect that nurses took gifts from the patients in the men's ward, and reproved the guilty party (presumably the then nurse in the men's ward, Mary Lea) but also found that 'the low wages of the nurse had given birth to this practice'.[39] It was immediately ordered that if she behaved herself in future, she would receive two guineas per annum gratuity from the hospital. Incidentally Lea's successors enjoyed a higher basic rate of pay, perhaps to obviate the cause of soliciting or accepting patient gifts permanently. Therefore, the hospital board in Stafford was gradually recognising a structural problem with low wages rather than seeing Lea's failure as particular to her due to poor character. Naturally the proffering of gifts could also be cited as evidence of a nursing job well done, from the patients' perspective.

The average tenures of nurses in provincial infirmaries were not wildly different from one another, but it is still clear from a combination of calculated tenures and from the board minutes that different infirmaries evolved very different working cultures for nurses that were not predicated solely or wholly on salary levels. The average tenure of the women's service at Stafford was approximately three years and ten months. This generalisation conceals some important texture, because multiple short-term appointments were balanced by six women who worked at the hospital for more than ten years each. There was notable stability in the nursing staff during the early years of the infirmary when two women remained in their posts throughout the 1770s and for most of the 1780s. The tenure of assistant nurses in the 1810s was, in comparison, very brief. There is no real indication of why this was, but we might speculate that assistant nurses felt less affiliation to the institution than the full nurses, and that short tenures betray a speedy disenchantment with the working environment offered by the infirmary in comparison with other domestic service settings. It is also feasible that, having secured experience in the infirmary, they left to take up better-paid nursing roles in other institutions or in private homes.

Liverpool saw a brisk turnover of nurses, but this was not necessarily owing to dissatisfaction on either side. Instead, the hospital drew on a pool of local women who might experience multiple short stints as nurses (presumably indicating that their behaviour was either good, or not so objectionable as to preclude future re-employment). The cohort of nurse employees was almost certainly influenced by the infirmary's close physical proximity to the city's workhouse, which (as noted above) employed fourteen nurses in the 1790s. The presence of a larger employer of sick-nurses on its doorstep, albeit for women probably drawn from the workhouse paupers, meant the infirmary was competing for the available women, and perhaps motivated to offer better working conditions. While it is not inevitable that Hannah Lucas, appointed to Liverpool in 1759 and working until 1762, was the same

Hannah Lucas employed between 1764 and 1766, at least seven women with this name served successive terms of office as nurse. Furthermore, Christiana Dunwoodie worked in Liverpool until the time of her marriage and was rehired the following year under her married name Christiana Pearson, raising the prospect that other women were rehired invisibly (where their names before or after marriage were less distinctive). Similarly, in Gloucester Mary Lyman or Lemon was first employed in 1771, and at her two subsequent appointments her designation as 'Nurse' Lemon seems to confirm that it was the same woman serving three separate stints in the infirmary. She was one of at least four women re-employed at Gloucester in the 1770s. These patterns of rehiring strongly imply that infirmary governors were glad to regain some women's services, even if their earlier period of employment at their institution had been brief.

Infirmary trustees could certainly prove flexible when women's circumstances changed. In Gloucester, nurse Mary Richards was allowed leave for one month for her health, having found her own replacement.[40] Elizabeth Jones at the Shropshire Infirmary left her post to get married, but was re-employed as Elizabeth Pearce after she had been abandoned by her husband. The pregnant Pearce worked until her confinement, and then returned after effectually taking maternity leave.[41] This speaks of an institution which, despite the problems with nurse recruitment and retention highlighted by Howie, was nonetheless supportive of nurses when they worked well.

Anne Borsay found, on the basis of staff experiences at the Bath Infirmary, that the hospital 'gave little credence to the disorderly view of the Georgian Infirmary'.[42] She was able to reach this conclusion by putting instances of misbehaviour into context: the nurses at Bath were not alone in being subject to discipline, because the cooks, maids, and even matrons were among those discharged, but importantly the rate of female staff turnover by these means was modest over time. Bath saw one nurse dismissal approximately every five years. The tenor of relationships between nursing staff and others in Stafford was apparently quiescent, as only one nurse was categorically dismissed for misbehaviour in a 55-year period.[43] This indirect testimony to satisfactory nurse behaviours is confirmed by the 'visitors'. Infirmaries invariably appointed visitors to call on the hospital unannounced and discover whether there were any problems with the smooth running of the institution. Unfortunately the visitors did not always keep meticulous records, so evidence of petty conflicts involving the female staff may be scant.[44] The 'complaints book' kept by the weekly hospital visitors at Stafford, however, was kept regularly and only once noted disputes between one of the nurses and the patients, whereas the patients as a group were much more prominent and frequently objected to the food.[45] The visitors' books for the Chester Infirmary only survive from 1802 onwards, but tell a similar story up to 1820. One explicit complaint against a female nurse must be read in the context of otherwise repetitive satisfaction with the cleanliness of the wards, and frequent reports of the patients grumbling about the quality and quantity of hospital provisions.[46]

At the end of a long infirmary career, nurses might expect to be looked after in their old age. Individual women secured a pension or a permanent place in the house until their deaths. Nurse Jones of the Chester Infirmary, for example, became unequal to her work in January 1767, but was permitted to continue as an assistant to the other nurses and obtain her bed and board at the infirmary indefinitely.[47] Nurse Jones's role later mutated (uniquely, among the eight institutions studied here) into that of hospital porter in 1770.[48] Nurse Nash at Worcester was even more fortunate, retiring in 1799 after twenty-eight years of service on a pension of six guineas per year.[49] There were no guarantees, of course, and financially pressed infirmaries could prove quite dismissive. Worcester summarily sent an aged night nurse to the city's House of Industry when she could no longer work, but it is worth noting that this took place late in the period, concerns a (possibly non-residential) night nurse, and identifies the only nurse in these infirmaries known to have been ejected into the remit of the Poor Law.[50]

As this information suggests, and as the data for the nurses at St Bartholomew's Hospital in London hinted, nurses were perhaps just as likely to leave their employment of their own volition as be sacked. In Shrewsbury nine nurses left the hospital to get married. At the same time, the negative stereotype of the nurse given to drink, for example, receives little confirmation from provincial sources.[51]

On a consistent survey of these infirmaries' minutes, accusations of nurses being drunk crop up quite rarely. No nurses were reprimanded or dismissed for drunkenness from either Stafford or Liverpool infirmaries, and only one night nurse was implicated in Gloucester. Even Shrewsbury, the focus of Howie's critique, only dismissed two nurses for drinking. This suggests either that the minutes frequently omitted to mention dismissal arising from drink or that the stereotype was inaccurate.

Even if infirmary minutes routinely neglected to mention reprimand or dismissal of female ward staff as drunk, we might now interpret nurses' behaviour in the light of their age, gender, and social status rather than anachronistically against the criteria for nursing after calls for reform. For some nurses, as for other women, permissible or 'normal' levels of alcohol consumption were not enough. There are at least two possible structural reasons why drinking among infirmary nurses might have been a visible and habitual practice. First, even if any propensity to drunkenness (or as we might say now addiction to alcohol) was no more marked than that among other women from similar backgrounds and with similar wages, it might have been that a nurse's role as a representative of (and resident in) the institution meant that repeated inebriation carried a higher social penalty than in private life or her own home. Second, perhaps the rigours of nursing took their toll on women who lived and worked under undeniably difficult circumstances and undertook some repellent duties such that drinking became a form of coping mechanism. The risks of domestic nursing were surveyed in Chapter 1: the remainder of this chapter considers the drawbacks of nursing in an institutional environment for the women's toleration of physical experience and their accommodation of threats to social status.

Working conditions, risks to infirmary nurses, and the implications of 'dirty work'

Carol Helmstader and Judith Godden have alluded briefly to the discomforts of nursing work as noise, confusion, and odour, but the impacts of these factors have been substantially underestimated.[52]

Nursing was hard work, and this took some women who were recruited to provincial infirmaries by surprise. Ann Mainwaring, formerly the matron of the St Alkmund's Workhouse in Shrewsbury, was recruited as nurse in the men's ward at the infirmary in 1784 (when the town's new House of Industry threw former workhouse servants out of employ); however, she found life as the men's nurse too tiring, and owing to fatigue sought an internal transfer after eight months. She went first to the upper ward (in charge of venereal patients) and later to the women's ward, but left the hospital after two years and nine months (so shorter than the average tenure at Shrewsbury) to live with her son in London. Shrewsbury went on to experience a small crisis owing to the physical limits of its staff in 1792, a year which saw the appointment of seven nurses (for an institution of three wards). Three of the appointees served only a fortnight or a month by reason of fatigue, being insufficiently active, or otherwise unfit for the post.[53]

In addition to the patients, nurses had to tolerate each other. They were separated by their wards but brought together to eat and to sleep.[54] Enmities between nurses might have been reported in infirmary minutes if they resulted in disciplinary action, while friendships would have gone unnoticed. Notably (and in contrast to the experiences of female ward staff at St Bartholomew's Hospital) not one instance of conflict between female nurses is reported by these hospitals, whereas disputes between staff and patients, or between other staff including matrons and porters, are referenced.[55]

Furthermore, nurses collectively had to experience the same aspects of infirmary life as the patients, a working and living environment that challenged the five senses.[56] Victims of accidents were frequently admitted as infirmary patients, and presented repeatedly gory sights to infirmary staff. Transport accidents involving carriages and wagons were reported consistently in the local press, necessitating emergency hospital admission.[57] Accidents in industry and construction, plus injury by fires and animal bites, were also noted.[58] Intentional wounding with guns and knives was particularly likely to attract public attention, especially where (despite infirmary treatment) an inquest proved necessary. At Liverpool Infirmary in September 1820, nurses were confronted by butcher Lewis French who had purposely stabbed himself in the stomach with his own carving knife to a depth of five or six inches before being brought to the hospital: the coroner reported a verdict of suicide under temporary insanity.[59] Craig Spence has attempted to consider the impact that accident, injury, and fatality had upon those who encountered them (rather than those who experienced them).[60] We know that medical students in this period could find hospital scenes and anatomical study depressing.[61] Lay people were possibly more alarmed by drastic wounding than their medical contemporaries, as implied whenever newspaper reports found the injuries of accident victims too dreadful to describe.[62] We do not possess equivalent nurse narratives, but this does not mean we can assume that witnessing serious injury and death made no difference to them.

Similarly, there is no evidence about how nurses reacted to touching patient bodies. There are clues about the occasions when other creatures touched nurses, however, because any vermin plaguing the house were as likely to bite nurses as well as patients.[63] Bedbugs were a ubiquitous nuisance for the provincial infirmaries, and the timing of concern about bugs tended to reflect their prevalence in the hotter summer months.[64] There was no guaranteed way to eliminate institutional bedbugs permanently, which meant that infirmaries might have to make repeated efforts to eradicate them by in-house cleansing or by employing an external contractor to kill them. In July 1783, for instance, the matron of the Gloucester Infirmary was instructed to place six bug traps in every ward, and other rooms at her discretion.[65] The discomforts caused by infestations of bugs and lice were typically addressed by disposing of wooden bedsteads in favour of iron ones (sometimes specifically to the benefit of infirmaries' female staff).[66] Yet bugs were more than just a physical nuisance: by the mid-eighteenth century they were the cultural 'canary in the coal mine' of social differentiation.[67] Infirmaries joined the monied classes in trying to get rid of bedbugs. The continued presence of these vermin arguably became a marker of infirmary residents' vulnerability and of the charity's unwanted association with dirt and decay.[68]

The nurses were generally expected to share in the patients' diet. On paper this followed the monotony of other institutional diets, being dominated by porridge and other sloppy dishes that were easily served and easily eaten.[69] It is important to note, though, that the Stafford Infirmary, for example, had its own garden (and gardener from 1776) while the Gloucester infirmary apparently grew a variety of crops on extensive grounds so, as in recent parallel research on English workhouses, there was more food on offer in infirmaries than may be apparent from their dietary schedules.[70]

Surgeries without anaesthetic were intensely painful and therefore noisy procedures.[71] Patients' shrieks distressed the men and women in adjacent beds or wards, and while nurses may have become more accustomed to the nature of surgical noise it was certainly loud, repeated, and expressive of distress. John Buchanan was one of the first physicians of the Stafford Infirmary and deprecated smallpox hospital wards (let alone surgical ones) where 'the cries of one disturb and offend the others'.[72] Yet it was only in 1808 that the Stafford Infirmary, for instance, gave official notice to the 'inconvenience' of not having an operating room separate from the wards, and even then it was the inconvenience of patients which was paramount.[73] Sounds made by patients were augmented by the unusual noises associated with electrical shock treatments. Most infirmaries bought an electrical machine where shocks were designed to remit or cure palsy, giving rise to 'sparks drawn from it and the greatest blows' to paralysed limbs.[74] In this way infirmary nurses became even more exposed to the aural excesses of illness and death than would have been the case for nurses outside institutions, if only by dint of the number of patients in infirmaries in comparison to the number of inhabitants of most domestic houses.[75]

The relatively close confinement of flatulent patient bodies, undergoing vomits and purges in addition to the symptomatic production of pus or the occurrence of post-operative infection, rendered infirmaries noisome even under repeated cleaning.[76] The heat of summer augmented the offensiveness of the air and, at their worst, infirmaries harboured stinking wounds all year round.[77] Nurses' complaints about the smell of their patients are rarely recorded nationwide, but they can be found, and infirmary visitors and trustees who experienced short-term exposure to offensive odours made recommendations for improvements.[78] Infirmaries also gave specific rewards to nurses for their attention to cases that proved 'very offensive'.[79] The most consistent suggestion for a hospital's better management was that windows be kept open at all times, only to be ignored by patients who often preferred warm smells to chilly fresh air.[80] John Howard deprecated the Leicester Infirmary where none of the windows were open, while wards at the Radcliffe Infirmary in Oxford and the Worcester Infirmary were judged positively offensive for similar reasons.[81] Nurses could take the blame for what might have been patients' preferences: surgeon Edward Alanson wanted to fine nurses for a failure to keep windows open.[82] Even so, the stench from 'necessaries' was the most likely inducement to decisive, and even costly, action by governors in the form of building works.[83]

Smells were not just a problem for institutional management: they were also indicative of physical risk in the last quarter of the eighteenth century.[84] The domestic sick room was thought to be filled with 'noxious vapours' that were dangerous to people exposed to them.[85] These poisons might arise from the patient's symptoms, or from the customary conditions in which the sick were treated involving warm rooms and heightened perspiration. The resulting 'disagreeable smells' were dubbed by medicine as 'putrid miasmata'.[86] The advice to visitors that they hold their breath was hardly applicable to a nurse in regular or constant attendance.[87] Nurses were advised instead to stop their nostrils with tobacco or herbs and sprinkle the room with vinegar.[88] These reflections on household sickness were no less applicable to infirmaries. Even so, there is no evidence of infirmary nurses being encouraged to filter their breathing in any way, nor did infirmaries tend to invest in equipment to aid the circulation of fresh air.[89] Hospital architecture could be adapted to facilitate ventilation for all occupants, but where this occurred it generally took place after 1820.[90]

In addition to challenges around sensory perception, nurses also had to manage an ill-defined workload. Cleaning wards was one of the few jobs allocated to nurses by most infirmary rules, requiring sweeping, dry-sanding or washing floors, but they might also be called upon to clean beds and patients, involving the removal of excreta and other bodily waste. The disposal of soiled bandages and wastewater could prove a particular problem. In April 1780, only a few months after opening, the Birmingham hospital visitors registered a complaint that patient dressings were being thrown onto the fire in the wards, when they should be removed and buried.[91] Cleaning may have been required by statute but not, it seems, if it was judged a lesser responsibility than patient care. In Birmingham in 1782 the matron asked that patients 'be employed in cleaning the rooms instead of the nurses whose duty in attending the patients seems to have been neglected in consequence of their doing such business'.[92]

Yet the range of duties hinted at by collective infirmary minutes indicate a more demanding roster of activities requiring some organisational capacity. Nursing duties cohered around the ward for which they were responsible, but the nurse's functions took her away from her ward and into other parts of the building. In this respect the nurse had something of a roving brief within the institution and cannot have undertaken constant observation of patients. They might be called to support medical staff in dressing wounds or conducting procedures. At the same time they might be responsible for, or assistants in, the hospital's laundry which of necessity did not take place on wards. In Stafford the domestic staff were augmented by a laundry maid, and in Liverpool by a washerwoman, suggesting that the nurses in those places did not have sole responsibility for keeping linen clean, but the picture was more complicated elsewhere.[93]

The role of laundry when seen from the nurse's point of view was as a diversification of their role. Infirmaries might employ a laundry maid, but these domestics did not necessarily carry out all of the laundry alone, and (the sufferings of habitual washerwomen notwithstanding) nurses might welcome the chance to escape from their patients, move around the infirmary, and carry out non-nursing tasks.[94] The nurses at the Gloucester infirmary were reproached for absenting themselves from their wards on the 'excuse' of being employed in washing 'to the detriment of the patients'.[95] This is a clear example of former requirements on nurses being withdrawn, and the liberties they entailed being recast as a form of misbehaviour. The Chester nurses were also withdrawn from washing in the early nineteenth century.[96]

The nurses came into contact with townspeople at the infirmary baths. Most hospitals acquired their own hot and cold baths at some point after opening, and nurses were sometimes detailed to take the money from paying users.[97] This work offered an opportunity to meet people beyond the confines of the ward; it also gave nurses another sphere in which to 'fail'. In 1774 the Chester trustees received information that 'the women's nurse who has hitherto attended the hot bath has behaved impertinently to some ladies who have bathed there, by demanding presents from them for her trouble'.[98] The unnamed nurse was forbidden to attend anyone at the baths other than patients in future, and the matron was deputised to collect any gratuities from users of the baths to be distributed to servants based on their civility to strangers.

Nurses' time was therefore stretched and official duties specifically required women to leave their wards on occasion. This notional breadth of duty either generated time conflicts for nurses or, depending on their attitude to their work, gave them leeway to juggle preferred tasks with less appealing ones. A measure of autonomy may well have been welcome given the physical risks of their employment and the stresses of the job.

As infirmaries were not supposed to admit infectious patients, there was relatively little risk of catching fevers (although this did occur in hospitals with fever wards).[99] Possibly the most obviously vulnerable woman in the late eighteenth-century was Lowry Thomas, fever nurse at Chester. Thomas fell ill several times and eventually died after exposing herself to infection 'more than was necessary or useful'.[100] Thus, when working conscientiously, a nurse could be castigated for working too hard. The propensity to blame nurses for failing to maintain their own good health has been noted for the early twentieth century.[101]

Nurses routinely shouldered the task of making sure patients took their medicines, but were promptly reproached if they showed any initiative, such as at Shrewsbury in 1783 when nurse Sarah Ward was dismissed at the request of a surgeon for administering an opiate to one of his patients.[102] Nurses laboured under a double bind: doctors required obedience to their instructions on the basis that nurses could not be expected to understand the theory behind dosages, yet at the same time depended heavily on nurses' attentiveness to patients to understand the progress of a case.[103] It seems likely that physician Thomas Fowler, who published accounts of cases at the Stafford Infirmary on the effects of (variously) tobacco, arsenic, and bloodletting, relied on nurses' reports on patient progress while making scant mention of input by female ward staff in his publications.[104]

Remaining awake overnight might be asked of nurses for a variety of reasons, including continuation of treatment, observation of a patient's condition, or companionship for the dying. Patients in Liverpool were asked to 'assist in attending or watching each other', but there is little evidence that patients anywhere watched each other at night.[105] Only pressing necessity, such as the occurrence of patients' fits at night, could mean that 'the whole ward is often employed in keeping Epileptics from hurting themselves'.[106] Nonetheless infirmaries were generally careless of their nurses' exposure to nightwatching, despite the fact that at least one matron reported such watch-nursing 'has been prejudicial to their healths'.[107] Instead hospitals offered salaried nurses the chance to earn more money for each night they sat up with patients, usually at the rate of six or eight pence per night.[108] In Stafford remuneration increased from six pence to one shilling in 1807. This compared very favourably with the three pence which was the effective going rate for day nursing on a salary of £4 plus £1 gratuity per year (the latter payable only on confirmation of good behaviour), and so constituted a substantial inducement. Unfortunately, it might also become routine: at Worcester nurses' increase in salary in 1808 was predicated on their sitting up as night nurses every fourth night.[109] Night nursing by existing staff was supposed to be undertaken in addition to daytime duties, which risked making the working day a continuous twenty-four hours. No infirmaries made explicit concessions to women who had been awake at night (in the form of stated permission to sleep during the day), although the matron of Gloucester was allowed to have a special flannel gown made for the nurses who sat up with patients at night; presumably this was warmer than a standard nightgown.[110] Regular salaried night nurses gradually became part of the standard infirmary's staffing in the late eighteenth or early nineteenth century.[111] Therefore the women employed only at night might have the chance to sleep during the day, but still be burdened with the charge of the whole hospital at night.[112] Infirmaries' attitude to night nursing becomes explicable if we see the nurses as subject again to a form of occupational double jeopardy. By accepting the job of watcher, they may have inadvertently signalled to their employers that they were already hardened women, impervious to the dangers of wakefulness and watchfulness. If or when they failed in their task, either through inattention or being guilty of a hard-hearted attitude from lack of rest, it was therefore their own fault and not automatically attributable to the nature of the work.[113]

While night nursing in an institution presented a physical challenge, the charge of a ward offered an emotional and conceptual one. Anne Borsay has argued there was little social differentiation between nurses and patients and there is good reason to confirm this view: nurses were probably drawn from the same backgrounds as patients and might have earned comparable amounts to their charges (when the latter were in employment rather than in hospital).[114] Unlike nurses at London hospitals like St Bartholomew's, the women were not differentiated from their patients by costume.[115] But the infirmary's smooth running was predicated on an assumption of important divisions between the two.

Nurses were placed in an anomalous position in relation to patients. On the one hand infirmary rules typically enjoined nurses to treat patients with tenderness, while urging patients to assist nurses in their duties wherever physically possible.[116] In this sense patients were the de facto deputies and assistants of salaried nurses. Joseph Wilde's poem, quoted at the start of this chapter, appears to confirm this reliance of patients on one another, signalling high approval for peer-to-peer care (in contrast to his critique of the paid ward nurses).[117] Individual inpatients were less tractable, like the man at Leeds who 'says he did not come here to work'.[118] On the other hand, nurses were responsible for exerting authority in wards to ensure appropriate patient behaviour and adherence to proscriptions of trustees, honorary medical staff (physicians and surgeons), and household managers (the matron and house apothecary). The moral and social control components of infirmaries' business in the eighteenth century, in the rules designed to eradicate swearing, gambling, and other ostensibly problematic behaviours, were aimed squarely at patients and their visitors.[119] Nurses faced with rebellious patients called in the matron, who in turn called in the governors. In October 1777 the patients of Berkeley ward in the Gloucester Infirmary refused to make their beds or clean the ward. The orders of first the nurse and then the matron were ignored, so the governors 'reproved the patients and admonished them to behave better for the future on pain of dismission'.[120] In Shrewsbury the governors commiserated with one 'poor old nurse' in the face of patient rudeness.[121] Birmingham and Chester infirmaries deployed the ultimate sanction against patients by discharging them for insolence or ill behaviour to a nurse.[122] Inappropriate behaviour by patients' visitors, in contrast, was not recorded in the minute books, perhaps because it was of necessity a time-limited problem, but nurses might still be expected to control their access to patients. John Howard thought that at all hospitals 'the nurse, and proper persons, should always be present to preserve order and quietness' during visits.[123]

The ward hierarchy was further complicated by the fact that patients might become nurses and nurses become patients. Both transitions were logical. Able patients were recruited to assist in wards and thus became familiarised with the tasks and the personnel, while proving their own capacity to take on the work. This process is best recorded in Shrewsbury where, between 1772 and 1784, five patients stayed on to work in the wards where they had formerly been treated, two of them male patients. Most did not remain in post for long, undercutting the average tenure for Shrewsbury.

Nurses became patients in old age or sickness, sometimes while retaining their job. Anastasia Power was a nurse at Liverpool between 1780 and 1787, but was repeatedly bled with leeches during her employment.[124] Rachel Atwood was highly esteemed by the trustees of the Gloucester Infirmary, as they gave her extra gratuities for her care and diligence in most years between 1779 and 1785, and when she fell ill she was admitted as an inpatient. Her job was kept open temporarily until it became clear that she would not recover sufficiently to return to work, and she was then permitted to remain in the infirmary for much longer than the average patient. In September 1786, twenty months after falling ill, Atwood was judged in 'a situation not to be relieved by medicine', but even so she was not sent home until January 1787.[125] Even Sarah Wright, discharged for accepting presents from the patients in Shrewsbury in 1815, was allowed to stay on as a patient herself.[126]

Additionally, the employment of relatively able-bodied patients provided plenty of opportunity for conflict between the infirmary's different vested interests. Nurses wanted extra pairs of hands, but medical men had other priorities, expecting ward staff to regulate patients primarily with a view to cure. In this era, practitioners' directions always won out: in Birmingham, for example, a patient of Mr Vaux had 'been employed improperly [by the nurse] so as to retard the cure of his sore leg', ensuring that surgeons' permission for patient employment became the rule thereafter.[127] At the point of their discharge, patients could be asked to report on nurses, to establish whether they had been well treated.[128] In institutions which had made a point of posting the rules for nurses in every ward, literate patients had every inducement to hold their carers to account.[129]

In this complicated mesh of obligation and deference, nurses probably found it quite difficult to manage the boundaries between themselves and patients. Certainly, the task of being tender carer, work supervisor, and disciplinarian with only limited powers put infirmary nurses in a highly ambiguous position in the eighteenth and early nineteenth centuries.

A focus on human waste brings this problem into sharp relief. Emptying and cleaning chamber pots was a routine part of the job for nurses.[130] At Manchester Royal Infirmary, rules of 1791 specified that nurses should scald the chamber pots every morning and scour them twice per week.[131] Chamber pots were a fact of institutional life, and part of the furniture that needed to be maintained. Pots were replaced very frequently in St Clement Danes Workhouse, for example, perhaps owing to breakages, but plausibly because cheap pots absorbed fluids and released odours.[132] In addition to their physical properties, chamber pots were also heavy with significance. Beyond their institutional use, Mark Jenner has argued that throwing waste from chamber pots was illustrative of tensions in the social structure of the parish, where excrement became a weapon of the weak and the basis for assertion of authority from an ostensible position of dependence.[133] Nurses cannot be presumed to have had access to literary models of the late seventeenth and early eighteenth century that deployed human effluent to comical or satirical effect, but they may nonetheless have apprehended the general principle of contact with waste as a source of denigration.[134] The management of chamber pots by people other than their immediate users could be similarly problematic, and in the context of infirmaries gave rise to conflict around nursing duties and the exaction of fees.

Unlike the female ward staff at St Bartholomew's Hospital discussed in Chapter 2, infirmary nurses were forbidden by the rules of their institutions from taking presents or money from patients. This did not prevent nurses in practice from requiring payments of three pence or more from each incoming patient for 'earthenware' or, in other words, the supply of a chamber pot.[135] The ubiquity of this practice is rendered all the more distinctive because there was no means for the nursing staff of different institutions to communicate with one another, unless they happened to be friends, relations, or women who secured work at more than one institution over the course of their working lives. Nurses could augment their collective wages by these means: the female ward staff of each infirmary shared an average of £5 18s between them per annum (if the annual patient numbers given in Table 3.1 are a reasonable guide).[136] It might take a long time for infirmary management boards to realise this exaction was taking place if patients did not speak up and complain (and if infirmary visitors did not happen to run across the practice). Such was the case at Gloucester where managers discovered in 1791 that money had been taken from patients for these purposes 'for many years'.[137] Viewed from the patients' perspective this could be seen as extortion, a racket to ensure that chamber pots were both present under beds and not permitted to overflow.[138] Trustees might be of the same opinion when nurses' practice came to light, but official reactions to nurses who took these payments were complicated because no infirmary wanted to be in dispute with its entire nursing staff at once, and long-standing earthenware payments could be characterised as legitimate custom. The alternative to sudden application of neglected rules or wholesale dismissal was specifically to forbid nurses from requesting payments for earthenware in future, but to accompany this injunction with an acknowledgement of nurses' consequential loss of income. In Gloucester, a payment of three pence per new patient was ordered to be paid to nurses out of the hospital's funds in compensation for the loss of this customary perquisite.[139]

Why would an infirmary placate its nurses over money for chamber pots but not over other sorts of rule breaking? The answer may have lain in the dire challenge to self-respect represented by dealing with human waste. Margaret Pelling has highlighted the 'extreme loss of status involved in nappy washing' in the early modern period and proximity to the smell of excrement was flagged as occupationally problematic in early eighteenth century European writing.[140] Twentieth-century ward domestics have been construed as needing 'a kind of shock absorber against the more polluting aspects of the work'.[141] Nurses in the twentieth century were supposedly 'purified' by the qualification process, protecting them from the pollution that would otherwise have been inevitable from their contact with waste.[142] The modern association of the nurse with the bedpan has been construed as nurses conferring on patients the 'social sanction and conceptual space within which he can pollute', whereby the loss of control over bodily fluid is endorsed and managed.[143] Conferring this sanction is authorised for modern nurses by the presence of a uniform and the possession of training, but the scope for barriers to pollution was undoubtedly more restricted in the long eighteenth century. Infirmaries' tolerance of nurses' exactions on patients may have been a tacit acknowledgement of this need to mitigate the stigmatising impact of processing excretions, in modern sociological terms to ensure that dirty work did not inevitably produce dirty workers, and to recognise the physical manifestation of differential self-control between patients and nurses.[144]

Whether or not nurses felt personally aggrieved or undermined by the task of removing ordure, they had an additional motive to take money if in doing so they were better able to differentiate themselves from the patients (over and above pecuniary gain). In a ward where patients and nurses were dressed similarly, inhabited the same spaces while performing similar tasks, ate the same food, and slept under the same roof, a customary payment on admission was one slender way to assert a form of authority over patients by somewhat unscrupulous means. Servants were paid small gratuities by employers for additional or unusual services, but as the infirmary nurses were essentially drawn from the same social groups as patients, there was no employment or status-based justification for nurses expecting payment from people of equivalent standing. Similarly, there is no simple equivalence between the nurses who exacted fees in infirmaries and the gaolers who did so in prisons at this time. Gaolers were entitled to their fees as their chief source of income, and salaries for them were at best occasional.[145]

In the twentieth century, one response to challenged authority identified by Arlie Hochschild was the practice of making 'small tokens of respect a matter of great concern.'[146] This fits very well with nurse behaviour in infirmaries around the exaction of small sums of money in exchange for the provision of a chamber pot to each patient. The practice allowed an assertion of status in the absence of any other means. The evidence gathered here suggests that patients needed much more persuasion of nurses' authority than did the nurses' employers. And a postscript to the situation in Gloucester: in 1809, eighteen years after the institution agreed to pay nurses three pence per patient for earthenware, the chamber pots were still being used as part of a power play by ward staff, because in that year the matron was instructed to tell nurses that pots were to be supplied *'immediately'* to the bed of every patient.[147] This strongly suggests the nurses had been delaying the delivery of chamber pots in a continued attempt to differentiate themselves from patients and that delaying tactics might have been in action for years after the patients ceased to pay their three pence in person. The money was less important than the conferral of authority on nurses who were seeking to differentiate themselves from patients.

Infirmary nursing was therefore considerably more complex and varied than has been implied by either hospital rules or institutional histories. It was rendered even more difficult by the stretching of their working day, and by their responsibilities for managing (as well as nursing) patients both as the objects of policing and as social competitors for authority.

Hospital governors may well have been unaware of the full range of these difficulties, but they were cognisant in general terms of the hard work and dangers involved for nurses. Rebecca Robinson worked at Liverpool Infirmary from early 1778 until later 1781 when she was found no longer capable.[148] She was given five guineas in recognition of her faithful service. Margaret White, a contemporary of Robinson, received ten shillings for giving 'extraordinary attention' to patient George Begaley from whom she caught a fever.[149] An outbreak of gangrene at the Gloucester Infirmary placed unusual demands on the nurses in terms of cleaning and fumigating bedding: every one of the seven nurses was given a guinea in addition to their wages for their trouble.[150] Beyond the infirmaries surveyed here, nurses could just occasionally secure tangible recognition from the medical practitioners they had worked alongside. In 1792 the members of the Lincoln medical society held a charitable assembly for the benefit of Elizabeth Scholey, a poor older woman who had formerly worked at the Lincoln County Hospital: the collection for her raised twenty guineas.[151]

After 1820, the task of nursing in a general hospital changed substantially. The rise of hospital infections like gangrene, and a gradual withdrawal of the expectation that patients would act as nurses' deputies, meant that the nursing job description became more rigorous even before increased scientific requirements (attendant on, for example, the use of anaesthetic from 1847 onwards). Helmstadter and Godden have argued that the requirements of 'new' medicine, whereby hospital practice evolved even in advance of the introduction of anaesthetics and antiseptic surgery, meant that medical practitioners found the old-style nurse increasingly unsuited for the work.[152] This might have been the case in London, but is not particularly evident in the provinces before 1820, albeit the ability to read was sometimes required.[153] The only shreds of evidence of additional requirements being placed on nurses among these institutions relate to Shrewsbury, where one incident is particularly telling.

In October 1789, the Shropshire Infirmary board reported:

> It having been found that some of the patients frequently neglect taking their medicines, and that others take it irregularly and in improper quantities, Ordered that in future the nurses take the charge of the several medicines from the apothecary and that they be directed to be particularly careful in seeing it duly administered to each patient, agreeably to the directions upon the respective labels.[154]

This was a very significant addition to nurses' responsibilities in Shrewsbury, and it was not long before someone fell foul of the new rule. In May 1790 nurse Martha Bevan of the women's ward was discharged for failing to dispense medicines to patients accurately.[155] She had been given written directions and could apparently read, so she was accused of carelessness. This is a clear instance of the ground moving beneath nurses' feet, and their former adequacy in post becoming recast as inadequacy, but it is the only example of such a dismissal from one of these provincial infirmaries in the period up to 1820. As such it falls well before either the advent of 'new' medicine or the requirement for nurses to 'read writing' laid down elsewhere.[156]

Conclusion

Returning to Joseph Wilde's indictment of the nurses at the Devon and Exeter Infirmary in light of the discussion above, we can now surmise that one of the reasons he was he so negative about the female ward staff was because he was affronted by the nurses' attempts to claim authority, and to put social distance between themselves and their patients. His own status as an actor was far from certain, sitting somewhere on a spectrum from vagrant to reduced gentleman, with a troubling proximity to 'low' art.[157] His humble economic position was essentially confirmed by his hospital admission. This mix may have rendered Wilde especially sensitive to perceived slights from nurses. He may also, of course, have been the witness to bad temper on the part of ward staff occasioned by overwork, lack of sleep, and anxiety about responsibilities for patient medicine.

Close examination of the working experiences of nurses, with more attention to the women's working experiences than Wilde was prepared to consider or than has been undertaken since, provides a more secure basis for evaluation, and offers the opportunity to adjust our assumptions. Female nurses could perform well in the eighteenth-century context. Nurse tenures, reappointments, support from employers or rewards in service, and reasons for leaving all speak to a good measure of governor contentment. We can only appreciate the fact that nurse reputations changed for the worse, and the speed of the alteration, if we understand that routine nursing practice for the eighteenth-century provincial infirmary was generally endorsed, only to be rebadged as faulty in the nineteenth.

Of particular importance for the nursing context was the women's responsibility for dirty work. The supply and emptying of chamber pots was a universal feature of the infirmary nurse's duties, and the cause of contention between nurses and governors across different institutions. Nurses attempted to mitigate their exposure to human waste, and secure recognition from patients, by levying informal fees at the point of patients' admission. Hospital committees were apparently mystified and angered by nurses' repeated contravention of institutional rules against taking money, but not so obdurate that they did not typically find ways to forgive transgressors. The provincial infirmary was perhaps the first venue where both ward staff and their managers perceived the need for an increase in nurses' authority, albeit reacting to the realisation in different ways.

The combination of physical risks and social abrasions for nursing staff rendered the environment of infirmaries somewhere on the spectrum of distasteful to harrowing. Yet some women tolerated these conditions for protracted periods. Sixteen nurses served in their respective infirmaries for more than a decade each, while seven more died in service.[158] Nurse Hadley was noted to have exhibited 'exemplary deportment' over a career lasting thirty years at Birmingham.[159] Long service in a hospital or responsibility for one ward over several years may have given the infirmary nurse a sense of identity and job control, although this is not demonstrable for women with shorter tenures in provincial locations: only the longer careers of nurses at Barts or (as in the next chapter) at the Royal Hospital Chelsea can give proof of this sense of belonging.[160]

Notes

1 Portions of the first half of this chapter have been published in A. Tomkins, 'Stafford Infirmary and the "unreformed" nurse, 1765–1820', I. Atherton, M. Blake, A. Sargent, and A. Tomkins

(eds), *Local Histories: Essays in Honour of Nigel Tringham* (Stafford: Staffordshire Record Society, 2022). I am very grateful to the editors for permission to use extracts here.

2 J. Wilde, *The Hospital: A Poem in Three Books* (Printed for the author, 1809), p. 58.

3 W.B. Howie, 'Consumer reaction: A patient's view of hospital life in 1809', *British Medical Journal* 3: 5879 (1973), 534–6.

4 R. Ernest, *The Origin of the Sheffield General Infirmary* (Sheffield: C. and W. Thompson, 1824), p. 5.

5 J. Lucas, *A Candid Inquiry into the Education, Qualifications, and Offices of a Surgeon-apothecary* (London: [no details], 1800), pp. 304–5.

6 W.B. Howie, 'Complaints and complaint procedures in the eighteenth- and early nineteenth-century provincial hospitals in England', *Medical History* 25: 4 (1981), 345–62. Hospital histories have been egregiously dismissive of nurses' behaviour: A. Rook, M. Carlton and W.G. Cannon, *The History of Addenbrooke's Hospital, Cambridge* (Cambridge: Cambridge University Press, 1991), p. 43.

7 A. Borsay, *Medicine and Charity in Georgian Bath* (Aldershot: Ashgate, 1999), pp. 352–6.

8 There were also new general hospitals in or around London, namely Guy's, St George's, the Westminster, the London, and the Middlesex Infirmary. Nurses at these institutions are not considered in this book.

9 The exception to this rule was the first hospital at Bath, which was specifically designed to cater for the poor from beyond the usual orbit of the hospital. Dispensaries which had no inpatient population are not included in this total.

10 A. Tomkins, *The Experience of Urban Poverty 1723–82: Parish, Charity, and Credit* (Manchester: Manchester University Press, 2006), pp. 163–4; I. Krausman Ben Amos, *The Culture of Giving: Informal Support and Gift Exchange in Early-Modern England* (Cambridge: Cambridge University Press, 2008); B. Croxson, 'The price of charity to the Middlesex Hospital, 1750–1830', M. Gorsky and S. Sheard (eds), *Financing Medicine: The British Experience Since 1750* (London: Routledge, 2006).

11 N. Goose, 'The chronology and geography of almshouse foundation in England', N. Goose, H. Caffrey, and A. Langley (eds), *The British Almshouse: New Perspectives on Philanthropy ca 1400–1914* (Milton Keynes: Family and Community History Research Society, 2016). The significance of almshouses for nursing careers is discussed briefly in Chapter 4.

Nursing provincial infirmaries 1735–1820   163

12 For example see S.T. Anning, *The General Infirmary at Leeds, Volume 1: The First Hundred Years 1767–1869* (Edinburgh and London: E.S. Livingstone, 1963), p. 81. In these respects, the infirmaries were akin to their medieval predecessors which excluded pregnant women, lepers, people who had been crippled, and the insane on the grounds that people were expected to 'leave' promptly when they were either cured or dead: M. Rubin, *Charity and Community in Medieval Cambridge* (Cambridge: Cambridge University Press, 1987), pp. 157–8.

13 M.E. Fissell, *Patients, Power, and the Poor in Eighteenth-Century Bristol* (Cambridge: Cambridge University Press, 1991), chapter 4.

14 Shropshire Archives, 3909/1/1 minute of 30 September 1749; H.E. Boulton, 'The Chester Infirmary', *Chester and North Wales Architectural Archaeological and Historical Society Journal* 47 (1960), 9–19, on pp. 11–12.

15 For example, see Staffordshire Record Office, D685/2/7 minute of 1 July 1808; Gloucestershire Archives, HO 19/1/7 minute of 28 January 1802.

16 Since 208 women were appointed to the Liverpool, Shrewsbury, and Stafford infirmaries between 1747 and 1820, and these three infirmaries represented an eighth of the general hospital capacity in provincial England by 1782, then at least 1,664 women should have been employed across the twenty-four charities that were open by 1782 and which remained open up to 1820. Eleven additional provincial hospitals opened in the period 1783–1820, and the non-standard Bath Hospital was open throughout 1742 to 1820, so it is quite likely that 2,000 women or more worked as provincial infirmary nurses between 1745 and 1820, when none had done so before.

17 *Medical Register for the Year 1783* (London: Joseph Johnson, 1783). See also Borsay, *Medicine and Charity*, pp. 65, 239 and G.H. Anderson, 'The house of recovery and board of health – from the archives of the Lancaster Medical Book Club', *Morecombe Bay Medical Journal* (originally the *Lancaster and Westmorland Medical Journal*) 2: 4 (1995), 84–7.

18 Cheshire Archives, ZH1/24 Chester Infirmary minutes of the board of economy 1801–06, including statistics of other infirmaries 1787–1817. For inpatient numbers at the Durham Infirmary see *Monthly Magazine or British Register* 23 (1807), p. 91. For inpatient numbers in Lancaster see Anderson, 'House of recovery', p. 85. For the inpatient numbers in North Staffordshire see Stoke on Trent City Archives, SD 1321/3 North Staffordshire Infirmary annual reports 1804–33, report of 1819–20. For approximate inpatient numbers in

Colchester see J.B. Penfold, *The History of the Essex County Hospital, Colchester* (published by the author, 1984), p. 54. For inpatient numbers at Canterbury see F.M. Hall, R.S. Stevens, and J. Whyman, *The Kent and Canterbury Hospital 1790–1987* ([Canterbury]: Kent Postgraduate Medical Centre, 1988), p. 58.

19 Chester recorded 749 patients, whereas Reinarz gives 663 for 1787 and 687 for 1788; J. Reinarz, *Birth of a Provincial Hospital* (Dugdale Society, 2003), p. 34.

20 Chester Archives, ZH1/1/6 minute of 25 April 1786; for common restriction of beds see Borsay, *Medicine and Charity*, p. 65.

21 For ending the practice of more than one patient per bed see Birmingham City Archives, MS 1423/5 minute of 29 April 1814.

22 Birmingham City Archives, MS 1423/2 minute of 25 September 1779; Cheshire Archives, ZH1/1/3 minute of 4 October 1768 and ZH1/1/5 minute of 29 September 1778.

23 *The Statutes and Rules, for the Government of the General Hospital, near Birmingham* (Birmingham: Pearson and Rollason, [1779]), p. 26; *The Statutes of the General Infirmary at Chester* (Chester: Elizabeth Adams, 1763), p. 26; *Rules and Orders for the Public Infirmary at Liverpool* (Liverpool: John Sadler, [1749]), p. 24; *Rules and Orders of the Public Infirmary at Manchester* (Manchester: R. Whitworth, 1752), p. 22; *Rules and Orders for the Government of the Salop Infirmary* (Shrewsbury: [no details], 1746), pp. 21–2; *The Statutes of the Stafford General Infirmary* ([Stafford: no details, 1766]), p. 22; *An account of the publick hospital for the diseased poor in the county of York* (York: C. Ward and R. Chandler, 1743), p. 22.

24 W. Brockbank, *The History of Nursing at the Manchester Royal Infirmary 1752–1929* (Manchester: Manchester University Press, 1970), p. 9. Shropshire Archives, 3909/1/4 minute of 17 June 1786.

25 *Rules ... Manchester*, p. 21; *The Statutes and Rules for the Government of the General Infirmary, at the City of Salisbury* (Salisbury: Benjamin Collins, [1767]), p. 47; *Statutes and Rules, for the Government of the General Kent and Canterbury Hospital* (Canterbury: Simmons, Kirkby and Jones, 1793), p. 50; *Rules ... Salop*, p. 21; *The Statutes ... Chester*, p. 25; *The Statutes ... Birmingham*, pp. 27–8; *Rules and Orders for the Government of the Gloucester Infirmary* (Gloucester: [no details], 1790); *Rules ... Liverpool*, p. 23; *The Statutes ... Stafford*, p. 21; *Rules and Orders for the Government of the Worcester Infirmary* (Worcester: [no details], 1760). The directive to tenderness could feasibly be construed as an early instance of the prescriptive mode of emotions management, only recognised in the early twenty-first

century: S. Bolton and C. Boyd, 'Trolley dolly or skilled emotion manager? Moving on from Hochschild's Managed Heart', *Work, Employment, and Society* 17: 2 (2003), 289–308, on pp. 291, 295, 299–303.
26 *The Statutes of the Salop Infirmary* (Shrewsbury: J. and W. Eddowes, 1792), pp. 33–7.
27 *An Account ... York*, p. 20. York did not insist on its nurses behaving with tenderness towards patients but did enjoin them to account to the housekeeper for their use of cloth and 'rowlers', p. 22. Leeds Infirmary copied its near neighbour, perhaps, in adopting the 'upper' nurse designation: Anning, *Leeds*, p. 77.
28 J. Woodward, *To Do The Sick No Harm: A Study of the British Voluntary Hospital System to 1875* (London: Routledge & Kegan Paul, 1975), p. 32. Most such advertisements were less specific: see *Gloucester Journal*, 6 December 1784.
29 Nottinghamshire Archives, PR Addit 9739 St Mary vestry minutes 1807–33 including details of the parish's annual income for poor relief, which stood at approximately £24,000 in 1814–15; see also A. Tomkins, 'Workhouse medical care from working-class autobiographies, 1750–1834', J. Reinarz and L. Schwarz (eds), *Medicine and the Workhouse* (Rochester, NY: Rochester University Press, 2013), pp. 91–2.
30 F.M. Eden, *The State of the Poor*, volume II (London: J. Davis, 1797), pp. 195–200, 330.
31 M.E. Fissell, 'The disappearance of the patient's narrative and the intervention of hospital medicine', R. French and A. Wear (eds), *British Medicine in an Age of Reform* (London: Routledge, 1991).
32 Gloucestershire Archives, HO 19/1/5 minute of 11 August 1779.
33 Their wages were lower than their domestic service equivalents in London during the first half of the eighteenth century: T. Meldrum, *Domestic Service and Gender 1660–1750: Life and Work in the London Household* (Harlow: Longman, 2000), p. 188.
34 K. Snell, *Annals of the Labouring Poor: Social Change and Agrarian England 1660–1900* (Cambridge: Cambridge University Press, 1985), pp. 411–17.
35 Cheshire Archives, ZH1/1/1 minute of 18 January 1757.
36 Cheshire Archives, ZH1/1/5 minute of 15 January 1782.
37 J. Howard, *An Account of the Principal Lazarettos in Europe* (London: J. Johnson, C. Dilly, and T. Cadell, 1791), p. 154.
38 J.J. Hecht, *The Domestic Servant Class in Eighteenth-Century England* (London: Routledge & Kegan Paul, 1956), pp. 157–8.

39 Staffordshire Record Office, D685/2/6 Stafford Infirmary weekly board minutes 1795–1803, minute of 22 December 1797.
40 Gloucestershire Archives, HO 19/1/4 minute of 24 February 1774. See also a similar case HO 19/1/9 minute of 20 April 1820 when the infirmary contributed to the nurse's expenses.
41 Shropshire Archives, 3909/1/4 Salop Infirmary board minutes, minutes of 25 September 1790 and 11 February 1792.
42 Borsay, *Medicine and Charity*, p. 353.
43 Staffordshire Record Office, D685/2/7 minute of 23 February 1810.
44 Visitors' books seem not to survive for the Birmingham, Gloucester, Liverpool, Manchester, Shropshire, or Worcester infirmaries for this period.
45 Staffordshire Record Office, D 685/18 Stafford Infirmary visitors' book 1766–1811.
46 Cheshire Archives, ZH1/88 visitors' book 1802–14, where the complaint against a nurse is noted on 31 December 1805; ZH1/89 visitors' book 1814–57.
47 Cheshire Archives, ZH1/1/2 minute of 20 January 1767.
48 Cheshire Archives, ZH1/1/3 minutes of 15 May 1770, 26 June 1770, 26 March 1771.
49 Worcestershire Archives, BA5161/1 minute of 28 June 1799.
50 Worcestershire Archives, BA5161/2 minute of 30 December 1808.
51 Borsay, *Medicine and Charity*, pp. 440–1 where only two of nineteen nurse dismissals between 1742 and 1830 arose because the women were 'disguised in liquor'.
52 C. Helmstadter and J. Godden, *Nursing before Nightingale, 1815–1899* (Farnham: Ashgate, 2011), p. 22; considered at more length by C. Jones, *The Charitable Imperative: Hospitals and Nursing in Ancien Régime and Revolutionary France* (London: Routledge, 1989), pp. 143–5.
53 Fatigue and most if not all of the conditions and risks considered below also pertained for nurses in the two ancient London hospitals, but they are nonetheless discussed here as the collective experience of institutional sick-nurses.
54 For communal eating, see for example *Rules for the Government of the Glocester Infirmary* (Gloucester: [no details], 1755), p. 16; for sleeping see Birmingham City Archives, MS 1423/2 minute of 22 Jan 1780; *Account … York*, unnumbered pages at the end of the pamphlet; the Devon and Exeter Infirmary's floor plan showing nurses' rooms is depicted in H. Richardson, *English Hospitals, 1660–1948: A Survey of their Architecture and Design* (Swindon: Royal Commission

Nursing provincial infirmaries 1735–1820 167

on the Historical Monuments of England, 1998), p. 22; Cheshire Archives, ZH1/1/12: Chester reported the existence of three nurses' rooms in a minute of 20 May 1817, at a time when nurse numbers are unknown but there were probably five nurses, see the salaries reported in a minute of 11 June 1816. NB one nurse at Liverpool died in December 1783 in her bedroom which lacked a chimney, suggesting she had an individual room; see T. Houlston, *Observations on Poisons* (London: R. Baldwin, 1784), p. 17.

55 For example Shropshire Archives, 3909/1/4 minute of 18 August 1787 and Gloucestershire Archives, HO 19/1/4 minute of 17 May 1770 for tensions between porters and other members of staff.

56 J. Reinarz, 'Learning to use their senses: Visitors to voluntary hospitals in eighteenth-century England', *Journal for Eighteenth Century Studies* 35: 4 (2012), 505–20.

57 'Sunday's Post', *Bury and Norwich Post*, 20 October 1802 for a transport accident victim admitted to Stafford; *Felix Farley's Bristol Journal*, 9 June 1787 and 21 February 1789 for admissions to Gloucester Infirmary following carriage accidents.

58 'Country news', *Felix Farley's Bristol Journal*, 14 February 1789; *Memoirs of the Literary and Philosophical Society of Manchester* (London: T. Cadel, 1785), volume IV, p. 486 remarked on forty applications to the Manchester Infirmary in 1794 for treatment following mad-dog bites.

59 [Untitled], *Liverpool Mercury*, 29 September 1820.

60 C. Spence, *Accidents and Violent Death in Early Modern London 1650–1750* (Woodbridge: Boydell, 2016), chapter 7.

61 See B. Cozens-Hardy (ed.), *The Diary of Sylas Neville 1767–1788* (London: Oxford University Press, 1950), p. 143; W. Brockbank and F. Kenworthy (eds), *The Diary of Richard Kay 1716–51, of Baldingstone near Bury: A Lancashire Doctor* (Manchester: Chetham Society, 1968), p. 73.

62 'Melancholy catastrophe', *Morning Post*, 28 April 1819.

63 Bedbugs were not the same as the lice which clung to hair and bodies: L. Falcini, 'Cleanliness and the poor in eighteenth-century London' (PhD thesis, University of Reading, 2018), p. 152 onwards.

64 J. Southall, *A Treatise of Buggs* (London: J. Roberts, 1730), pp. 27–8.

65 Gloucestershire Archives, HO 19/1/5 minute of 31 July 1783.

66 Perhaps following the advice of S. Sharp, *Letters from Italy* (London: Henry and Cave, 1767), p. 239. Staffordshire Record Office, D685/2/5 Stafford Infirmary board minutes 1789–95, minute of 28 March 1794, although both wood and textiles were blamed for

harbouring bugs; Southall, *Treatise*, pp. 34–6. Shropshire Archives, 3909/1/5 minute of 13 June 1801 when the matron asked for new iron bedsteads.
67 L.T. Sarasohn, '"That nauseous venemous insect": Bedbugs in early modern England', *Eighteenth-Century Studies* 46: 4 (2013), 513–30, on p. 513.
68 Sarasohn, 'Venemous insect', p. 515.
69 Tomkins, *Experience of Urban Poverty*, p. 53; C. Williams, *The Staffordshire General Infirmary: A History of the Hospital from 1765* (Stafford: Mid Staffordshire General Hospital, 1992), p. 23.
70 Staffordshire Record Office, D685/2/3 minute of 1 November 1776 onwards; Gloucester Infirmary's garden is depicted in Richardson, *English Hospitals*, p. 24; P. Collinge, '"He shall have care of the garden, its cultivation and produce": Workhouse gardens and gardening c.1790–1835', *Journal for Eighteenth-Century Studies* 44: 1 (2021), 21–39.
71 NB patients could be noisy without the aggravation of surgical pain: Gloucestershire Archives, HO 19/1/9 minute of 7 December 1820; Cheshire Archives, ZH1/88 minute of 6 January 1811.
72 P. Kopperman (ed.), *'Regimental Practice' by John Buchanan, MD: An Eighteenth-Century Medical Diary and manual* (Abingdon: Routledge, 2016), p. 65.
73 Staffordshire Record Office, D685/2/7 Stafford Infirmary weekly board minutes 1803–12, minute of 1 July 1808.
74 T. Percival, 'A palsy arising from the effluvia of lead, cured by electricity', *London Chronicle*, 6–8 December 1774 for treatment with electricity at Stafford; Cheshire Archives, ZH1/1/7 minute of 15 January 1788. The quote is taken from C. Hart, 'Part of a letter from Cheyney Hart, MD to William Watson FRS giving some account of the effects of electricity in the county hospital at Shrewsbury', *Philosophical Transactions of the Royal Society* 48 (1753–54), 786–8.
75 Modern domestic assistants in hospitals have reported a process of acclimatisation to such ward conditions; L. Hart, 'A ward of my own: Social organisation and identity among hospital domestics', P. Holden and J. Littlewood (eds), *Anthropology and Nursing* (London: Routledge, 1991), p. 100.
76 There is no equivalent for the eighteenth century to match K. Thomas, 'Bodily control and social unease: The fart in seventeenth-century England', G. Walker and A. McShane (eds), *The Extraordinary and the Everyday in Early Modern England* (Houndmills: Palgrave Macmillan, 2010), pp. 9–30.

77 Birmingham City Archives, MS 1423/2 Birmingham General Hospital trustees' minutes 1766–84, minutes of 5 and 12 August 1780; Gloucestershire Archives, HO 19/1/9 Gloucester Infirmary minutes 1814–21, minute of 30 June 1814. NB in addition to biting, bedbugs also smelled: Sarasohn, 'Venemous insect', p. 516.

78 G. Hartman, *The True Preserver and Restorer of Health* (London: T.B. for the author, 1682), p. 45; Old Bailey t17411014-8: www.oldbaileyonline.org (accessed 11 May 2020); P.P. *Report from the Committee on the Prisons within the City of London and Borough of Southwark* (1818), p. 103.

79 Gloucestershire Archives, HO 19/1/8 minute of 11 July 1811.

80 For example, see Shropshire Archives, 3909/1/4 infirmary minutes 1784–99, minutes of 15 November 1788 and 21 November 1789.

81 Howard, *Account*, pp. 160, 171, 173.

82 C. Lawrence, P. Lucier, and C.C. Booth (eds), *"Take Time by the Forelock": The Letters of Anthony Fothergill to James Woodforde 1789–1813* (Medical History Supplement number 17: London: Wellcome Institute for the History of Medicine, 1990), p. 34; E. Alanson, *Practical Observations on Amputation* (London: Joseph Johnson, 1782), p. 97.

83 Cheshire Archives, ZH1/1/2 Chester Infirmary weekly minutes 1763–68, 14 February 1764 and 23 December 1766; Gloucestershire Archives, HO 19/1/9 minutes of 15 July 1819 and 25 August 1819.

84 The evidence in this paragraph contradicts the notion that the medically deleterious effects of smell were being disavowed at this time: W. Tullett, *Smell in Eighteenth-Century England* (Oxford: Oxford University Press, 2019), p. 2.

85 J. Armstrong, *Medical Essays* (London: T. Davies, [1773]), p. 23.

86 *The Complete Family Physician: being a perfect compendium of domestic medicine* (Newcastle upon Tyne: Matthew Brown, 1800–01), p. 160; W. Grant, *An enquiry into the nature, rise, and progress of the fevers most common in London* (London: T. Cadell, 1771), p. 66.

87 *Information for Cottagers* (London: Society for Bettering the Condition and Increasing the Comforts of the Poor, 1800), p. 23.

88 *Complete Family Physician*, p. 161.

89 'An account of a machine for changing the air of the room of sick people', Mr Baddam (ed.), *Memoirs of the Royal Society* (London: G. Smith, [1738–41]), p. 98. Worcester considered, but did not apparently purchase, ventilators: W.H. McMenemey, *History of Worcester Royal Infirmary* (London: Press Alliances, 1947), p. 67. Chester

bought ventilators that are only acknowledged because they did not work: ZH1/88 visitors' book 1802–14, minute of 2 January 1810.
90 Borsay, *Medicine and Charity*, p. 349.
91 Birmingham City Archives, MS 1423/2 minute of 22 April 1780. It is not clear how or where the burial of rags would have been carried out.
92 Birmingham City Archives, MS 1423/2 minute of 6 July 1782.
93 For the earliest indications of employment of laundry maids or washerwomen in addition to nurses, see for example Shropshire Archives, 3909/1/1 minute of 13 January 1747; Liverpool Archives, 614 INF/1/1 minute of 1 September 1755; Chester Archives, ZH1/1/3 minute of 27 December 1768; Staffordshire Record Office, D685/2/3 minute of 9 July 1778.
94 Falcini, 'Cleanliness and the Poor', pp. 98, 108, 111–12.
95 Gloucestershire Archives, HO 19/1/8 minute of 24 December 1812.
96 Cheshire Archives, ZH1/1/10 minute of 28 April 1807.
97 W.B. Howie, 'Finance and Supply in an Eighteenth-Century Hospital 1747–1830', *Medical History* 7: 2 (1963), 126–46, on p. 135.
98 Cheshire Archives, ZH1/1/4 minute of 18 January 1774.
99 J. Currie, *Medical reports, on the effects of water, cold and warm, as a remedy in fever and febrile diseases* (London: Cadell and Davies, 1797), pp. 19–20.
100 J. Haygarth, *A Letter to Dr Percival on the Prevention of Infectious Fevers* (London: Cadell and Davies, 1801), pp. 102–3.
101 P.J. Wood, 'Sickening nurses: Fever nursing, nurses' illnesses, and the anatomy of blame, New Zealand, 1903–1923', *Nursing History Review* 19: 1 (2011), 53–77.
102 W.B. Howie, 'The administration of an eighteenth-century provincial hospital: The Royal Salop Infirmary 1747–1830', *Medical History* 5: 1 (1961), 34–55, on p. 44.
103 J. Carré, 'Hospital nurses in eighteenth-century Britain: Service without responsibility', I. Baudino and J. Carré (eds), *The Invisible Woman: Aspects of Women's Work in Eighteenth-Century Britain* (London: Routledge, 2005), p. 96.
104 T. Fowler, *Medical Reports on the Effects of Tobacco* (London: J. Johnson and William Brown, 1785); T. Fowler, *Medical Reports on the Effects of Arsenic* (London: J. Johnson and William Brown, 1786); T. Fowler, *Medical Reports on the Effects of Blood-Letting* (London: J. Johnson, 1795) is the only work by Fowler to mention a nurse, at p. 46. The same omission of nurses can be alleged of John Wall at the Worcester Infirmary: J. Wall, *Experiments and*

Observations on the Malvern Waters (London: R. Lewis, [1763, 3rd edition]), pp. 33–5.
105 Liverpool Archives, 614 INF/1/1 minute of 18 Sep 1752.
106 McMenemey, *Worcester Infirmary*, p. 58.
107 Shropshire Archives, 3909/1/1 minute of 25 Feb 1749/50. For the risks of night watching, see Chapter 1. The Salisbury Infirmary allowed for the employment of separate 'supernumerary' nurses for any patients requiring around-the-clock attention: *Statutes ... Salisbury*, p. 47.
108 G. McLoughlin, *A Short History of the First Liverpool Infirmary 1749–1824* (London: Phillimore, 1978), p. 42; Staffordshire Record Office, D685/2/7 Stafford Infirmary weekly board minutes 1803–12, minute of 4 December 1807 when the rate was raised from 6d to one shilling.
109 Worcestershire Archives, BA5161/1 Worcester Royal Infirmary order book 1800–28, minute of 30 December 1808; in Shrewsbury the nurses shared night-watching duties with the other female servants and the male porter (see Shropshire Archives, 3909/1/2 minute of 23 January 1767), a system apparently still in operation on 21 May 1808: Shropshire Archives, 3909/1/5.
110 Gloucestershire Archives, HO 19/1/5 Gloucester Infirmary minutes 1777–86, minute of 26 February 1778.
111 Hall et al., *Kent and Canterbury*, p. 79 for night nurses from 1795; Worcestershire Archives, BA5161/1 Worcester Royal Infirmary order book 1800–28, minute of 26 December 1817. Irregular 'watch' nurses sometimes appeared earlier in the wages books as being paid by the night; see Liverpool Archives, 614 INF/1/1 minutes of 2 December 1776 onwards.
112 The single night nurse at the Lock Hospital in London, for example, was required to 'visit the several wards every hour'; A. Highmore, *Peitas Londinensis: The History Design and Present State of the Various Public Charities in and near London* (London: C. Cradock and W. Joy, 1814), p. 149. The physical health challenges to nurses from night-shift work are now being researched: see for example E.S. Schernhammer et al., 'Rotating night shifts and risk of breast cancer in women participating in the Nurses' Health Study', *Journal of the National Cancer Institute* 93: 20 (2001), 1563–8, E.S. Schernhammer et al., 'Night-shift work and risk of colorectal cancer in the Nurses' Health Study', *Journal of the National Cancer Institute* 95: 11 (2003), 825–8.
113 C. Cappe, *Thoughts on the Desirableness and Utility of Ladies Visiting the Female Wards of Hospitals and Lunatic Asylums* (London: [no

details], 1816), p. 8 for a contemporary author's assumption that lack of sleep contributed to a hardening of nurses' hearts.
114 A. Borsay, 'Nursing 1700–1830: Families, communities, institutions', A. Borsay and B. Hunter (eds), *Nursing and Midwifery in Britain since 1700* (Basingstoke: Palgrave, 2012), p. 38.
115 G. Yeo, *Nursing at Barts: A History of Nursing Service and Nurse Education at St Bartholomew's Hospital, London* (Stroud: Alan Sutton, 1995), p. 7.
116 In Liverpool, patients were answerable to the matron and apothecary rather than the nurses, making nurses' authority even more unstable; Liverpool Archives, 614 INF/1/1 minute of 1 December 1777.
117 Wilde, *Hospital*, pp. 27–31.
118 Anning, *Leeds*, p. 91.
119 J. Stonehouse, *A Friendly Letter to a Patient admitted into an Infirmary* (London: John and James Rivington, 1748).
120 Gloucestershire Archives, HO 19/1/5 Gloucester Infirmary minutes 1777–86, minute of 30 October 1777.
121 Howie, 'Administration', p. 44.
122 Birmingham City Archives, MS 1423/4 minute of 4 April 1802; Cheshire Archives, ZH1/1/11 minute of 4 January 1814.
123 Howard, *Account*, p. 81.
124 Liverpool City Archives, 614 INF/1/1 Liverpool Royal Infirmary quarterly board minute book 1749–96, minutes of 1 September 1783 and 7 June 1784.
125 Gloucestershire Archives, HO 19/1/6 Gloucester Infirmary minutes 1786–95, minute of 11 January 1787.
126 Shropshire Archives, 3909/1/6 Salop Infirmary weekly minutes 1814–27, minute of 16 December 1815.
127 Birmingham City Archives, MS1423/2 Birmingham General Hospital trustees' minutes 1766–84, minute of 2 January 1790.
128 Brockbank, *Manchester Royal Infirmary*, p. 12 for Manchester rules of 1791.
129 *Statutes ... Salop Infirmary* (1792), p. 33.
130 The evidence for female nurses' engagement with human waste beyond institutional settings is extremely rare but see C. Nourse, 'XXV An extraordinary cure of wounded intestines', *Philosophical Transactions of the Royal Society* (1776), 426–38, on pp. 431, 435–6, 438.
131 Brockbank, *Manchester Royal Infirmary*, p. 11.
132 Falcini, 'Cleanliness', p. 169.
133 M. Jenner, 'Chamberpots at Dawn', seminar paper, Keele University, 6 March 2019.

134 S. Gee, 'The sewers. Ordure, effluence, and excess in the eighteenth century', C. Wall (ed.), *A Concise Companion to the Restoration and Eighteenth Century* (Malden: Blackwell, 2005).
135 The custom was formally curtailed at Manchester in 1785 and at Chester in 1792: Brockbank, *Manchester Royal Infirmary*, p. 10; Cheshire Archives, ZH1/1/7 minute of 27 November 1792.
136 Calculated on the assumption that the 'average' infirmary treated 473 inpatients per year, and every inpatient was charged three pence for earthenware.
137 Gloucestershire Archives, HO 19/1/6 minute of 27 January 1791.
138 P. Williams, 'Religion, respectability and the origins of the modern nurse', R. French and A. Wear (eds), *British Medicine in an Age of Reform* (London: Routledge, 1991), pp. 234–5.
139 Gloucestershire Archives, HO 19/1/6 minute of 27 January 1791.
140 M. Pelling, *The Common Lot: Sickness, Medical Occupations, and the Urban Poor in Early Modern England* (London: Longman, 1998), p. 192; A. Corbin, *The Foul and the Fragrant* (London: Picador, 1994), p. 145, concerning rag-pickers rather than nurses.
141 Hart, 'A Ward of my Own', p. 104.
142 J. Littlewood, 'Care and ambiguity: Towards a concept of nursing', P. Holden and J. Littlewood (eds), *Anthropology and Nursing* (London: Routledge, 1991), p. 177. Care staff, lacking the nurse's exemption, may still feel polluted; I. Eyers and T. Adams, 'Dementia care nursing, emotional labour and clinical supervision', T. Adams (ed.), *Dementia Care Nursing: Promoting Well-being in People with Dementia and their Families* (Basingtoke: Palgrave Macmillan, 2007), pp. 189–90.
143 Littlewood, 'Care and ambiguity', pp. 170, 180.
144 B.E. Ashforth and G.E. Kreiner, '"How can you do it?": Dirty work and the challenge of constructing a positive identity', *Academy of Management Review* 24: 3 (1999), 413–34, on pp. 413, 417. Sydenham associated disease with dirt too, but there is no evidence for nurses' reactions to symptomatic dirt rather than to routine excretion; quoted in N. Cotton, *Observations on a Particular Kind of Scarlet Fever* (London: R. Manby and H.S. Cox, 1749), p. 7.
145 M. DeLacy, *Prison Reform in Lancashire, 1700–1850: A Study in Local Administration* (Stanford, CA: Stanford University Press, 1986), p. 35.
146 A.R. Hochschild, *The Managed Heart* (Berkeley, CA: University of California Press, 2012), p. 180.
147 Gloucestershire Archives, HO 19/1/8 minute of 10 August 1809.

148 Liverpool City Archives, 614 INF/1/1 Liverpool Royal Infirmary quarterly board minute book 1749–96, minute of 2 September 1782.
149 Liverpool City Archives, 614 INF/1/1 Liverpool Royal Infirmary quarterly board minute book 1749–96, minute on 7 December 1778.
150 Gloucestershire Archives, HO 19/1/9 Gloucester Infirmary minutes, minute of 25 August 1814.
151 'Lincoln, June 7', *Stamford Mercury*, 8 June 1792.
152 Helmstadter and Godden, *Nursing Before Nightingale*, pp. 4–6.
153 Borsay, 'Nursing 1700–1830', p. 36.
154 Shropshire Archives, 3909/1/4 Salop Infirmary weekly minutes 1784–99, minute of 10 October 1789.
155 Shropshire Archives, 3909/1/4 Salop Infirmary weekly minutes 1784–99, minute of 1 May 1790.
156 Borsay, *Medicine and Charity*, p. 354: nurses at Bath were only required to read handwriting from 1829.
157 K. Straub, *Sexual Suspects: Eighteenth-Century Players and Sexual Ideology* (Princeton, NJ: Princeton University Press, 1992), p. 10; D.S. Sechelski, 'Garrick's body and the labor of art in eighteenth-century theater', *Eighteenth-Century Studies* 29: 4 (1996), 369–89, on p. 371.
158 Two women worked for more than ten years and died in service, but they are only counted once here, for long service, i.e. Ann Cooper at the Salop Infirmary, who was appointed in 1792 and died in 1804, and Elizabeth Williams who died in 1819 after 'near fourteen years' in the fever ward.
159 Birmingham City Archives, MS 1423/6 minute of 25 June 1819.
160 Hart, 'A ward of my own', p. 107 for experience conferring a sense of job control for cleaners in modern hospital wards. See also Chapters 2 and 4.

4

Nursing in the Royal Hospital Chelsea[1]

If the ancient *Britons* and *Gauls* should come out of their Graves, with what amazement wou'd they gaze on the mighty Structures every where rais'd for the Poor! Should they behold the Magnificence of a *Chelsea College* ... and see the Care, the Plenty, the Superfluities and Pomp which People that have no Possessions at all are treated with in those stately Palaces, those who were once the greatest and richest of the Land would have Reason to envy the most reduced of our Species now.[2]

As this exaggerated quote from Bernard Mandeville's satire *The Fable of the Bees* indicates, the English state began to accept responsibility for limited provision of welfare, visible in the erection of a new type of hospital exclusively for superannuated servicemen. The archetype of this institution originated in France in the 1670s and inspired innovation across Europe. The resulting establishments were of much higher status than other types of residential welfare such as English workhouses, for example, and were built on a vast scale compared to almshouses. They served at least three different agendas, namely care of the serviceman disabled in action, containment of the disruptive former soldier, and aggrandisement of the Crown. The state's debt to its male military servants, and the desire to recognise men's suffering of personal damage and undermined prosperity, were accompanied by an ambition to contain the former soldier within structures requiring deference and forestalling desertion during active service (and given the stereotype of chaotic, drunken, or criminal soldiers, particularly following demobilisation).[3] An institutional welfare scheme met all of these objectives and was typically augmented by an out-pension scheme making regular payments to men who were not (or not yet) admitted to the physical hospital.[4]

The continental exemplar was the Hôtel des Invalides in Paris which was built in the 1670s to accommodate 3,000 men.[5] This was followed rapidly by Kilmainham Hospital in Dublin, opened 1684 albeit with a much smaller capacity, while the Chelsea Hospital for 450 soldiers and the Greenwich Hospital intended to house 2,044 sailors opened in 1692 and 1705 respectively.[6] Investment in soldier hospitals was not confined to western Europe. Pest in Hungary, under Habsburg rule, opened a hospital in 1729 that by 1743 held 1,400 residents.[7] Despite their capacity, however, centralised hospitals for populations of these sizes were more effective as statements of intent than as welfare safety nets for all men who might have been eligible. In Chelsea, for example, the hospital residents were drawn from the recipients of Chelsea out-pensions, and the latter rose in number from 4,740 in 1715 to 20,150 in 1792.[8] This means that in 1715 the hospital accommodated the equivalent of 9 per cent of out-pensioners, and by 1792 just 2 per cent.

This chapter will consider the Chelsea military hospital as Mandeville's place of 'Care' and as an employer/home of nurses. Unlike the ancient London hospitals and provincial infirmaries, Chelsea was firstly a place of residence, aligning with the contemporary identification of a hospital as an almshouse. Nonetheless, it accommodated men with an acknowledged physical problem (owing to age, disability, or a combination of the two), contained an infirmary ward for the men when they fell ill, and appointed female staff identified as 'matrons' to look after the men either in their dormitories (the 'long wards') or infirmary beds, a seventeenth-century echo perhaps of those pre-Reformation hospitals that cared for the sick.[9] It also attracted a good deal of controversy in contrast with charities solely directed at the sick, and while its state funding meant that there were no subscribers to appease the whole nation could regard itself as interested in the management of the hospital. This chapter will first consider the Chelsea Hospital briefly as a variety of almshouse, and as a source of conflict over philanthropic goals when the 'objects' of charity were adult men. This backdrop provides the context for longer discussion of the matrons' recruitment and tenure, their occupational experiences in comparison with other hospital nurses, their marital experiences, their behaviour in post, and their place in the hospital community. The chapter argues that, unsurprisingly, Chelsea offered secure employment and some status to its 'matrons', but that the hospital was not so important to the women that it stood in the way of their forming new family ties by marriage, in contravention of the institution's rules. It concludes with a short discussion of the Chelsea 'community', which included both the hospital's military beneficiaries and its officers, and with an example of domestic nursing within the institutional setting, carried out for an ageing member of the hospital's salaried staff. I argue that the concentrated nature of the Chelsea Hospital, dedicated to older and disabled soldiers, plus its financial wealth and concomitant facilities, gave rise to a distinctive microclimate of care.

The almshouse model and its relationship to nursing[10]

Early modern England was accustomed to the almshouse as a site of residential welfare. These charities were typically established by bequest to commemorate the name of their founder, and offered dwellings for beneficiaries who met certain criteria. They were small-scale, accommodating between four and fifty people at a time, and often incorporated the word 'hospital' in their name. Almshouses might be directed to support men or women, local people, members of designated congregations, or representatives of certain occupational groups. One thing that almshouse charities had in common when it came to recruiting inmates was their desire to relieve people who were older or in declining health. The threshold for old age or admissible age might vary, but the almshouse was a place for the shelter and support of people whose earning power was reduced or ended by age or infirmity.[11]

Beyond these generalities, almshouses differed dramatically in their provisions. Some were richly endowed and gave residents comfortable accommodation with additional benefits like cash pensions, handouts of food, or deliveries of fuel. Others were short of money, forcing inhabitants to find alternative sources of income.[12] Even the buildings might be insufficient. If they were in disrepair or built in problematic locations, the almspeople might choose to live elsewhere, as in the case of St Bartholomew's Hospital in Oxford.[13]

When the Chelsea Hospital was opened, it was therefore a very large version of a pre-existing welfare type, and one which harked back to the pre-Reformation hospital for the sick, but where funding was underwritten by the state and was therefore comparatively secure. It was devoted to men formerly in military service on the grounds of their age or disability. It differed from the seventeenth-century almshouse model in one essential respect only: extensive delivery of care. Almshouses tended not to have numerous staff, and only a minority specified that care for the ageing should be available at all (either from other members of the residential community or from a paid carer).[14] This created a problem for older people who entered almshouses with good health and mobility but whose capacity to care for themselves declined markedly before their death. If there was enough space and the rules allowed, residents could invite a younger relation to live with them in the almshouse to deliver assistance, but this was a personal arrangement rather than an institutional one. It was not unknown for almshouse charities to release or expel men and women who fell into the need for constant care, leaving families and parish relief systems to meet the requirements of chronic debility.[15]

Chelsea differed from the almshouse template in its staffing structure. Some of this was necessary to provision the full range of almshouse-type benefits that the hospital guaranteed, including small cash pensions, food, fuel, clothing, and impressive accommodation that would be kept in good repair. Unlike most almshouses, Chelsea also appointed a physician and built an infirmary ward for the reception of men who were sick or dying. Nonetheless it was the constant presence of female nurses, both on the accommodation wards and in the infirmary, that permitted a diffusion of care and comprised the key feature distinguishing the charity from its forebears. Men appointed to a Chelsea ward were safe in the knowledge that, no matter how ill, immobile, or frail they became in their older age, they would not be ejected on these grounds. If men were thought to be 'insane' they were sent to a private house in Hoxton, but otherwise they remained in the house until their deaths. The security this conferred on the in-pensioners was simultaneously a source of reassurance to the men themselves, and a target for concern by the wider public.

Chelsea, charity, and conflict over masculinity

Chelsea, like other military state hospitals, had a physical authority denied to other charities, visible to historiography in the architectural studies of their buildings and decor.[16] The hospitals' symbolic presence also offered something new for impoverished masculinity. In other contexts, male poverty and supplication were at best problematic and at worst repudiated.[17] The military hospitals like Chelsea were instead surrounded by rhetorics of sacrifice and dignity, enabling honourable withdrawal from labour, albeit under appropriate circumstances. In France, for example, war minister Saint Germain saw access to Des Invalides as a concluding component in a lifetime of honourable military service, but only if it rewarded those decisively unable to serve (as opposed to providing extravagant benefits to those still capable but unwilling).[18] At best, the activity of war was inherently ennobling, transforming the young, untried, or unruly soldier into a veteran worthy of veneration.[19] Nonetheless, at Chelsea the criteria for admission were defined around the facts of a service record, and a man's physical condition or diagnoses, rather than looser judgements about men's characters. Service was ideally of fifteen or more years, preferably twenty, where age should be over 50, or where incapacity had been accelerated by severe disability.[20] The widespread assumption that people might be regarded as old around the age of 60 was thus adjusted downwards for former military personnel.[21]

At the same time, both Des Invalides and Chelsea were potentially 'ripe targets for critics of fiscal abuses' despite or plausibly because of their serving as sites of suitable reward for incapacitated older men.[22] Chelsea Hospital's staff, beneficiaries, and supporters soon had to combat concerns around the cost of the charity and the consequences of its existence. One voice, for example, feared that inmates were supported in 'affluence and idleness', or unjustified dependence.[23] The charity had to counter the suspicion that the hospital caused as many problems as it solved, particularly if the resident men's virility was intact. Anecdotally a young man of 25 who was severely wounded at Bunker Hill, and who lost both of his eyes and both of his arms, was given dedicated one-to-one nursing by a young woman of about his own age. She was supposed to feed him, and ensure he took sufficient exercise, for a supernumerary payment of half a crown per week. This institutional pairing allegedly inspired a sexual relationship that yielded twins, and the removal of the mother and children from Chelsea at a cost to the parish poor rates of over £50: even if the story was apocryphal, it was indicative of ratepayer concerns.[24] Additionally, and more definitively, wives of the inmates could not expect to subsist on the benefits issued to their husbands. Among many settlement cases in the parish of Chelsea concerning the wives and families of hospital inmates, the case of Isabella Corbett offers a salutary reminder of the limits of state provision. Isabella had married her husband Walter in Ghent in approximately 1709, but his election to a place in the hospital did not permit the subsistence of both. In 1755, Isabella was 'found wandering and begging in the parish of Chelsea'.[25]

Anxieties about Chelsea Hospital reached a critical point in 1784, when the Tory MP Sir Cecil Wray proposed the abolition of the hospital, and removal of accommodation, in exchange for cost-effective pensions. The arguments raised in defence of the hospital, the voices in support of Wray, and the contemporary written and visual satires about this issue in the election contest tended to reinforce stereotypes of Chelsea as, respectively, a haven for the deserving or a sinecure for the undeserving ex-serviceman.

Wray's opponents operated in prose and verse. The poem 'The Old Chelsea Pensioner to Sir Cecil Wray' for example represented the hospital resident as of advanced age, both directly as 'old' and by reference to physical signs; 'our locks are grey'. This idealised pensioner was quiescent and not attempting to imitate the disorderly behaviour of the young recruit, so it was claimed that if ejected from the hospital building there would be no resistance as 'soldiers must obey'. The result would be homelessness, threatened with 'cold winds' and being 'expos'd on the highway'.[26] The poem was therefore an unalloyed defence of the hospital men, using sentimental tropes to paint a picture of the former soldier as a vulnerable, frail person.

Those in favour of hospital closure tended to avoid any detailed reference to the old men who risked eviction. Instead, their critique circled around the high cost of maintaining an in-pensioner, where each man was an abstract unit rather than a disabled or older serviceman. Men were reduced to their per capita cost of £51 per annum who, it was alleged, 'could be better subsisted, and with more content to themselves, for one third of the sum'.[27] Since Chelsea Hospital already paid out-pensions of £7 12s 1d per annum, the argument could viably have suggested a sixth.[28]

The satirical response to the involvement of the hospital in the election contest did not necessarily portray anyone in a good light, again with implications for the masculinity of old soldiers. The soldiers themselves were allegedly the authors of a published petition to Wray. In addition to age and poverty, the petition alluded directly to men being crippled and helpless, 'shattered carcases at sixty'. Nonetheless it also raised sly questions about the sexual continence and physical frailty of resident pensioners.

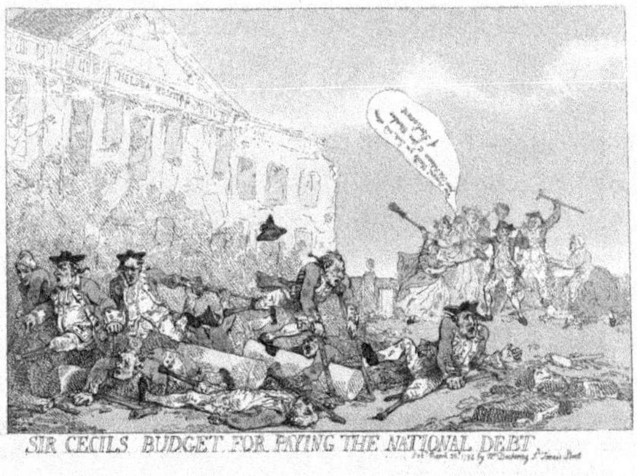

Figure 4.1 T. Rowlandson, 'Sir Cecils Budget for Paying the National Debt' (1784): courtesy of the Metropolitan Museum of Art, New York

The seven named signatories (all apocryphal) refer to their sons and grandsons 'mostly got on Maid Servants'.[29]

Most telling was the significance accorded to loss of limbs, both in the spurious petition and in cartoons of the period. The petition estimated 200 residents without legs and 89 without arms (or a third of the alleged total of 800, nearly double the number of actual residents). Any images of Chelsea inmates ensured heavy representation for loss of limbs, particularly by the depiction of crutches as ubiquitous pieces of equipment, and even hospital organist Charles Burney flippantly called it 'the wooden leg hospital'.[30] Dismemberment became a handy way to signify the ex-serviceman in pictures, being more readily depicted than other forms of disability such as blindness or deafness, and ensured a coherent visual image for 'typical' pensioners. This had the advantage (from the point of view of the charity's male beneficiaries) of presenting a pretty unequivocal case for support. The loss of a limb in service to one's country was both an undeniable barrier to prosperity in later life (if not a complete barrier to employment) and a guarantee of their deserving philanthropic assistance, even if the experience of wearing a prosthesis gave 'about the same kind of satisfaction which a dog does when he gets a tin kettle tied to his tail'.[31] Interestingly and additionally, the image 'Sir Cecil's Budget' by Thomas Rowlandson also avoids the stereotypes of disabled people as 'pitiful, criminal, perverse, or "brave"' because here the pensioners are righteously angry about the threatened loss of their home.[32] Rowlandson's image is a vigorous rejection of the idea that all disabled soldiers were broken spirited and unmanned at the same time that he implies that all of the Chelsea veterans were missing at least one limb. The truth was more prosaic and ambiguous than the engraving suggests. Chelsea Hospital did admit men who had lost arms and legs, but they did not comprise a third of entrants. A modest 15 per cent of men had lost a limb at the time the hospital opened.[33] The women appointed to care for them would therefore have become familiar with dismemberment yet were more heavily exposed to less obvious forms of physical damage.

Recruitment, tenure, and terms of service for Chelsea's 'matrons'

Since the Royal Hospital Chelsea catered for men permanently disabled or worn out in military service, caring for them in disability, sickness, and older age required a specific skill set from the women employed to look after them. The hospital's documentation persistently lists the female ward staff as 'matrons'. The women themselves, their male patients, and others all preferred the label 'nurses', as evidenced by wills throughout the period. Therefore, this chapter refers to the women collectively as nurses. Muster rolls permit initial identification of nurses, and other sources of information provide the resources for a prosopographical history of the women. It is not possible to offer full biographical details for all of them, but a collective biography of women working across the long eighteenth century certainly goes beyond the typical characterisation of such women as simply 'soldiers' widows'.[34]

The women's effectual job description was brief. In addition to generally civil behaviour and attendance at divine service, the nurses were enjoined to 'keep the Wards and Roomes under their care always Clean and Sweet, That they mend the Linnen belonging to the said Wards and Roomes when torn or rent, That they empty and scoure the Brass Pales'.[35] Chelsea nurses were thus not exempt from the same associations with domestic service and human waste that characterised service in hospitals for the sick. Nonetheless, they may have secured startling success in this aspect of their work. John Macky found 'The little Rooms also where the Soldiers lie are kept very clean' in 1724, while a French visitor to London in 1765 judged that the Chelsea invalids 'are kept with a cleanliness which appears altogether astonishing to strangers in a house of this sort'.[36]

The women's lives before appointment as nurses are not easy to recover, but some shreds of evidence emerge from institutional and other sources. One of the earliest appointments was the widow of Francis Johnson, Master of University College in Oxford.[37] Her successors had not necessarily enjoyed any such former status. Faith Mills, the wife of soldier Benjamin Mills, was prosecuted for assault and imprisoned in 1716 before becoming a nurse in 1733.[38]

The Chelsea nurses may even have been former battlefield scavengers, a stereotype of the camp followers on campaign which is challenged below in Chapter 6.

After recruitment, the muster rolls for Chelsea Hospital contain annual lists of the nurses, giving first name, surname, and occasionally other details.[39] The rolls survive from the early years of the hospital between 1703 and 1711 and then from 1728 to 1820 (missing only four years from the latter decades, i.e. 1750, and 1760–62). In 1703 there were twenty-four women denoted matrons in the annual list, but by 1820 the number had risen to twenty-eight: two more women had been recruited specifically to serve in the infirmary in the 1780s, and two women were needed for new wards after 1800. By collating the names of women in the rolls, it is possible to identify the vast majority of individual women working at the hospital in a nursing capacity between the early eighteenth century and the end of the period. It is also possible to infer where in the hospital they worked. The earliest lists and the latest within the period (1703–11 and 1818–20) indicate the wards to which women were allocated, and circumstantial details suggest that the women were listed in ward order even in years when the wards themselves were not specified.[40] Women who served on one of the sixteen to eighteen 'long' wards were 'promoted' to the Light Horse or Officer wards (long-serving nurses literally moved up the list to these postings) or were allocated to the infirmary ward (a hospital within the hospital). The musters permit an estimation of the number of months or years of women's service, and sometimes record the occasions when nurses experienced periods of sickness or if they died in post.

The addition of extra datasets yields more information for selected groups of the nurses. Burials of women in the Chelsea grounds were recorded in the Chelsea Hospital burial register, giving a specific date of end of service (rather than the blunter indication of presence or absence from an annual muster roll).[41] Inventories of hospital wards list the equipment routinely associated with a nurse's duty and salary lists give their remuneration.[42] Wills from a very small proportion of women and a larger selection of their male charges point towards the women's material lives and circles of acquaintance. Lastly intensive searching of all of the sources available to genealogists can unearth longer chains of family connection including women's spouses and children. Family histories are easier to secure for Chelsea nurses than for their counterparts at either the ancient London hospitals or at the provincial infirmaries because of the intended institutional relationship between nurses and deceased servicemen: if nurses were the widows of soldiers who had been resident in the hospital, their surnames could be matched to the men listed in earlier musters. This means that, in selected cases, it is possible to trace the marriage of the man named as a soldier to a woman who later became a nurse.

The muster lists, burial registers, and wills, when combined, yield the names of 266 women who worked as nurses at Chelsea Hospital between 1693 and 1820. The average tenure of service (for 126 women whose period of employment can be calculated) stood at over twelve and a half years, akin to that for nurses at Chelsea's sister institution Greenwich Hospital where ten or fifteen years of service was common.[43] The Chelsea nurses also served for substantially longer than their counterparts at St Bartholomew's Hospital whose maximum tenure (on the basis of 108 women) stood at between six and seven and a half years.[44] The gap in the musters between 1712 and 1727 will mean that some women's names have been missed: any women whose full service fell between these two dates will not have appeared on any surviving musters. Even so, the lengthy average tenure of the women means that the Chelsea list of ward staff is much closer to a full roster than that calculable for Barts and used in Chapter 2.

Burials at Chelsea can be found for 157 women, meaning that a minimum 59 per cent of all nurse employees died in service (and therefore did not choose to leave their employment or suffer removal for wrongdoing).[45] Others may of course have died in service but been buried elsewhere at their own or their family's request without confirming their occupational status in the relevant burial register (and therefore leaving the burials of nurses outside of Chelsea non-confirmable). Again, this is much higher than the observable death-in-service rate at Barts of 19 per cent. For the majority of women, then, securing a post as a Chelsea 'matron' was a job for life.

For most of the period under study, women received a salary of £8 per year in addition to their bed and board.[46] There was an increase of salaries across the hospital's staff in 1806, and the nurses received an additional £2 as a result.[47] Each woman was issued with 'a Grey Colour Cloth Gown and Petticoat', a tradition which continued to at least 1870.[48] Equipment associated with their duties was purchased out of other hospital funds. Cleaning materials, for example, were bought and stored by the hospital and collectively allocated to the nurses, including in the early 1780s twenty-four hair brooms, forty-eight birch brooms, and twenty-four mops.[49] Each ward also had cleaning and fire-lighting equipment listed under the nurse's responsibility, including scrubbing brushes and tinder boxes. Ward nurses remained responsible for sweeping and cleaning their wards, and possibly keeping the fires, as well as for tending to the male residents. The inventories of the 1770s also show that the nurses slept in twelve rooms, two women per room, each with her own bedstead, mattress, three blankets and one coverlid (or bedspread).[50] The nurses of the Captains, Light Horse, and Infirmary wards were initially privileged in being given feather beds, but the flock mattresses of the nurses for the 'long' accommodation wards were upgraded to match in 1791.[51]

The nurses of the infirmary ward were granted additional leeway over and above the other women beyond the early allocation of a feather bed (sometimes after they had been effectually demanded by the women in post). In 1738 the infirmary nurses 'assumed a perquisite' of coals technically allocated to their patients. The hospital's illustrious surgeon William Cheselden at first complained about this behaviour, but on further reflection he came to see the nurses' point of view.[52] Cheselden petitioned the hospital's commissioners in 1739 to grant the infirmary nurses an extra allowance, given their increase in business, which was eventually agreed.[53] Similarly a special case was made on behalf of the infirmary nurses in 1743 in relation to the rules about their access to food. The hospital's surgeon and apothecary desired that the four infirmary nurses be allowed additional wages for their board as

> they cannot conveniently leave the sick to dine at ye Nurses Hall that their business is sometimes so great that they are forced to hire

helpers at an expense more than they can afford which makes all the nurses in the house refuse the Infirmary when a nurse is wanted.[54]

This led on to additional money being reserved in the short term for both the surgeon and apothecary of the infirmary to remunerate nurses, although whether for the employment of temporary unnamed nurses, or for additional benefits to the existing four infirmary nurses, is not known. The 'College', as it was known in Chelsea Parish, did recruit women casually to support the nurses, including two women from St Luke's Workhouse in 1784 and 1791 (neither of whom were ever listed in musters).[55] By 1797 these largely anonymous women could expect a retainer of £4 per annum plus six pence per week worked, which was not enough to tempt many: 'it is very difficult to get helpers' presumably because unlike the 'matrons' the helpers did not live in and have their residential costs met by the Hospital.[56]

Incidentally, Chelsea was an early adopter of dedicated night nursing, but not by the 'matrons'. Cheselden petitioned the governors in 1739 for nightwatching by men 'to attend ye sick men all night in ye part of ye Infirmary under his care, to assist ye poor men that are lame & weak on occasion of any accident that may befall them'.[57] Extra money was allocated to Cheselden, who appointed two or more watchmen from among the Chelsea in-pensioners (who signed for their additional cash allowances for a short period, between 1740 and 1744). It is not clear whether nightwatching by men continued throughout the remainder of the eighteenth century.

The physical capacity of the infirmary became a problem in the 1780s, at which time the nineteen beds were regarded as too few.[58] The hospital's governors realised that this created a point of pressure on the sick-ward's womanpower too.[59] The number of infirmary nurses was increased, and their additional remuneration formalised in the accounts.[60] By a new hospital warrant of 1809, the matrons all received a flat rate of £10 per year, and each of the six infirmary nurses at that time received an additional £2.[61]

Women's employment was maintained during their own perhaps repeated periods of sickness. Elizabeth Berry was first listed in the muster of 1805, but was denoted as 'sick' in 1806, 1808, and 1818.

Her service only ended with her death in 1836 when she was buried at the hospital. Frances Downs worked at the hospital for thirty years from 1754 to 1784, but her declining health was tolerated by the hospital as she was first sick, then lame, and finally sick *and* lame from 1782 onwards. Similarly, women were not expected to serve on their allotted wards when severely ill. Muster rolls might list women as 'absent with leave', typically in the year or years before their death, and the benefit could be extended to long-serving women and newcomers alike. Mary Newman was only listed in one muster, 1803, where she was also described as absent with leave. She was buried by the hospital in December 1803. Nurses were even allowed to visit their friends who lay ill outside of the hospital, at least in the early years. In July 1714, Mary Owen and Mary Overton visited their friend Mary Whitton who was suffering terminal decline at the house of Mrs Wade at King Street near Bloomsbury. All three of these Marys were nurses at the hospital, and a trip from Chelsea to Bloomsbury must have entailed notable absence from duty for Owen and Overton: it was not merely a question of visiting a house next door to the hospital.[62]

Medicine and nursing for older people: comparison of Chelsea's matrons with other hospital nurses

Medical understanding of ageing bodies underwent only modest change in the period 1660 to 1820. At first it was assumed that people died from disease, not from old age alone, and that disease was understood in terms of an imbalance in the four bodily humours. In the mid-seventeenth century, orthodox medicine in England which accommodated continental authors may have accepted the distinction made by François Ranchin between 'natural senescence' arising from a loss of bodily heat consequential on ageing and 'accidental senescence' caused by disease.[63] More radically, Francis Bacon's contemporaneous treatise of 1623 about the prolongation of life moved away from humoralism and towards an understanding of aging based on the observable features of decay in the natural world (plus its avoidance in humans by moderate living). Neither Ranchin nor Bacon seems to have made much immediate impression on a medical profession still committed to traditional Galenic interpretations of ill health. Even so, Bacon provides a summary of the behaviours of patients undergoing end-of-life nursing that might indicate the contemporary perception of approaching dissolution:

> The *Immediate preceding Signes* of *Death,* are; *Great Unquietnesse,* and *Tossing* in the Bed; *Fumbling* with the *Hands; Catching,* and *Grasping* hard; *Gnashing* with the *Teeth; Speaking hollow; Trembling of* the *Neather Lip; Palenesse Of* the *Face;* The *Memory* confused; *Speechlesnesse; Cold Sweats;* The *Body shooting in Length; Lifting* up the *White of* the *Eye; Changing of* the whole *Visage;* (As, the Nose sharp, Eyes Hollow, Cheekes fallen;) *Contraction,* and *Doubling of* the Tongue, *Coldnesse* in the *Extreme Parts of* the Body; In some, shedding of *Bloud,* or *Sperme; Shriking; Breathing thick,* and short; *Falling of* the *Neather Chap;* And such like.[64]

In cases of loss of consciousness or seeming death, Bacon recommended the use of water, wine, or cordials, bending the body forwards, rubbing of parts especially the face and legs, or putting rose water, vinegar, or burning feathers to the nose.[65]

During the long eighteenth century, nurses taking medical direction might just have detected a slow drift away from a solely humoral interpretation of the complaints of old age and towards an appreciation of conditions generic among (if not exclusive to) older people. John Floyer's *Medicina Gerocomica* engaged directly with Bacon in its preface, but is better at surveying existing remedies than breaking new ground. What this book does, however, is to organise its material somewhat according to the perils of 'Decays' in old age, including 'Rheumatic hot Pains', 'Gout', 'Loss of Memory', and other conditions symptomatic of the ageing body. Floyer spends most time recommending specific interventions in, for example, cases of memory loss when the patient's constitution is either cold and moist or hot and dry in accordance with humoral thinking: in a short but telling paragraph, however, he also admits that memory may fail entirely by dint of old age.[66] Half a century later, Buchan's *Domestic Medicine* betrayed some of the same assumptions about inherent connections between old age and diagnoses of rheumatism, diabetes, and palsy, albeit he devoted lengthy sections of his book to children, and none to older people.[67]

By 1820, the humoral trappings of medical commentary around age had gone. There was instead a new optimism and confidence about the ability of medicine to tackle the consequences of ageing or delay their onset. Susannah Ottaway says that the confluence of a more diagnostic approach with the delivery of medical care in workhouses established some of the understandings which later informed old people's care homes (albeit these understandings were not recognised as such at the time).[68] The Chelsea Hospital was even more focused on old age than were workhouses, and so constituted a distinctive microclimate of care.

The physicians, surgeons, and nurses attached to the Chelsea and Greenwich hospitals had their attention repeatedly focused on the disabled, the sick, the ageing, and eventually the terminal residents. If the men were not expelled from these hospitals for misbehaviour, or did not suffer a diagnosis of madness, they died there.[69] In this context, Geoff Hudson has speculated that Robert Robertson, physician at Greenwich in the late eighteenth and early nineteenth centuries, was one of the first authors to tackle geriatric medicine in a modern sense on the grounds that he was made a specialist by circumstance.[70] This may be too emphatic given Robertson's extensive investigations of fever (in patients of any age) and his rather judgemental perception of cases at Greenwich (that he frequently ascribed to intemperance). Even so Robertson's *Observations on Diseases Incident to Seamen*, first published in four volumes in 1807, made a modest continuation of Floyer's work by emphasising his own exposure to clusters of patients with common complaints like pleurisy, apoplexy, paralysis, and rheumatism.[71]

In a pragmatic sense, the governors of both the Greenwich and Chelsea hospitals had to make judgements about men's physical capacity to mediate their transfer into the hospital or the allocation of an out-pension. This entailed dealing with the presentation of specific men and their sufferings in ways that gave practical endorsement to the idea that the afflictions of age deserved special treatment.[72] The governors of Chelsea, for instance, recognised sciatica and visual impairment as grounds for higher out-pensions.[73] They were also aware that the resident men might frequently suffer from conditions such as hernia, or 'rupture' in contemporary terminology.[74] They went to some lengths in the 1750s to secure specialist treatment for this class of patient, unfortunately without success.[75] It is unsurprising that one of the next major interventions in the literature on disease in ageing in England after Robertson was written in 1863 by the then physician to Chelsea Hospital.[76]

The Army Medical Board devised regulations for regimental and general hospitals in the 1790s which indicate the intentions for medical provision and care (considered further in Chapter 6). Coincidentally, they also flag the types of condition which were anticipated to arrive for treatment in temporary or fixed establishments, revealing assumptions about military-style illness beyond the emergency requirements of battle. The 'Monthly Return of the Sick' form shows that, as for the general population, fevers were at the head of the list followed by chronic pulmonary complaints. Living in close quarters such as barracks meant that dysentery was also prominent. Thereafter the 'return' gives priority to the conditions which would have influenced soldiers' mobility, like rheumatism or hernias, plus disorders of the eyes. Fractures, fits, tumours, and contusions concluded the roster.[77] Chelsea, however, catered for the subset of men whose conditions became chronic and debilitating, or whose battle injuries were severe. Nurses were therefore less likely to encounter fevers or dysentery, and were instead more regularly exposed to rheumatism, hernias, and tumours.

Extreme cases of ill health or innovative treatment among the residents of Chelsea were reported by attendant medical men in line with the tradition of publishing case notes, as in the case of Laurence Welch aged 75. Welch was admitted to the hospital in or before 1728 and died in the infirmary in July 1739 following treatment for bladder stones. His case was made remarkable to surgeon William Cheselden by the combination of Welch's response to treatment with lixivium saponis and the discovery of 214 stones in his bladder when subjected to a postmortem.[78] The same account can be read differently from the point of view of the attending nurses who had to deal with the consequences of Welch's symptoms and treatment. These included vomiting from taking so much saponin internally, pain occasioned by the voiding of stone fragments via the urethra (requiring some use of opiates), urine characterised by the discharge of fetid mucus, and on one occasion Welch's manual manipulation of his penis for two hours to extract large stones.

The personal and intimate nature of his experiences meant that nurses were required to witness, to commiserate, and to clean up his excretions. Furthermore, it is unlikely that Cheselden sat with Welch continuously during his illness, and therefore nurse testimony was essential if uncredited in the composition of the published case.

Welch's circumstances are a reminder that the Chelsea Hospital's infirmary nurses faced some of the same assault on the senses as was experienced by the nurses of provincial infirmaries in terms of sight, touch, sound, and smell. There is little confirmation for the first three of these categories, but the issue of odour receives inadvertent confirmation from the hospital journals and (as with the risks of sensory disturbance in infirmaries) the focus is on patient inconvenience rather than the nurses. In April 1801 the hospital received a report of the infirmary bedding required which, in addition to textiles, included six straw and six feather 'beds' (meaning mattresses):

> Three of the above Beds with the blankets etc have been removed to the wardrobe keepers store room in consequence of their offensiveness, the remainder are in the different infirmaries but so dirty that they cannot with propriety be used again.[79]

Concern is expressed about the reuse of 'beds' from deceased patients, to extend the infirmary's accommodation to those in need, rather than the habitual exposure of ward staff to noisome bedding.

These institutional sidelights imply that, despite the delay to recognising geriatrics as a medical specialism, the nurses in the infirmary at Chelsea would have become familiar with, and adept at responding to, the needs of ageing bodies. Their charges collectively suffered impairments of perception, restrictions on mobility, disturbances of bodily function such as digestion, and undermined comprehension.[80] These features among the inmates contributed to an experience for nurses somewhat at odds with that for women in hospitals wholly dedicated to the sick. There were fewer acute cases at Chelsea, more chronic ones, and no categorical patient discharges (because men simply moved from the infirmary back to the 'long' accommodation wards). These features of work in the infirmary and the hospital at large meant that nurses' relationships with patients certainly lasted longer, and were potentially deeper, than those between other sick-nurses and their patients. They even led to marriage.

Nurses' experience of marriage

On 12 January 1761 a man living in the parish of Chelsea called Turner Desborough was buried at the Royal Hospital and, rather than give his trade or calling in the burial register, the clerk put him down as 'nurse's husband'.[81] This was probably not the first time in history that a man was identified by his wife's occupation, but it was a notable divergence from the eighteenth-century norm. It is possible to read this as either a mark of the high regard the hospital had for its employees, nurses included, or alternatively as a reflection on Desborough as a nonentity. Either way, the hospital's nurses had a secure occupational identity that (in Sarah Desborough's case) superseded that of their spouse to explain a husband's residence, settlement, and burial.

The nurses worked in a very specific marital environment at Chelsea. The hospital's population was male, of whom many would

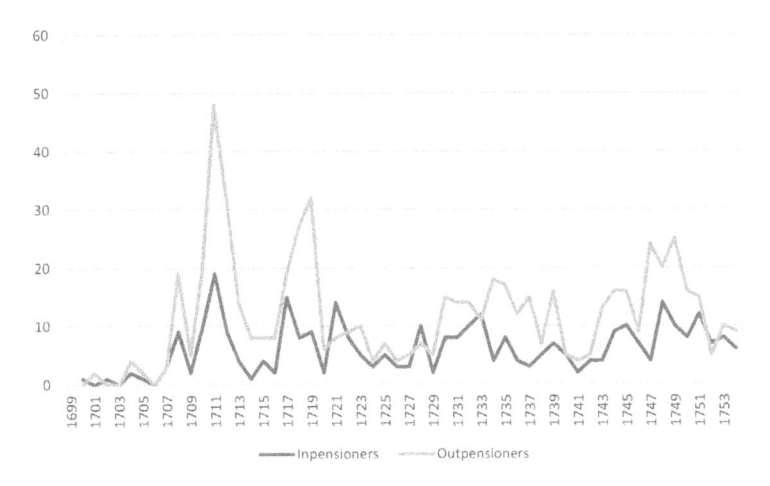

Figure 4.2 Chelsea Pensioner marriages by year 1699–1753

have been married before their admission, and inpatients were either strongly discouraged or forbidden to marry afterwards.[82] This did not mean that the men eschewed post-admission nuptiality in practice, as critics of the institution had feared. An analysis of the 'clandestine' marriages conducted at the Fleet between 1699 and 1754 (when Fleet marriages ceased) reveals that a small but steady stream of hospital men participated as grooms at this venue alone. An average of six such men per year conceals annual fluctuations of inpatient grooms numbering between nought and nineteen, equating to vital events for up to 5 per cent of the hospital's men per annum at the Fleet. Cumulatively, this gave rise to an array of institutional know-how around entering marriage against the rules and a pathway into marriage for the women who men had met as nurses.

Chelsea pensioners (in- and out-pensioners) were so numerous among Fleet spouses that they influenced the composition of all grooms for marriages solemnised at the Fleet during the first half of the eighteenth century. Chelsea was the most prominent place outside of London cited as the origin of grooms (accounting for between 1 per cent and 4 per cent of men who gave an address in 1711 and 1751) and the hospital was responsible for most of these proportions.[83] Chelsea men also contributed to the fact that 'the Fleet was indeed a popular place for remarriage'.[84] An analysis of all marriages at the Fleet among men giving Chelsea as their address, filtered to remove the names of out-pensioners and include only men who appeared in hospital musters as residents, yields 345 men who were living in the hospital at the time they were married between 1699 and 1753.

Table 4.1 Status of couples at the Fleet, where the groom was a Chelsea in-pensioner, 1699–1753

	Number	Percentage
Batchelor/Spinster	58	17
Batchelor/Widow	72	20
Widower/Spinster	35	10
Widower/Widow	159	46
Unknown	21	6

The Fleet already exerted a disproportionate pull upon widowers marrying widows, but these unions still only comprised 15 per cent of all Fleet marriages. The fact that 46 per cent of Chelsea inpatient spouses were widowers marrying widows means that the hospital's inmates made an influential contribution to this profile for remarriages. These events recorded at the Fleet hold a number of implications for the female staff at Chelsea, because they also imply that the hospital's widowers and widows were more likely to remarry than their peers outside the walls. More demographic research concerning rates of remarriage in London would be needed, however, to confirm this point.

The women who married Chelsea in-pensioners in these Fleet ceremonies were among the potential future nurses, because even if the hospital imposed penalties on men for their unauthorised relationships they did not go so far as to bar the wives of clandestine unions from employment. Phineas Dynes was an inpatient by 1704 and was one of the nine men who married at the Fleet in 1711. His wife was widow Joyce Gant (née Badham), first married in 1674. How the couple lived or accommodated their marriage in practical terms is not known. Phineas died in 1721, and Joyce was buried at the hospital in 1728. The absence of musters between 1711 and 1728 means that we do not know when Joyce became a nurse (i.e. during her marriage or after she was widowed for a second time).

It seems very likely that some women were brought to the hospital's attention as viable nurses explicitly because their inpatient husband had died. This was the case for Edith Foord, whose husband John Foord (of the 6th ward) died in 1704. The couple were originally from Bristol and had been married for twenty-five years.[85] John's residence in the hospital lasted only from April 1703 to May 1704, but Edith's spanned her appointment in 1704/05, relatively shortly after her husband's death, until her own death in 1717.

A higher proportion of women for whom data are available, at least nine out of thirty-seven confirmed marriages among Chelsea's female ward staff, entered the pool of possible nurses when their husbands were *admitted*. This was the case for Mary Fuljames, appointed in 1740 (after her husband William's arrival in 1739), and similarly for Fanny Fosmire, appointed in 1809 (after her husband Joseph's appointment to the 12th ward in 1808). This is notable because, by an Order of 1703, the hospital's female servants were supposed to be the widows of soldiers, or the wives of soldiers, 'not [wives of] Pension^{rs} in the said Hospitall'.[86]

The hospital may have favoured the employment of soldiers' widows as nurses, but this rule was clearly not applied rigidly, in relation to either husbands' military service or widowhood. Some nurses were the wives of other hospital officers, such as Elizabeth Lilly (née Stinson).[87] Elizabeth was married on 21 August 1811 to Abraham Lilly, variously listed in the muster rolls as a sweeper or under-scullery man at Chelsea (so a lower-ranking hospital servant). The couple had a son William, born on 14 June 1812 and baptised at the Chelsea Hospital, and a daughter Eliza, born on 13 May 1821, also at Chelsea.[88] Intriguingly Elizabeth senior's job as a nurse to the 17th ward began on 17 July 1818, so between the births of her two children and well before her husband's death in 1835. She remained employed at the hospital at the time of the 1841 census (when she was still the nurse of the 17th ward).[89] The appointment of an employee's widow was also possible, as in the case of Grace Howroyde. She was the widow of John Howroyde, the hospital's cellarman, and was appointed as a nurse to the infirmary three years into her widowhood in 1774.[90] Finally, nurses might also have been appointed from among the widows of Chelsea's out-pensioners (who were too numerous to permit checking against nurse surnames for the purposes of this chapter) or the widows of in- or out-pensioners of Kilmainham Hospital in Dublin. Rachel Pinkerton (née Hudson) was the widow of John Pinkerton, recommended as a proper object for a Kilmainham out-pension at the time of his discharge from the army in 1783.[91]

Nurses who were single or widowed at the time of appointment lived at close quarters with the male charges in their own ward and could establish familiarity with men in other wards. It is unsurprising, therefore, that a small but continuous cohort of women were appointed as nurses and subsequently married male inpatients. Unions between inpatients and serving nurses, both of which groups were supposed not to contract marriage, gave these couples particular reason to seek 'clandestine' marriage services. Nurses may be aligned (again) with domestic servants in their marital behaviour in this regard: servants were generally overrepresented at the Fleet, which Field argues was expressive of servants' liability to dismissal if their marriage became public.[92] Again, the case of Grace Howroyde is relevant, albeit her example postdates the Fleet as a site of marriage. One year after her appointment as a widowed nurse in 1774 she married Serjeant Edward Fairy of the 6th ward. It took a while for the hospital journals to refer to her under her new name (i.e. to be denoted Nurse Fairy rather than Nurse Howroyde) and even longer for her married status to show up in the annual musters where she was listed as 'Grace Howroyde' until 1793/94. Regardless of her fortunes in marriage – she was quickly widowed for a second time in 1778, inheriting all of Edward Fairy's property – she served as a nurse in the infirmary for forty years until her death in 1814.[93]

How did the hospital's governors react when such a marriage was discovered? There is no discernible commentary in the hospital journals.[94] We can, however, see the movement of women across different wards in ways which may be expressive of the governors' disapprobation. Hannah Archer, for example, was appointed in the early years of the hospital's existence and in the course of her work met Richard Goddard of the 13th ward. The couple were married in July 1707, Hannah being decisively identified in the Fleet registers as being of Chelsea Hospital, 'a nurse in ye same'. The following month Archer was moved from her post in the hospital's infirmary to the 16th ward. The timing is suggestive: was this effectively a demotion, signalling the hospital's disapproval but imposing a penalty short of dismissal? Richard died later the same year and Hannah remained at the hospital in the 16th ward until the time of her death in service. At her burial she was named Hannah Archer, not Goddard. Yet ward changes could have been predicated on ability, preference, or other circumstances rather than as a means of chastisement, and marriages had to be discovered before the hospital could act. Mary Roe, for example, was appointed as a nurse in 1739 to the 11th ward, and remained there until her death in 1757. In 1744 she had married Francis Busby/Buzby in Westminster. Francis was admitted to Chelsea's 10th ward in 1752, but still Mary continued to be listed in the musters as Roe. She was buried, however, as Nurse Busby.

Marriage patterns included women who experienced marriage to more than one inpatient, and men who were married to more than one nurse. Mary Mitchel's first marriage was to William Fuljames in 1705. He became an inpatient in 1739, and she was appointed as a nurse in 1740. After William's death in 1743 Mary was seemingly demoted from the high-profile Light Horse to the modest 8th ward for reasons unknown. Following four years of widowhood Mary Fuljames married a second inpatient, John Miller, in 1747 without being moved from the 8th ward. She died and was buried as Nurse Miller in 1754. A similar profile with less available detail is shown by Elizabeth Lander (née Perram), first the widow of inpatient Joseph Lander and later the wife/widow of James Marshall. At least one man, George Phiffen, was married sequentially to two nurses. He married Mary Jones in 1794, and she secured a job as a Chelsea nurse in 1800. George was admitted as an inpatient in 1803.[95] Mary died in March 1804, and George remarried in 1805 to Judith Keld. How Judith Phiffen survived in the succeeding years is not known, but a decade later she too was appointed as a nurse, responsible for the 15th ward from 1816. These examples suggest that nominal disapproval for marriages between nurses and inpatients was expressed mildly if at all. Instead, one spouse's association with the hospital could lead to tangible benefits for the other, at least in this period.

There is no visible pattern to suggest that single or widowed women appointed as nurses went on to prefer marriage to the men on their own wards, so it was not necessarily a simple matter of affection arising from immediate proximity, but there is fragmentary evidence that an existing marriage encouraged the hospital's management to place men in their wives' wards (or that chance would place them there). Lydia Walker was appointed to 12th ward in 1708 and remained there until at least 1711, whereas her husband Dennis was transferred there from the 5th ward between July and October 1710. The exigencies of men's ageing also played their part. Ruth Hands was appointed to the hospital's infirmary in 1810 and remained there throughout her career until her death in 1837. Her husband, James Hands, was almost forty years older than his wife, and died in 1818 aged 96 in the Chelsea Infirmary (perhaps directly under his wife's care).

These partial biographies for nurses and their husbands raise questions about the nature of a marriage when both parties lived within an institution which did not offer married quarters and where no independent household was envisaged. The marriages may have indicated a commitment to sexual exclusivity, albeit in a context where sexual activity for inpatients, nurses, and other employees was perforce constrained but not impossible (as the experience of Elizabeth Lilly above shows). The purpose of marriage aside from the prospect of progeny may simply have been a statement of affection and pooled resources among men and women who lacked their own marital home. A further rationale relates to gendered identity. Nurse and in-pensioner marriages conferred a measure of autonomy on both parties which allowed them to express their sense of self. These relatively poor women had a preference to be a wife rather than a widow in the context of an uncertain world, even given the apparent security of employment at Chelsea and despite the paucity of resident men's daily cash allowance. At the same time men living in Chelsea had of necessity been accustomed in their earlier life to see their identity bound up with their physical capacity. Loss of youth, physicality, or both were simultaneously pathways to admission and blows to manly independence.[96] Marriage, even without the maintenance of a separate household, offered a modicum of proof that not all of the markers of male adulthood were beyond reach.

Were women more likely to deliver good care as paid institutional nurses if they had themselves experienced nursing in an institution? It is not possible to know for certain. Nonetheless, Chelsea nurses did have this breadth of experience among their number by the end of the period (where the proof is tied to knowledge of their married life). Elizabeth Gillett was married in Taunton in 1785 to Edward Whitecomb when she was about 19. The marriage remained fertile for over two decades, because the couple had at least five children born at the British Lying-In Hospital in Holborn between 1798 and 1807.[97] Edward had been admitted to a pension in 1798 having been wounded at St Vincent, and was given a room at Chelsea in 1811. This means that when Elizabeth was first listed as a nurse in the muster of 1818, when in her early fifties, her life experience included the receipt of nursing care at the hands of female employees in a different caring institution. At the very least this lay in the background to her employment at the hospital and at most it may have influenced her delivery of care to others.

The 'matrons' were supposed at the time of their appointment to be once-married women, but they are better described in practice as much-married women who gave priority to their marital relationship before, during, and after their nursing appointment to the hospital. This suggests that the institution placed a high value on its nurses that was not quite matched by the value nurses placed on their occupation (namely compared with their value for status as wife).

Misbehaviour and dismissal

Marriage by a nurse was demonstrably not grounds for automatic dismissal. The journals of Chelsea Hospital are not at all revealing, unfortunately, about what infractions might result in women losing their job. This is in contrast to the journals and other record-keeping at Greenwich where monitoring of the (much larger) pool of nurses gives rise to a detailed picture of behaviour adjudged as misdemeanour.[98]

Rare evidence about the likelihood of nurses' discharge from Chelsea is offered by a staff list of 1795.[99] The twenty-nine separate women listed that year (two each for the Captains and Light Horse wards, four for the old infirmary, two for the new infirmary, sixteen women for the numbered wards and three additional women appointed to vacancies during the year) were dominated by examples of nurses who died in post, twenty-two in all. The fate of two women is not recorded, probably because their employment stretched beyond the terminal dates of the document. The five remaining women's employment records were marked as discharged, four of whom left the hospital in the week between 14 and 21 November 1798. This was apparently a one-off campaign to rid the hospital of 'superannuated' nurses, meaning women who were either too old or too weak to manage the work and who (for once) were not permitted to remain in the hospital's employment until their own demise.[100] One of those discharged, Mary Catherine Wood, was quickly admitted to the Chelsea Workhouse, so hospital employment did not always give women the chance to save against future hardship.[101] Overall, though, this snapshot suggests that 17 per cent of nurses might have been liable to end their hospital career with dismissal, the equivalent of less than half the 38 per cent of women who did not obviously die in post.[102]

There is only one well-documented instance of a Chelsea nurse being discovered in unequivocal wrongdoing. In November 1779 the hospital board was informed that Nurse Bradford had been turned out of the hospital for 'grossest misbehaviour and unpardonable insult offered to the Lt Governor'. Adding injury to insult, as it were, the unusually named Benedict Bradford and two other nurses (the latter two recently deceased) were found to have embezzled hospital property including blankets, pillows, chamber pots, candlesticks, and one chair. Nurse Bradford seems not to have been prosecuted, though, for the losses during her employment. Instead money owed to her for salary was withheld to the value of the missing goods.[103]

As remarked in Chapter 2 concerning the St Bartholomew's nurses, there is scope for petty conflict in any institution which may on occasion escalate to something more public. It is a shame that it is not possible to trace the nature of the disagreement between hospital adjutant Mr Grant and the former nurse Siddina Williams, pursued in the Middlesex county court (for which no relevant records survive).[104] Whatever it was, the hospital gave Grant ten guineas 'in consideration of the abuse & trouble he has had in this matter'. If there were disputes between the nurses, these are not now visible to the historian's eye. A fatal disagreement between two hospital inmates in 1801, however, provides a coincidental sidelight on the voice accorded to nurses. William Lamb was admitted to the hospital in 1795, and two years later James Legg was similarly admitted.[105] On the morning of 2 October 1801 James Legg shot fellow ward resident William Lambe in the Chelsea Hospital, killing him immediately. The 73-year-old Legg was subsequently tried at the Old Bailey, and among the witnesses called to give evidence was Ann Grant, nurse to the hospital's infirmary. She testified to Legg's being in the infirmary from approximately January to

May 1801, and undergoing a discernible change in character. He developed 'a lowness, a melancholy, a deranged state' and when she asked him the reason for his mood Legg replied that 'his mind was confused; that he had no rest night or day; that he was hurried from place to place, and could not tell what he was doing'. Grant became concerned that he might commit suicide, but thought he was harmless to others. She confirmed that Legg's confusion of mind seemed to persist until the time of the murder.[106] Despite this clear attempt by his nurse to secure mercy Legg was found guilty, sentenced to death, and hanged at Newgate on 2 November 1801. In this way the nurse's testimony was sought as valid, but ultimately disregarded as a route to greater leniency.

The hospital community from testamentary evidence

Only a small proportion of the Chelsea nurses have extant wills. These are spread across the period, with fifteen wills found representing women who died between 1704 and 1818, and one will surviving for Frances Fosmire, appointed 1810 and serving the hospital until her death in 1854.[107] The wealthiest of these nurses was Catherine Burchill (who worked on the Light Horse ward) who left £210 to her daughter Catherine junior in 1803, cannily specifying 'her husband John Ramsey nor eldest son James Ramsey to have any part or share thereof'.[108] As in the wills left by the nurses of St Bartholomew's Hospital, the most interesting details allude to ties of friendship and affection within the hospital community. Burchill named two of her fellow nurses, Rachel Lucas and Mary Ballantine, as trustees for her daughter (who lived in Scotland). This sort of reliance on female colleagues was not confined to the end of the period. Sarah Cobb in 1712 and Sarah Bishop in 1762 both made a friend and fellow nurse their legatee and sole executrix.[109] Frances Burnham, in contrast, wrote a will which evidences a wide circle of hospital friends and acquaintances. In 1733 she left £1 10s to be distributed among all of the residents of the 4th ward where she had been nurse (with different amounts allocated to the privates, serjeants and corporals), in a will witnessed by two nurses.[110]

The nurses even claimed bonds of friendship with women whose status within the hospital was much higher than their own. Rose Laisne was the wife of the hospital's Master Butler John Laisne, gentleman: this did not stop nurse Mary Sterry from leaving her silk gown to Rose and claiming John as her friend and as an executor. Furthermore, Sterry was Dutch by birth, providing just a shred of evidence for a diversity of heritage among Chelsea's nurses.[111]

The male inmates of Chelsea Hospital made wills too, and given the much larger number of men compared to nurses the surviving examples are more numerous. Sixty-one wills can be identified across the period 1700–1820 from men who were certainly or very probably in-pensioners of Chelsea (rather than members of staff or out-pensioners who gave Chelsea as their address for convenience). The majority, nearly two-thirds, of these wills do not give further details about friendships between either men or staff, but the remainder do offer additional snippets of information about community contact and fifteen make clear reference to nurses. The patterns of references to nurses in men's wills exhibit two discernible trends. First, evidence for personal recognition of nurses by men dries up the further up the hospital's social hierarchy the male testators sat. Of the twenty-five wills left by Captains and Light Horse men, for example, only one mentions a nurse. Second, the incidence of men's recognition for nurses was largely confined to the years 1752 and earlier. Only five wills after this date mention nurses in any capacity.

Nurses acted as witnesses for the men, as Jane Hogg did for Hugh Butterfield in 1722, but were not made executrixes unless they were the wives of the men concerned (as was the case for Grace Fairy on the death of her inmate husband Edward). Nurses were beneficiaries wherever men named them as the recipients of small bequests. William Ballard left his nurse half a crown in 1716, as did James Lile in 1741. Thomas Lee in 1787 generously gave his nurse Elizabeth Dale five guineas.[112] The will of Nathaniel Neale is particularly notable for demonstrating the further scope for men's personal connections across the male in-pensioners of multiple hospital wards, alongside his gift of a guinea apiece for two named nurses. A third nurse witnessed the will.[113] This suggests that, just as men regarded their military comrades as a part of their family, so too did Chelsea's inmates and employees sometimes become knitted together by shared experience into fictive kin, in much the same way as for the nurses at St Bartholomew's Hospital described in Chapter 2.[114]

A final intriguing factor about the men's wills is that they provide fragmentary evidence of moneylending by inpatients to nurses. Alexander Duglis's will of 1723 permitted nurse Elizabeth Prideaux to keep the 2s 6d of his which she already had in her hands.[115] Nearly a century later, Richard McConnell's will of 1820 referred to ten pounds that was owed to him by Elizabeth Walker, one of the nurses in the hospital's infirmary (alongside other small debts owed by men among the inpatients and Chelsea out-pensioners).[116] This means that while the hospital inmates may have been indebted to their nurses for care, they may simultaneously have been their creditors for cash. The web of connections that was possible in a residential institution with a relatively stable population was potentially dense in both emotional and material terms.

A Chelsea denouement: an alternative view of nursing for older people within the institution[117]

The experience of multiple nurses as members of the hospital community given above is lacking insight into the emotion work involved. There is one parallel source for the trials of nursing older people in the same location, if not for a patient in the same circumstances as the in-pensioners. Chelsea Hospital conferred free accommodation on its beneficiaries and on any officers who chose to live there. From 1787 the roster of live-in officers included the musician and composer Charles Burney, appointed as the organist of the hospital. The co-residential nature of Chelsea Hospital, in terms of the proximity of higher-status staff to the male inpatients, was sometimes uncomfortable. An auditory portrait of the hospital's infirmary in 1798 gives a vivid sense of movement and activity among the room's occupants, and the inconvenience incurred to Burney who occupied rooms directly below the infirmary. He was not sure of one hour's stillness, out of the 24: as the changing the places of bedsteads, without wheels – rolling rumbling of ponderous chairs, with & without casters – together with the poor men's wooden legs & crutches marking their painful steps – & the nocturnal occupations of the Nurses – render the bedroom & study of Dr B a very unfit residence for a hermit.[118]

Two of Charles Burney's daughters, Frances and Sarah Harriet Burney, were both novelists – Frances famously so – and were very well connected. The Burney family had contact with both London's intellectual and creative leaders (lexicographer Samuel Johnson, actor David Garrick) and royal patronage: Frances herself was second keeper of the robes to Queen Charlotte for a five-year period. Frances and Sarah were half-sisters who each called Chelsea home at different periods of their lives. They were also both drawn in to the task of nursing their father and his second wife (Sarah Harriet's mother) in older age or at the end of their lives. The literary spinsters whose narratives proved so useful for Chapter 1 have their equivalents in Chelsea: for Frances, the role of parental carer seems to have been relatively brief.[119] For Sarah, it was a work of years and a matter of protracted, if narrow, reflection.

Sarah lived at Chelsea in her father's hospital apartments acting as her mother's nurse during the latter's last illness in 1795–96 and (after an absence from the hospital between 1798 and 1807) Charles's companion, amanuensis, and nurse in the final years of his life between 1807 and 1814 (when he was aged 81 to 88). What is distinctive about Sarah's letters is that they give no appreciable insight into the practicalities of nursing, despite the fact that she certainly spent hours and days at her parents' bedsides. It is just possible that the hospital's 'matrons' undertook some of the physical nursing needed by appointees like Charles Burney, in addition to their duties on the wards, but if this is the case there is no clear evidence of it happening.[120] Instead, Sarah's surviving correspondence speaks solely about her father's physical state and the emotional burdens of care work.

Charles Burney's health in the final years of his life was beset by a number of the maladies common to old age. A seizure in 1806 when he was 80 probably accelerated his withdrawal from social life, and from then onwards his biographer judges that he adopted the lifestyle of a permanent invalid.[121] Alongside the chronic complaints of old age, he suffered from bouts of acute ill health. In 1809 he had a severe sore throat which inhibited his swallowing, characterised by Sarah as 'a thrush, and a spasmodic hiccup, which, almost without cessation lasted four days and nights!'[122] The drug regime which was prescribed on this occasion was itself heroic, including opiates, and Sarah attributed her father's loss of appetite during his convalescence to the action of drugs on his stomach.

In his final year of life, Charles Burney suffered from low mood, giving Sarah an additional task. She wrote to her half-brother Charles junior in December 1813 urging him to visit and help her in raising their father's spirits: 'He has had for some time a very severe cold, and other teasing complaints have followed it which render him so low that it is shocking to see him. I want you to come and cheer him up a little.'[123] Sarah's own attempts had proved less than effective, she thought, owing to her easily being silenced (as a familiar member of the household, and possibly as a younger female with a negligible authority).[124] There are no surviving letters from Sarah between the end of January 1814 and September of the same year, a gap occasioned by Charles's death in April.

The rather tangential reflections on nursing contained in Sarah's letters were expanded somewhat in her fictional writing. Her novel *Traits of Nature* (1812) sees the heroine Adela Cleveland defining her emergent womanhood somewhat in terms of an aptitude for nursing, and subsequently becoming a nurse to her father in the desperate hope of winning his affection.[125] In return, Adela is treated to an object lesson in emotional blackmail. Her father 'would acknowledge no pleasure in receiving her attentions: but the attentions of any other were not even permitted'.[126] In the novel, then, to nurse a manipulative older parent is to suffer chilling emotional isolation at the same time as physical domination. Sarah's editor Lorna Clark characterises the outcome of the novel, whereby Adela secures no obvious display of affection from her father but discerns the growth of her own fondness for him as the result of habits of self-denial at a huge emotional cost for questionable gains.[127]

It would be glib to assume too close a relationship between Adela's yearning toil and Sarah's lived experience. Yet there are grounds to suppose that echoes, at least, of Sarah's parental nursing found their way into her fiction, because while she is largely silent about the mundane aspects of care she is less reticent about the affective strain of living with an ageing parent who exerts authoritarian control in the expression of his own interest. In 1811, for example, it was agreed that Charles Burney would temporarily be moved from his own bedroom into Sarah's room, to allow for thorough cleaning. This left the problem of where Sarah should sleep in the interim, and she allowed herself the luxury of imagining she might be permitted to travel to Richmond to stay with her favourite niece. This arrangement did not at all suit her father, who apparently resented this modest show of independence and preferred that Sarah sleep in the accommodation of a Chelsea neighbour. When Charles was presented with the Richmond plan, he 'grumbled ... and wondered so much at my fickleness and caprice, that I told him I would give up the plan, & came out of his room quite sick'. Sarah construed her father's preference for her staying nearby to his liking for her reading the newspaper to him every evening, a routine she characterised as 'the sickening dose'. The difference in opinion rumbled on between the older parent used to obedience and the adult daughter keen for a change of scene. It was concluded only when the former 'told me last night in a pet, that if I had set my heart upon the Richmond jaunt, he would not oppose it: - "I never set my heart upon any thing, Sir".'[128] Sarah's self-denial may not have reached the same melodramatic pitch as that of her character Adela yet still have been a tangible accompaniment to the tenor of her life at Chelsea, to the extent that it evidently invoked metaphors of her own consequential sickness. The emotional conflict she experienced in 'playing a part' is an early illustration of the penalties on women who tried to retain a sense of self, or the exercise of choice, while subordinating themselves to older, petulant patients.[129] This raises the question of whether the hospital's paid nurses felt similar pressures in the same ways. Unlike Burney, the 'matrons' were sometimes the same age as their patients, or older, among men who were not their fathers and subject to the authority of hospital managers who were not also patients. Even so, the evidence of this volume so far suggests that it would be wrong to assume that paid, unrelated nurses felt none of the same emotions as unpaid family members. The discussion begun in Chapter 1 with female nurses and continued in Chapter 5 in relation to male nurses strongly supports the argument that both domestic and institutional settings challenged nurses' autonomy and identity in powerful ways. Rather the Burney evidence suggests that, when under pressure, unpaid children nursing sick parents were willing to submit to their patient's will under almost any circumstances, potentially having been trained in their duty from an early age, whereas paid nurses (in performance of contractual service, and lacking the same emotional investment in their patient) might have been less ready to bend entirely to patient authority, particularly if the necessary flexibility would have jeopardised their own sense of duty or self.

Conclusion

This chapter has focused on the care conferred on the residents of Chelsea Hospital from the perspective of the chief carers. The 266 women identified working as 'matrons' up to the end of 1820 are a near maximum figure, unlike the roster of nurses and Sisters at St Bartholomew's Hospital, giving the chance of a more comprehensive picture of their experience. Chelsea clearly offered secure employment and accommodation to its nurses, comprising reliable benefits to working women that were unusual and distinctive. A study of these women's careers within the hospital, and retrieving shreds of data for their previous or subsequent lives, provides some unexpected sidelights on the prehistory of professional nursing, and the social milieu of Chelsea's nurses.

The concentration of nursing care on damaged and ageing bodies gave rise to routine exposure of nurses to rheumatism, 'palsy', gout, and similar conditions in the context of patients with fading memories and failing eyesight. Nurses as well as doctors could become specialists by circumstance, as the lengthy tenures of some infirmary nurses confirm. I argue that this concentration and continuity of personnel comprised an unusually focused climate of care, one perhaps only mirrored at the time by Chelsea's sister hospital at Greenwich. Allegations about the charity's 'corruption' might even be read as the perception of this quality of care by some contemporaries: from the outside, the care taken on behalf of the men looked like a scheme for the enrichment of officers via their generous salaries, whereas from the inside the integration of comfortable accommodation, medical attention, and healthcare was a recipe for institutional expertise.[130]

The nurses were to some extent parallel beneficiaries of the wider hospital's care, in that they routinely died while in service and were rarely identified for expulsion. This atmosphere engendered a strong identity for nurses, and a confidence among them, which was expressed in their taking opportunities to marry the hospital's residents (despite rules to the contrary) and to collaborate with them in forging other forms of personal connection. Friendship and trust underlay the men's referencing nurses when they were devising their wills. The emotion work this may have entailed for the women concerned is unknown. Sarah Harriet Burney's experience of nursing her father, however, illustrates some of the penalties that could arise in nursing older men who became testy and domineering as their physical capacities declined. The pressures felt by Burney may perhaps have been experienced in attenuated form by women who were not related to their patients, and in similar terms by the nursing wives of resident husbands.

Military service gave men theoretical access to nursing in the Chelsea Hospital in the event of their becoming disabled and unfit for service, or in older age. It is necessary to look beyond physical care institutions to find evidence of nursing by men, which will be the subject of Chapter 5.

Notes

1 An initial draft of this research was published as a short work-in-progress piece: A. Tomkins, 'Chelsea Hospital nurses 1703–1820', *UK Association for the History of Nursing Bulletin* 7: 1 (2019). I am very grateful to the editor for permission to expand on the article in this chapter.
2 B. Mandeville, *The Fable of the Bees* (Harmondsworth: Penguin, 1970), p. 190.
3 J. Childs, 'War, crime waves, and the English army in the late seventeenth century', *War and Society* 15: 2 (1997), 1–17. Like most stereotypes, these judgements may well have been unfair; O. Brittain,

'Subjective experience and military masculinity at the beginning of the long eighteenth century, 1688–1714', *Journal for Eighteenth-Century Studies* 40: 2 (2017), 273–90.
4 C. Nielsen, 'The Chelsea out-pensioners: Image and reality in eighteenth-century and early nineteenth-century social care', (PhD thesis, University of Newcastle, 2014).
5 I. Woloch, *The French Veteran from the Revolution to the Restoration* (Chapel Hill, NC: University of North Carolina Press, 1979), p. 24.
6 L. O'Dea, 'The hospitals of Kilmainham', *Dublin Historical Record* 20: 3–4 (1965), 82–99, on pp. 92–4; D. Ascoli, *A Village in Chelsea* (London: Luscombe, 1974), pp. 61–2; P. Van de Merwe, *A Refuge for All: A Short History of Greenwich Hospital* (London: Greenwich Hospital, 2010), pp. 2–3.
7 S. Jesner, 'The world of work in the Habsburg Banat (1716–51/53): Early concepts of state-based social and healthcare schemes for Imperial staff and relatives', *Austrian History Yearbook* 50 (2019), 58–77, on p. 64.
8 Nielsen, 'Chelsea out-pensioners', p. 131.
9 M.K. Mackintosh, *Poor Relief in England 1350–1600* (Cambridge: Cambridge University Press, 2012), chapter 3. By 1535 only thirty-nine hospitals remained that offered medical care; see M. Carlin, 'Medieval English hospitals', L. Granshaw and R. Porter (eds), *The Hospital in History* (London: Routledge, 1990), p. 36.
10 The almshouse model has already been noticed in the literature as applicable to Chelsea's sister institution, the Naval Hospital at Greenwich; G. Hudson, 'Internal influences in the making of the English military hospital: The early eighteenth-century Greenwich', G.L. Hudson (ed.), *British Miltary and Naval Medicine, 1600–1800* (Amsterdam: Rodopi, 2007), p. 253.
11 For the material lives of almshouse-dwellers, see A. Tomkins, 'Retirement from the noise and hurry of the world? The experience of almshouse life', J. McEwan and P. Sharpe (eds), *Accommodating Poverty: The Housing and Living Arrangements of the English Poor, c.1600–1850* (Basingstoke: Palgrave Macmillan, 2011).
12 A. Tomkins, 'Almshouse versus workhouse: Residential welfare in 18th-century Oxford', *Family and Community History* 7: 1 (2004), 45–58, on p. 49.
13 A. Tomkins, *The Experience of Urban Poverty 1723–82: Parish, Charity, and Credit* (Manchester: Manchester University Press, 2006), pp. 92–4.

14 A. Nicholls, *Almshouses in Early Modern England: Charitable Housing in the Mixed Economy of Welfare, 1550–1725* (Woodbridge: Boydell, 2017), p. 159 for an example of ad hoc payments to a nurse by a Warwick almshouse.
15 N. Goose and L. Moden, *A History of Doughty's Hospital Norwich, 1687–2009* (Hatfield: University of Hertfordshire Press, 2010), p. 42 for an almsman allowed to leave so that his children could take care of him; A. Clark (ed.), *Sherborne Almshouse Register* (Dorchester: Dorset Record Society, 2014), p. xliii for an almsman 'turned out for indisposition'.
16 J. Bold, *Greenwich: An Architectural History of the Royal Hospital for Seamen* (New Haven, CT: Yale University Press, 2000); D. Cruickshank, *The Royal Hospital Chelsea: The Place and the People* (London: Third Millennium, 2004).
17 A. Shepard, *Meanings of Manhood in Early Modern England* (Oxford: Oxford University Press, 2003), pp. 192–5; A. Shepard, *Accounting for Oneself: Worth, Status, and the Social Order in Early Modern England* (Oxford: Oxford University Press, 2015), pp. 118–36.
18 Woloch, *French Veteran*, p. 10.
19 C. Kennedy, *Narratives of the Revolutionary and Napoleonic Wars: Military and Civilian Experience* (Basingstoke: Palgrave Macmillan, 2013), p. 20.
20 Nielsen, 'Chelsea out-pensioners', pp. 133, 197–9.
21 I. Devos, 'Population', S. Ottaway (ed.), *Bloomsbury History of Old Age* (forthcoming).
22 Woloch, *French Veteran*, 3. For an insight into corruption at Chelsea on a grand scale see Ascoli, *Village in Chelsea*, pp. 88–92, 101–2, 116–17.
23 'Journal of the proceedings and debates of the political club', *London Magazine* 19 (July 1750), 297–307, on p. 297.
24 'Curious anecdote of Chelsea Hospital', *Gazetteer and New Daily Advertiser*, 25 January 1780.
25 T.V. Hitchcock and J. Black (eds), *Chelsea Settlement and Bastardy Examinations, 1733–1766* (London: London Record Society, 1999), p. 99.
26 'The Old Chelsea Pensioner to Sir Cecil Wray. A New Song', *Morning Chronicle*, 5 April 1784.
27 J. Hartley, *History of the Westminster Election* (London: Debrett, 1784), p. 218.
28 Nielsen, 'Chelsea out-pensioners', pp. 1, 113.
29 Hartley, *Westminster Election*, p. 145.

30 R. Lonsdale, *Dr Charles Burney: A Literary Biography* (Oxford: Clarendon, 1965), p. 335.
31 E. O'Keeffe (ed.), *Narrative of the Eventful Life of Thomas Jackson, Militiaman and Coldstream Sergeant, 1803–15* (Solihull: Helion, 2018), p. 100.
32 D.M. Turner, 'Picturing disability in eighteenth-century England', M. Remis et al. (eds), *The Oxford Handbook of Disability History* (Oxford: Oxford University Press, 2018).
33 The National Archives (hereafter NA), SP 32/4, f. 13 for a stray list of in-pensioners dated 1692; see G. Hudson, 'Arguing disability: Ex-servicemen's own stories in early-modern England, 1590–1790', R. Bivins and J. Pickstone (eds), *Medicine, Madness and Social History: Essays in Honour of Roy Porter* (Basingstoke: Palgrave Macmillan, 2007), p. 112 for statistics relating to Chelsea's out-pensioners, among whom only 1 per cent had lost a limb.
34 C.G.T. Dean, *The Royal Chelsea Hospital* (London: Hutchinson, 1950), p. 128.
35 Quotation originally given in the hospital's book of instructions (1692) and cited by Dean, *Royal Chelsea Hospital*, p. 148. For comparison see the nurses' injunctions to clean wards and deal with foul linen at the military hospital in Kilmainham: E.G. von Arni, *Hospital Care and the British Standing Army, 1660–1714* (Aldershot: Ashgate, 2006), p. 196.
36 J. Macky, *A Journey Through England: In Familiar Letters* (London: John Hooke, 1724), volume I, p. 131; P.J. Grosley, *A Tour to London*, 2 volumes (London: Lockyer Davis, 1772), volume II, p. 47. J.W. von Archenholz, *A Picture of England* (Dublin: P. Byrne, 1791), p. 250 claimed that Chelsea pensioners were known to have a wager on the speed of vermin, but (if correct) this was not necessarily vermin sourced from within the institution.
37 Dean, *Royal Chelsea Hospital*, p. 128.
38 London Lives reference LMSMPS501550019, otherwise London Metropolitan Archives, Middlesex Sessions justices' working documents 3 September 1716 petition of Benjamin Mills: www.londonlives.org (accessed 26 January 2023).
39 Unless otherwise specified, all references to nurses' names and terminal dates of employment can be found in NA WO 12/11589-91 Royal Hospital Chelsea musters 1788–94, 1795–1808, and 1809–20, and WO 23/124-31 Royal Hospital Chelsea musters 1702–12, 1714, 1717, 1728–59, 1763–69, 1770–76, 1777–82, and 1783–89.
40 NA WO 23/124, 12/11591.

41 NA RG 4/4330 register of marriages (1691–1765), baptisms (1691–1796), and burials (1692–1797) at Royal Hospital Chelsea; RG 4/4387 baptisms (1797–1812) and burials (1797–1813) at Royal Hospital Chelsea.
42 NA WO 247/6, 7, 8, 9 inventories of Royal Hospital Chelsea 1754–60, 1761–65, 1775–76, and 1780–82; WO 245/57 Royal Hospital Chelsea salary books 1764–73, 1773–84, and 1782–89.
43 G. Hudson, 'Nursing disabled ex-servicemen in the Royal Greenwich Hospital, 1705–1800', paper given at the Society for the Social History of Medicine conference, Liverpool, July 2018. NB the duration of tenure in the case of Chelsea nurses is blunted by the fact that the musters were annual; for example, if a woman was first named in the muster of 1809 and last named in 1818, their service will have been computed at ten years when at the shortest possible duration it might have been nine years.
44 See Chapter 2.
45 NA RG 4/4330.
46 NA WO 245/4-7.
47 NA WO 250/467, Royal Hospital Chelsea journal 1806, see 8 May 1806 and 2 June 1806.
48 Dean, *Royal Chelsea Hospital*, p. 129.
49 NA WO 247/9.
50 NA WO 247/8.
51 NA WO 250/464 Royal Hospital Chelsea journal 1787–93, 14 June 1791.
52 NA WO 250/459 Royal Hospital Chelsea journal 1715–49, 25 October 1738.
53 NA WO 248/30 Royal Hospital Chelsea warrant to William Cheselden, 12 October 1739.
54 NA WO 250/459, 24 February 1742/3.
55 Elizabeth Dibble aged 60 was reported to be 'gone to be a nurse in the College' on 3 August 1784 but was back in the workhouse with the itch in October; Mary Simpson aged 55 went to be a 'helper' in the College in April 1791; St Luke Chelsea Workhouse admission and discharge registers via www.london.lives.org (accessed 26 January 2023).
56 NA WO 250/465 Royal Hospital Chelsea journal 1793–98 on 10 April 1797.
57 NA, WO 248/30, 12 October 1739.
58 NA WO 250/475 Royal Hospital Chelsea board minutes 4 August 1783. NB nineteen beds among four nurses meant that the Chelsea

Infirmary was in strict contrast to the provincial infirmaries, with much higher ratios, and more generous in its nursing provision even than St Bartholomew's Hospital.
59 NA WO 250/463 Royal Hospital Chelsea journal 1783–87 on 18 December 1783.
60 NA WO 245/7, see 1785 onwards for payment of the two new infirmary nurses.
61 P.P. *Commissioners of Military Enquiry: Nineteenth Report (Military Hospitals) Appendix* (1812), p. 425.
62 NA PROB 18/33/33 probate dispute Walker versus Kay 1714.
63 F. Ranchin, *Opuscula Medica* (Lyon: P. Ravaud, 1627) cited in A. Ritch, 'History of geriatric medicine: From Hippocrates to Marjory Warren', *Journal of the Royal College of Physicians in Edinburgh* 42: 4 (2012), 368–74, on p. 370.
64 F. Bacon, *Historie naturall and experimentall, of life and death: Or of the prolongation of life* (London: William Lee and Humphrey Mosley, 1638), pp. 361–2. These observations were not necessarily new in 1638.
65 Bacon, *Prolongation*, p. 365.
66 J. Floyer, *Medicina Gerocomica* (London: J. Isted, 1725), p 92.
67 For example the second edition: W. Buchan, *Domestic Medicine* (London: W. Strahan and T. Cadell, 1772).
68 S. Ottaway, 'The elderly in the eighteenth-century workhouse', J. Reinarz and L. Schwarz (eds), *Medicine and the Workhouse* (Rochester, NY: University of Rochester Press, 2013), p. 51.
69 Proof of in-pensioners' dismissal is very thin: NA WO 250/464, 1 February 1790 for one known case.
70 Hudson, 'Internal influences', p. 263.
71 R. Robertson, *Observations on Diseases Incident to Seamen: Whether Employed on, or Retired from Active Service, for Accidents, Infirmities, or Old Age* (London: T. Cadell and W. Davies, 1807) volume IV, pp. 789–804.
72 As Ottaway demonstrates, the Poor Law dealt with paupers in old age on a routine basis, but did not necessarily do so with the same range of motivation, facilities, or finesse as was displayed at Chelsea; Ottaway, 'The elderly'.
73 NA WO 250/463, for example on 21 June 1785.
74 P.R. Mills, 'Privates on parade: Soldiers, medicine, and the treatment of inguinal hernias in Georgian England', G.L. Hudson (ed.), *British Military and Naval Medicine, 1600–1830* (Amsterdam: Rodopi, 2007).

Nursing in the Royal Hospital Chelsea

75 These endeavours gave rise to a protracted dispute with Mr Lee, who had offered to treat ruptures; NA WO 250/460 Royal Hospital Chelsea journal 1750–71 on 16 January 1751, 24 April 1751, 2 April 1752, 8 February 1753, 14 March 1753, 27 March 1753, 14 June 1754, 13 February 1756, and 14 May 1756.

76 D. Maclachlan, *A Practical Treatise on the Diseases and Infirmities of Advanced Life* (London: John Churchill and Sons, 1863), cited in Ritch, 'Geriatric medicine', p. 371.

77 *Regulations to Regimental Surgeons &c for the Better Management of the Sick in Regimental Hospitals* (London: J. Jones, 1799), endpaper 'Form of a Monthly Return of the Sick of ____ Regiment'.

78 W. Cheselden, 'The effects of the lixivium saponis taken inwardly by a man aged 75 years, who had the stone', *Royal Society Transactions* (1746), 36–40. Lixiviation is a process to produce a solution by leaching, while saponins are substances occurring in plants such as soapwort which produce a lather.

79 NA WO 250/466.

80 The hospital musters took particular note of any male inmates who were blind or lame. See for example NA WO 23/129 muster roll of 1774 for William Wheeler and Samuel Howard of the 1st Company blind, and six other men in the same company lame; www.findmypast.co.uk (accessed 26 January 2023).

81 NA RG 4/4330; www.findmypast.co.uk (accessed 5 October 2022).

82 Depending on the year and perhaps on seeking the governors' approval; Dean, *Royal Chelsea Hospital*, pp. 150, 170.

83 J.F. Field, 'Clandestine weddings at the Fleet Prison, c.1710–1750: Who married there?', *Continuity and Change* 32: 3 (2017), 349–77, on p. 362.

84 Field, 'Clandestine weddings', p. 355.

85 Marriage of 20 May 1679 at Bitton St Mary, Bristol: www.findmypast.co.uk (accessed 12 June 2023).

86 Dean, *Royal Chelsea Hospital*, p. 169; *Papers Illustrative of the Origin and Early History of the Royal Hospital at Chelsea* (London: Eyre and Spottiswoode, 1872), p. 50.

87 Nurses probably married hospital officers throughout the period; see Anne Starlyn (died 1711), also married to a hospital sweeper.

88 NA RG 4/4387.

89 NA HO 107 census 1841. For a similar experience of maternity before and during appointment as a nurse see Benedict Bradford, first appearing in the muster of 1758, with sons baptised in 1755 and 1760.

90 NA PROB 11/973/277 will of John Howroyde 1771; for nurse appointments from among other employees' widows see for example Margaret Keynton (née Thornton, died 1767), presumed married to James Keynton the hospital's master gardener.
91 NA WO 23/133; www.findmypast.co.uk (accessed 26 September 2022).
92 Field, 'Clandestine weddings', pp. 366–7.
93 London Metropolitan Archives and Guildhall Library Manuscripts, DL/C/0366/0426/024 will of Edward Fairey 1778.
94 Searched for these purposes 1715 to 1806.
95 WO 23/134; www.findmypast.co.uk (accessed 26 September 2022).
96 Kennedy, *Narratives*, p. 76.
97 The combination of the parents' forenames with the unusual surname Whitcomb means that these births can be associated with the Taunton marriage with near certainty. The lying-in hospital's delivery books give Elizabeth's age.
98 Hudson, 'Internal influences', p. 259; Hudson, 'Nursing', reporting that of over 800 nurses at Greenwich between 1705 and 1805, 102 or approximately an eighth of the female workforce was expelled for wrongdoing.
99 NA WO 23/134 Royal Hospital Chelsea list of in-pensioners and staff 1794–1813, recording deaths 1795–1816.
100 NA WO 250/465.
101 St Luke Chelsea Workhouse admission and discharge registers 8 February 1799, via www.london.lives.org (accessed 26 January 2023).
102 A minute in the hospital journal of 17 December 1798 implies that superannuated nurses might be granted a pension of up to one shilling per day, and there is a reference on 13 December 1802 to the superannuated 'list' but it is not clear whether this allowance was ever paid before 1820; NA WO 250/465.
103 NA WO 250/462 Royal Hospital Chelsea journal 1778–82 on 24 November 1779.
104 NA WO 250/460, see 1 October 1768, 4 November 1768, and 3 March 1769. NB Siddina Williams does not crop up in any of the sources listing 'matrons', which suggests she was a short-term appointment or an otherwise anonymous helper.
105 NA WO 23/134.
106 Old Bailey, t18011028-39; www.oldbaileyonline.org (accessed 23 July 2018).
107 One of the wills is for a woman who does not otherwise appear in the musters or burial records for Chelsea; see LMA DL/AL/C/003/

9052/039/071, will of Margaret Lloyd 1719, nurse of the 10th ward.
108 NA PROB 11/1390/133 will of Catharine Burchill 1803.
109 NA PROB 11/529/406 will of Sarah Cobb 1712 and 11/872/387 will of Sarah Bishop 1762.
110 NA PROB 11/657/263 will of Frances Burnham 1733.
111 NA PROB 11/1205/128 will of Mary Sterry 1791.
112 NA PROB 11/1149/246 will of Thomas Lee 1787.
113 NA PROB 11/798/250 will of Nathaniel Neale 1752.
114 P.Y.C.E. Lin, 'Caring for the nation's families: British soldiers' and sailors' families and the state, 1793–1815', A. Forrest, K. Hagemann, and J. Rendall (eds), *War, Society, and Culture, 1750–1850* (Basingstoke: Palgrave Macmillan, 2009), pp. 112–13.
115 NA PROB 11/591/447 will of Alexander Duglis 1723; whatever the story behind this small bequest, Prideaux had a good year in 1723. She was also left £1 1s by in-pensioner John Batters/Battrs; see PROB 11/589/320 will of John Battrs or Batters 1723.
116 NA PROB 11/1636/13 will of Richard McConel otherwise McConell 1820.
117 Previously published as part of A. Tomkins, '"I helped to nurse": Unpaid care work by Georgian spinsters 1780–1820', *UK Association for the History of Nursing Bulletin* 10 (2022). I am grateful to the editor for permission to reproduce text here.
118 Lonsdale, *Burney*, p. 392.
119 J. Hemlow (ed.), *The Journals and Letters of Fanny Burney, Volume I: 1791–1792* (Oxford: Clarendon, 1972), pp. 221–3, for example, when a short period of nursing her stepmother does little to interrupt her social round.
120 Sarah's reference to 'heavy-bottomed young and old women' is presumed to be a description of her fellow hospital residents, the wives and daughters of employees, not the 'matrons'; L.J. Clark (ed.), *The Letters of Sarah Harriet Burney* (Athens, GA: University of Georgia Press, 1997), p. 197.
121 Lonsdale, *Burney*, pp. 460–1.
122 Clark, *Sarah Harriet Burney*, pp. 103–4.
123 Clark, *Sarah Harriet Burney*, p. 178.
124 Clark, *Sarah Harriet Burney*, p. 178.
125 For specific examples of Adela's conflation of nursing with good womanhood, either in expectation or in performance, see S.H. Burney, *Traits of Nature* (London: Henry Colburn, 1812), volume I, p. 155 and volume III, p. 189.

126 Burney, *Traits of Nature*, volume V, pp. 104–5.
127 L. Clark, 'Sarah Harriet Burney: *Traits of Nature* and families', *Lumen: Selected Proceedings from the Canadian Society for Eighteenth Century Studies* 19 (2000), 121–34. This looks very like an early example of the philanthropic operating state which renders emotional management in the workplace as a gift; S.C. Bolton and C. Boyd, 'Trolley dolly or skilled emotion manager? Moving on from Hochschild's Managed Heart', *Work, Employment, and Society* 17: 2 (2003), 289–308.
128 Clark, *Sarah Harriet Burney*, p. 137.
129 P. Smith and M. Lorentzon, 'Comment: Is emotional labour ethical?', *Nursing Ethics* 12: 6 (2005), 638–42, on p. 638.
130 NB officers' unjust enrichment and residents' access to care were not, of course, mutually exclusive options.

5

Nursing by men: an issue of identity[1]

Your Lordship hinted that you liked not men-servants about your person in your illness ... Male nurses are unnatural creatures![2]

The novelist Samuel Richardson has his character Sir Charles Grandison express this (at the time unexceptional) view of male nurses in order to underpin a paeon to the married state. Grandison promotes marriage to his ageing uncle Lord W on the grounds that wives make devoted nurses, and without a wife he will need to look to male domestics for care: 'There is such a tenderness, such an helpfulness, such a sympathy in suffering, in a good woman' in contrast with a male nurse where 'There is not such a character that can be respectable.' Richardson was unwittingly summarising the popular view of male caregivers for the next 260 years.[3]

Men also hold an unenviable place in the academic history of pre-1820s nursing, because their contribution has predominantly been represented by the male keepers of eighteenth- and early nineteenth-century madhouses who had a reputation for brutality.[4] This initial focus was a fair way to begin, given that such establishments provided employment for significant numbers of men. There were over one hundred public and private madhouses in England by the second decade of the nineteenth century, for instance, and work associated with them eventually underpinned the formation of the first proto-professional grouping to which male nurses could belong, namely the Asylum Workers' Association.[5] Exclusive attention to madhouses, though, does not do justice to the presence of men in paid and unpaid nursing roles.[6] This chapter aims to place men within the history of general nursing to demonstrate that they were not necessarily or always 'unnatural' holders of the role (as implied by the quote above) or conversely perpetrators of violence in the mould of the anti-nurse.[7] Instead, it draws on personal papers such as diaries, letters, and memoirs, plus British Parliamentary Papers, to establish patterns of activity by men in different contexts. The first half of the chapter establishes a baseline of nursing activity by men which yields an array of detail, with points of coherence across texts and by different authors. By collating accounts of nursing by men we may at least be able to see the parameters of acceptable stories about care given by men, beyond Richardson's jaundiced dismissal, and at best might gain insight into the nature of men's real-world actions.

The second half of the chapter addresses the negative male stereotype in nursing by an analysis of narratives concerned with male brutality within lunatic asylums. These accounts have been well-used for histories of institutions, or of the mad, but have not been subjected to the kinds of contextualisation for nursing that were undertaken in Chapter 1 for women.[8] This research sets men's alleged violence in caring roles against two related social and cultural phenomena: the reputational risks for men in undertaking paid work as a carer in light of the drivers of normative masculinity, and the impact of 'dirty work'. Men acted violently towards patients on occasion in ways that can be explained (if not necessarily mitigated) by reference to these factors.

The historiography of men in pre-professional nursing

Carolyn Mackintosh, Joan Evans, and others have recognised the historical precedents for men to undertake domestic nursing work, and the factors which have conspired to hide such work from historians.[9] Selected evidence of men's institutional nursing is easier to find.[10] Nonetheless, there is generally very little commentary on the practical dimensions of nursing by men in the period 1540 to 1800. Research on men expands from the second half of the nineteenth century onwards, such as in Linda Sabin's examination of family and community nursing by men in the American South during and after the Civil War.[11]

Nursing by men in contexts other than diagnoses of insanity were not so much anomalous as they were underreported.[12] This has been somewhat owing to the ideological construction of nurses as inherently female, a legacy from the Victorian era of nursing reform and concurrent assumptions about normative masculinity in the same period, but there are other factors to consider. In the late eighteenth century, masculinity came under the influence of 'sensibility' with the result that manliness could feasibly be consistent with personal sympathy and emotional display.[13] This shift might have provided a pathway for the performance of tender nursing as an accepted feature of masculine behaviour rather than a predictor of effeminacy, yet it did not. Historians may disagree about the infusion of Christian ideals and religiosity in manliness in the eighteenth and nineteenth centuries, but none of them have found that piety or the example of Christ led men into vocational nursing.[14] Instead nursing and medicine became very strongly gendered as female and male respectively by the second half of the nineteenth century: the term 'nurse' became feminised, while care work by men became known by other labels.

Mortimer reports for the seventeenth century that 6 per cent of the payments for nursing-type activity that he uncovered – denominated keeping or attending in probate accounts which he studied – was conducted by men. Men were paid to nurse other men, while women nursed both sexes.[15] Most of this male-nursing activity predates 1650, suggesting to Mortimer that nursing was either becoming femininized or that men's activity acquired descriptors other than nursing from 1660 onwards.[16] Even so, Samantha Williams found that in Campton, Bedfordshire between 1767 and 1834, 16 per cent of the carers paid from parish funds were men, who mostly attended other men.[17]

This chapter applies the model of nursing activity given in the Introduction which tries to typify the contexts in which care was demanded in the pre-professional era, namely as occurring one-to-one, one-to-many, or many-to-one.[18] Only the act of prioritising care over both location and payment allows us to appreciate the full range of men's nursing. It also allows us to get beyond an artificial separation between medical attention and nursing, because it is entirely possible to perceive nursing work by men with medical credentials. This might be located within the task of doctoring if it remained the case that 'care was inseparable from cure', as when the surgeon Mr Kent attended the Reverend Matthew Booker as both 'a nurse and a friend'.[19] Care was also the function of a practitioner who was both a male householder and family man. Eminent physician Robert Waring Darwin apparently helped his wife Susannah to nurse their numerous children during illness, for example, because Susannah mentioned nursing alone during Robert's absence from home.[20] Similarly, before nursing reform, there were low-level medical jobs held by men which required the performance of work (such as changing dressings) that in other contexts was performed by women.[21]

The boundaries of such working practices were blurred further by medical institutions which offered men remuneration for a form of delegated nursing. The provincial infirmaries discussed in Chapter 3 generally did not accept patients with infectious diseases, but would seek private lodgings for people suffering with infection if they also had a condition that would be treated by the infirmary. They were housed locally until the infection was gone, and then admitted to hospital for their non-infectious malady. People who let rooms to contagious patients could be either women (as illustrated in Chapter 1 by Mrs Canham) or men. Men in Gloucester who boarded and 'nursed' smallpox patients who could not yet be admitted to the infirmary included the apothecary Mr Mills.[22] This suggests that while caregiving was consonant with medical attention, it risked being subsumed into the more high-status tasks associated firmly with medicine whenever men thought about or described their own labour.

Nursing by male relatives, servants, and friends

Men were not thought to be good patients:

> what poor creatures men in general are, when necessity confines them to a sick chamber! ... I scarcely ever find a man, in sickness, support himself so well as a woman does. Men are, for the most part,

depressed in their spirits to the greatest degree when they are ill ... A good nurse will, in a great measure, alleviate our bodily infirmities, by supporting our spirits in time of sickness.[23]

Perhaps, as a result, there is relatively slight evidence to document one-to-one nursing by the male relations, servants, neighbours, and friends of the sick.[24] As one memoirist put it, 'The details of a sick bed are not interesting', and accounts in men's personal documents of nursing or being nursed tend to be reserved for moments of high emotion or extensive commitment.[25] The diary of Isaac Archer of Mildenhall in Essex, for example, gave a heart-rending account of his attendance on his small daughter when she lay dying in 1679. He and his father-in-law tended the child and her mother, ill at the same time and in the same room, where they 'helpt all night' and 'used all the meanes' they could, such as when the little girl 'slept with my arme under her'.[26] In the early eighteenth century Mr Thomas Ottway 'assisted' daily when two of his children and a niece were ill with the smallpox.[27] Similarly, the husband of Agnes Witt 'was up with' his son Edward at many times in the nights before Edward died.[28] Nor were these unique experiences:

> Contrary to common opinion, early modern men and women did not adhere rigidly to the prescribed spheres of masculine and feminine activity while their children were ill. During these anxious times, the boundaries delineating gender roles became blurred, and mothers, fathers, aunts, uncles, and grandfathers and grandmothers came to one another's aid. Perhaps when faced with the desperate reality of a sick child, the niceties of gender prescriptions seemed unimportant.[29]

This could also be true for servants; in 1802 when William Holland's children were ill with scarlet fever, his former servant William Tutton came back to give the family his assistance, when no one else would risk their proximity to the infection.[30]

Nursing by men was carried out for adults too, including for wives, parents, friends, and employers, albeit sometimes under pressure. Eliza Fay was nursed by her husband when there was no other source of care available (when the couple were in India).[31] John Stutterd looked after his mother when she was 'very poorly' in 1787: she had 'picked up abundance of tough yellow matter' which she perhaps vomited, since John had to 'hold her head' and 'empty her pot'.[32] John Macdonald gave a generally upbeat account of his life as a footman, but recalled the illness of his employer Colonel Keating in the early 1770s with feeling: 'He was so extremely ill that for twelve nights I never went to bed nor pulled off my clothes: he had no nurse but me.'[33] It may have been that female nurses were unavailable, given that Keating (like Eliza Fay) fell ill when in India. Macdonald probably overplayed his role in saving Keating's life, as the hero of his own narrative, but he certainly includes authentic details about the care he offered, including wetting the lips of his patient with a feather. Coincidentally, this illustrates that issues of intimacy between male servants and their employers need not be wholly concerned with sexuality.[34] We might deduce further that, given the status of male servants as luxuries expressive of conspicuous consumption, nursing by manservants would have carried higher social desirability than nursing by serving women.[35]

Nursing by male servants also offers the chance to perceive men of non-English heritage in a caring role. Francis Barber was born in Jamaica under enslavement and was taken to London in his youth. There he became the employee and friend of lexicographer Samuel Johnson, for whom he evolved into a carer.[36] The acceptability of Barber's nursing for the irascible Johnson must be inferred by the author's reactions to his replacement. As Johnson was dying:

> A man whom he had never seen before was employed one night to sit up with him. Being asked next morning how he liked his attendant, his answer was 'Not at all, Sir: the fellow's an ideot; he is as aukward as a turn-spit when first put into the wheel, and as sleepy as a dormouse'.[37]

Barber was one of the two men in attendance on Johnson at the time of the latter's death and was made Johnson's residuary legatee.[38]

A more specific account of a Jamaican man nursing both men and women tacitly uses the comprehensive delivery of care as a way to underscore the humanity of other races. Catherine Cappe, a philanthropic and well-connected woman in the Unitarian congregation, wrote an autobiography which naturally included details about the lives of her husband and step-children. Her husband's son Joseph and two of his unmarried daughters Mary and Anne sailed to Italy for Joseph's health, since the latter was suffering from consumption, but Joseph died in transit leaving his two bereaved sisters to travel home from Leghorn to Liverpool. They embarked in late December 1802 and their safety was threatened by both pirates and repeatedly by storms, yet they had the good fortune to be travelling in company with the black servant who had attended their brother. Cappe's gratitude to this man – 'to whose various talents, disinterestedness, and generosity it is difficult to do justice' – prompts her to give brief details of his life and capacities as a nurse.[39] John Hacket was born free in Jamaica in about 1779 but was recruited by the Cappe family in Liverpool in 1802.[40] Joseph confirmed John's 'unremitted, affectionate, and judicious attendance upon his dying master' by requiring his sisters, in his last request, to reward John accordingly. These general encomiums on John's abilities were augmented by his care for one of Cappe's step-daughters who suffered severely from sea-sickness:

> He anxiously and assiduously watched the intervals, when it was practicable for her to take nourishment; had it constantly ready prepared (for he was an excellent cook, as well as a judicious nurse) enforcing the necessity of her endeavouring to swallow it; and she is herself persuaded, that had it not been for these very minute attentions, she could not have survived the voyage.

His virtues were augmented for Cappe by his reading the Bible in preference to associating with the 'profane' sailing crew, and by his rapidly teaching himself to write under the tutelage of one of the Cappe sisters. In this way the story is mobilised as an emphatic support for abolitionism while coincidentally transmitting the otherwise uninteresting particulars of care to posterity.

The relationship between employers and servants was such that, as in Chapter 1 in relation to women, the former might need or want to care for the latter. This activity, too, might take place across racial lines. Olaudah Equiano reports that his friendly working relationship with English shipping captain Thomas Farmer was a factor in his recovery after Equiano, then working as a sailor, experienced a vicious beating at the hands of one Doctor Perkins. Equiano was unconscious and imprisoned when Farmer had him removed to lodgings, sought legal redress for the attack, and 'nursed and watched me at all hours of the night'.[41]

Literary men like Equiano were perhaps more likely to offer details of one-to-one nursing than their non-literary peers, an echo of the attribution in Chapter 1 of nursing insight committed to paper by literary spinsters. In most cases the details remain slender and, wherever the authors were also the nurses, can be read as anecdotes of self-approval under duress. In the memoirs of Thomas Holcroft, for example, the radical author recalled that in adolescence he had sat up with a school fellow who suffered a severe and unsightly injury because 'All the older boys expressed the terror it would give them' while he, Holcroft, pitied him.[42]

Rather more information is forthcoming for the Keats family in relation to terminal tuberculosis. The poet John Keats is known for his beautiful verse and his very early death.[43] This combination has made Keats one of the most biographised subjects in literary history. What is less often remarked is his experience of nursing tuberculosis, as both a supplier and a receiver of care. Keats nursed his younger brother Tom 'intensively' between August and December 1818 (when Tom died).[44] Keats's letters to family members during these months chiefly refer to Tom as either better or worse, and his own social life as curtailed by the need to remain in attendance given that Tom 'looks on me as his only comfort'.[45] His most revealing comment among this correspondence, however, offers a startling characterisation of the emotional penalties of nursing for a young man in his early twenties. He struggled to maintain a sense of self, writing of Tom:

> His identity presses upon me so all day that I am obliged to go out ... I am obliged to write and plunge into abstract images to ease myself of his countenance, his voice, and feebleness – so that I live now in a continual fever ... if I think of fame, of poetry, it seems a crime to me, and yet I must do so or suffer.[46]

In this way Keats was somewhat shamefacedly expressing perhaps a perennial problem for the emotionally invested nurse – the embarrassment of having any wants beyond those of the patient.

Keats's own health deteriorated in the following two years, such that by September 1820 he was travelling to Italy for his health. He was accompanied by Joseph Severn, a friend and painter also in his twenties. The two men settled in Rome, and Keats died there in February 1821.

Severn's letters from Rome dated November 1820 to February 1821 were much more detailed about the care offered to a terminal tubercular patient than Keats's own letters had been, in both practical and emotional terms.[47] He was tied to the patient's bedside: 'I sit by his bed and read all day and at night I humour him in all his wanderings', for Keats would not accept any substitute carers. The symptoms were grim, and unrelenting: for example, 'in an instant a cough seized him and he vomited near two cupfuls of blood'. Severn's response to the physical symptoms was kindly and ameliorative: 'I cool his burning forehead.'[48] He found the daily routine hard work, however, since it involved carrying and dressing Keats, making beds, lighting fires, and sweeping, plus cooking and washing up, namely 'all the menial offices' plus regulating the poet's intake of food on the instructions of Keats's physician.[49]

The frustrations of a sole attendance were described vividly in a letter of January 1821 to Mrs Brawne, mother of Keats's fiancée Fanny:

> What enrages me most is making a fire. I blow, blow, for an hour. The smoke comes fuming out. My kettle falls over on the burning sticks – no stove – Keats calling me to be with him, the fire catching my hands and the door bell ringing. All these to one quite unused and not [at] all capable.[50]

These material features of attendance were exacerbated by the anxieties Severn suffered over his friend's mental state, which he described as acute. On a particularly distressing day in December 1820, he recalled:

> What an awful day I had with him! He rush'd out of bed and said 'this day shall be my last', and but for me most certainly it would. At the risk of losing his confidence I took destroying means from his reach, nor let him be from my sight one minute.

In other words, in addition to nursing, Severn had to prevent Keats from achieving suicide, combating his 'despair in every shape ... I tremble through every vein in concealing my tears from his staring glassy eyes ... how can he be Keats again ... You cannot think how dreadful this is for me.' Severn too was concerned with identity, his patient's and his own, promising that if he [Severn] can receive good news from his family in England 'I shall take upon myself to be myself again.'[51] Emotional investment in nursing by these two young men challenged them in ways that threatened or distorted their sense of self. This feature of the correspondence by or about Keats gives us a hint of the resistances to nursing that might arise from contemporary masculinity, an unwillingness to surrender self except under immediate threat of losing loved ones.

In turn these intimations provide an echo of the nursing vocation which Nightingale was to promote a generation after Keats's death – i.e. not to resist the loss of self but willingly surrender one's identity to the role of nurse in a form of professional selflessness, whoever the patient or patients might be.[52] The challenge that nursing presented to the nurse's identity is one rarely surveyed explicitly in histories. The idea is expressed most cogently by Emily Abell in her history of nursing by American women in the period after 1850 and the ways that 'caregiving undermines autonomy'.[53] I argue in Chapter 1 that the delivery of care was largely congruent with women's broader identities, with failure to care an indictment of individuals on the grounds of normative femininity. In relation to men, the evidence from the Keats coterie suggests that the reverse was also the case: nursing conflicted with the masculinity of the group's members, and risked comprising an oppressive role which few external observers would have regarded as essential (in either personal or gender terms).

Admiral Lord Nelson and an elite experience

Many-to-one nursing was the experience of high-status patients surrounded by willing attendants and involved both men and women as nurses. The phenomenon is best documented for exceptionally wealthy and politically significant individuals, such as monarchs. It is possible to find examples of individuals of lower standing nursed by multiple people, but these are rarer and suggest a level of charisma or other cause of localised devotion.[54] A notable account of nursing by multiple men of a single male patient is found in the death of Admiral Horatio Nelson in 1805, as described by William Beatty (the surgeon on the ship *Victory*).[55] The poignancy of Nelson's success at the naval Battle of Trafalgar coinciding with his own death, and subsequently a lavish state funeral, ensured national interest in the minute circumstances of his demise. Beatty's narrative was first published in 1807 and ensured that the surgeon's name would be linked with that of the national hero in perpetuity.[56] The self-serving aspects of Beatty's account need to be acknowledged because they might tend to influence the way he depicted Nelson's final hours of life. A plethora of attention following a fatal wound from a stray musket ball was probably the minimum which was expected for a man of Nelson's standing, regardless of the fact that the battle continued (and other men were killed or wounded) after Nelson was taken below decks to die. A period of national mourning in 1805 can only have augmented expectations of attentive care. Yet the literal deployment of male carers around Nelson's dying body may not matter so much as the coherence of the tale told by the surgeon about the men's identities and behaviours.

Beatty's was a description of end-of-life care for a naval leader, performed on the lower deck of a warship during the latter parts of a sea battle. This required palliative attention in the form of making the patient as comfortable as possible in the approximately two hours and forty-five minutes it took for him to die. According to Beatty this included propping Nelson up into a semi-recumbent position, rubbing his chest, offering drinks of lemonade, wine, or water, and fanning his face. Nelson's high status was reflected in both the number and occupation of people attending him. Two named men, Alexander Scott and Walter Burke, were with him continuously, along with 'two of his lordship's domestics' (William Chevalier Nelson's steward and Gaetano Spedillo Nelson's valet) while others made periodic visits to Nelson's side to offer consolation.[57] Scott was a naval chaplain with a facility for languages, in his thirties in 1805, who had been appointed by Nelson as his foreign secretary. Burke was the purser on the *Victory* and in his late sixties at the time. The role of both as Nelson's final attendants was immortalised and idealised by painters such as Arthur Devis and Benjamin West, despite the artists' absence from the scene they depicted.

230 Nursing the English from plague to Peterloo

The latter's *The Death of Nelson* (1806) was viewed by thousands when first shown and remains a standard illustration of the event. The painter was candid about his ideological ambitions for the piece, depicting Nelson's death as 'extraordinary' to secure the correct emotional response from viewers.[58] A key to Devis's painting offers portraits of Nelson's male attendants and a stylised vignette of masculine attention, given the eyelines of the men concerned.

In Beatty's account and successive paintings, the men who attended Nelson as he died are not so much practical figures (despite their apparent delivery of practical service) as they are emblematic. Scott and Burke were perhaps the highest-status available non-combatants who could be spared for the constant care of Nelson. Furthermore, according to Beatty, they were the only two men on board who were aware of the hopeless nature of Nelson's injury

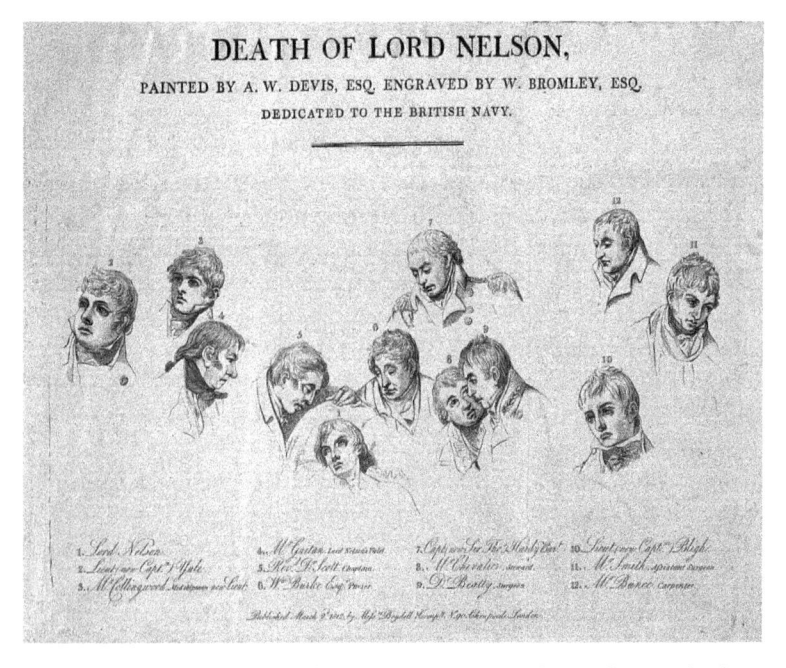

Figure 5.1 W. Bromley after A.W. Devis, detail from *The Death of Lord Nelson: key to the painting* (1812): engraving courtesy of the Wellcome Trust

aside from the surgeon and his two assistants. Therefore, the significance of these men lies in their allegedly single-minded devotion to Nelson, their exclusive knowledge of his fatal wound, and reportage of their demeanour and actions after life was extinct. Scott, for example, attended Nelson's remains when they were transported from the *Victory* to Greenwich Hospital in December 1805. Nelson's nurses were prominent players in the magnification of his glory, and their voluntary offering of tender masculinity augmented their role in this respect. The activity of the two domestics is less prominent for these ideological purposes, although they were both given mourning by the Lord Chamberlain's office to attend Nelson's funeral.[59] A multitude of afflicted male attendants was merely the due mark of respect following the death of a pre-eminent national hero and nursing one's betters allowed men to nurse while actively gaining prestige. This analysis conforms well with a twentieth-century view of nursing as an activity which restores the patient's worth (in the face of their helplessness) by dint of the willing and self-effacing service of their attendants.[60] This further suggests that the nineteenth-century development of a nursing vocation had some of its roots in the sacrifices made in the pre-professional era on behalf of very high-status patients.

Men's unpaid nursing in English prisons

There is good reason to suppose that in male-dominated or single-sex environments, mutual assistance was a necessity overriding any theoretical preferences by gender. Masculinity was arguably not threatened in these circumstances because all of the men present were in the same circumstances (potentially requiring nursing care, and there being no available women or insufficient access to female carers).[61] Following the model outlined in the Introduction, one-to-many nursing by men, which has so far been demonstrated in the historiography only in asylum contexts, will here be illustrated by evidence from gaols.

In the seventeenth and eighteenth centuries, prisoners awaiting trial, or long-term prisoners for debt, were heavily dependent on serendipity and context if they happened to fall ill. Nursing might feasibly be undertaken by employees like turnkeys or paid female nurses, or by relatives permitted to enter the walls.[62] In the absence of any of these options, prisoners of necessity relied on each other for care into the nineteenth century. Such nursing by men might have been mandated by the internal appointment of a male prisoner as a nurse, perhaps following their own illness as was the case for John Smith at Clerkenwell in 1791, or undertaken voluntarily.[63] A series of parliamentary reports on prisons published in the 1810s, designed to investigate the adequacy of infrastructure, offer shreds of insight into the unreliable world of prison nursing, if always from the point of view of medical men (and not the prisoners or nurses themselves).

Whitecross Street Prison, for example, was built between 1813 and 1815. It had an infirmary and a convalescent ward, sleeping ten and nine patients respectively. Dietary treatments, including alcohol, were allowed as a weekly bill paid by the prison keeper to the female 'nurse' (singular, serving both wards), whereas bandages and medicines were paid for by the surgeon from his annual salary. Parliamentary questioning raised the issue of institutional dampness, and the deleterious effects of the damp on prisoners' health and mortality.[64] In respect of the ratio of nursing staff to patients, therefore, the lone woman at Whitecross had more patients under her care than her equivalents at the ancient London hospital of Barts, but her workload was on a par with that of women serving in the larger wards of Guy's Hospital.[65]

Both female and male nurses appointed to London's prisons were drawn from among the prisoners. The surgeon of Newgate, testifying in 1814, reported that 'a decent woman' from among the female prisoners was given the management of the sick and convalescent wards in the female infirmary, with the support of a subordinate helper. A similar structure was observed in the male infirmary, managed by a wardsman and helper because 'it would be impossible amongst such a set [of prisoners], to have women to attend them'.[66] This distinction between male and female nursing was not observed in all prisons, though, because there was one female nurse for both male and female patients during the same year in Giltspur Street prison.[67] The nurses or wardsmen received modest remuneration for their work, such as the four shillings per week paid to a nurse on the felon's side at Newgate prison, or the extra rations given to the female nurse at Clerkenwell prison.[68] This ensured that, where they were given money, prison nurses received payment on a par with the women employed by provincial infirmaries at this date.[69]

If the sole stated criterion for a female appointment was decency, no equivalent characteristic was made clear for men. Nonetheless, the need to attend 'such a set' of men heavily implies that stereotypical masculine characteristics of physical strength and moral authority were required: a wardsman needed to manage the sick male prisoners in terms of both their bodies and their demeanour. An extreme interpretation of this assumption would be that wardsmen needed to be able to meet violence among male prisoner patients with superior strength. This evidence from prisons aligns with Len Smith's findings about recruitment of keepers to madhouses, that male nurses or keepers were designedly capable of throwing their weight around, although this may have been necessary for a display of strength rather than its use.[70] Any brutality which may have been ascribed to wardsmen was perhaps a side effect of their recruitment to a quasi-policing role.

Prisoners had different priorities to those in authority over them, and we can gain shreds of insight into the motives of men who offered themselves as nurses for their fellow prisoners. Sir John Acland, Chair of the Somerset Quarter Sessions, thought they acted initially from self-interest in the hopes of remitting part of their sentence, albeit his parliamentary testimony implied that compassion might overtake them in the performance of their duties:

> When we had typhus fever, two years ago, prisoners volunteered their services, at the hazard of their lives, to nurse the infected prisoners, and perform all the dangerous offices required of them, in hopes that they might meet with favour; they behaved extremely well; we were obliged to hire a house two miles distant from the prison, and our chief reliance for the security of our prisoners was from those men, because we had not servants enough for the different services required; those men knew it was not worth their while to try to escape; their better dependence for their liberation from prison was on the expectation that their good conduct and services would obtain them a pardon.[71]

Acland's observations were in fact illustrative of a long-standing tradition of mutual support between prisoners which was not wholly determined by the chance of judicial favour. In the Marshalsea Prison for debtors, for example, there was no regular nurse in 1815, but one was employed occasionally 'when they are seriously unwell, *and have no wife or friend that can pay attention to them* [italics mine], such as for taking care of the fire in the night, and giving them their medicines'.[72] The same witness, the surgeon at the Marshalsea, elaborated on his evidence in the following year: 'In common cases of illness ... they depend for assistance upon their fellow prisoners, and I have never found a want of attendance.'[73] Medical witnesses to Parliament might be supposed to have had an agenda of their own, to defend their actions in the light of potential complaints about care for sick prisoners. Even so, a consistent picture emerges of some shared acceptance of responsibility for nursing among male prisoners, confirmed anecdotally from other sources. Layton Smith, for example, was a debtor in the Fleet Prison in the years before he died, but during an outbreak of fever (possibly in 1765) he was remembered to have 'administered to the wants and necessities of the persons confined there'.[74]

This discussion of voluntary nursing by men in prisons, and the next section on asylum keepers, reinforces the idea that the critical distinction between the individuals who offered practical or even tender support, and those who were neglectful or worse, lies in whether they were acting spontaneously, or whether nursing activity was essentially the job for which they were paid. In this respect, male nurses were no different to their female counterparts at the same time, who suffered negative stereotyping for paid nursing and enjoyed praise for voluntary attendance.[75] Yet masculinity offered an additional challenge to men who were paid, because formal employment in a role demanding care meant either that post-holders must show tenderness to other men who were not their relations, or must find a way to counter suspicions of effeminacy (or potentially homosexuality) in willingly performing close bodily tasks for male patients.[76] This latter point may go some way to explain the stereotype of the asylum keeper as guilty of unrestrained brutality: a fierce and physically rough approach to paid work with the sick might have had the advantage of signalling distance between the individual employee and any apprehensions of their displaying willing kindness to their charges. Women were expected to fit roles as nurses, whether paid or unpaid, in ways that aligned with their femininity, whereas men who were paid as nurses risked their masculine identity if they looked like they enjoyed the job. Yet I argue that the conflicts for masculinity in tending to the mad were more complicated than this.

Madhouses, keepers, and the male anti-nurse 1790–1820

Asylum history has a protracted chronology in England. Bethlem, the national hospital for people thought to be insane, was exclusively catering for the mad by the fourteenth century and was joined by privately run commercial madhouses between 1600 and 1660.[77] The long eighteenth century encompassed a period of gradually rising interest in the incarceration of the mad, both as a physical practice with implications for individual liberty and as a prospect for entrepreneurial specialisation.[78] The result at the time was an expansion of public institutions from 1750 onwards, a growth in business ventures by people offering accommodation for the insane, plus an increased scrutiny on private madhouses which eventually gave rise to a change in the law and to parliamentary oversight.[79]

Government inquiries in the late 1810s generated comprehensive (if not reliably complete) listings of public and private facilities in 1819.[80] These are reproduced here with a small number of manual additions to the parliamentary publications (of large or well-known institutions which were otherwise obviously omitted from the 1819 lists).[81] The advantage of these listings was the inclusion of patient numbers, giving a snapshot of the total of people accommodated in specialist locations requiring distinctive staffing.

Just as there had been a desultory debate about the ratio of nurses to patients thought to be needed in provincial infirmaries, so there was a more concentrated discussion of the appropriate ratio of keepers to asylum inmates in the 1810s. That decade witnessed energetic inquiry into the supervision of mad patients, with commentators pointing out that the 'outrageous' mad might require two keepers to one person, while the quiescent mad might get along perfectly well with one keeper for twenty.[82] In practice The Retreat, for example, a private facility originally designed to receive patients who were among the Society of Friends (or Quakers), retained one keeper for every twelve patients.[83] Tables 5.1 and 5.2 divide the number of patients in each location by twenty, to secure an approximate minimum of the number of keepers recruited to attend them. Not all of the 69 or more keepers in public asylums nor the 129 or more keepers in private madhouses would have been men. Some institutions employed no men at all, as at Guy's Hospital where the Lunatic House had only a single female keeper for its twenty female inmates.[84] Even so, this rough-and-ready calculation provides a guide to the scale of employment available for keepers, male and female, by the end of the period under study here.

Table 5.1 Public asylums in 1819

Location	Founded	Patients	Keepers (min)
St Lukes	1750	252	12.60
Bethlem	1372	193	9.65
Lancashire county Lancaster	1816	129	6.45
York	1777	105	5.25
Manchester	1766	88	4.40
Norfolk county	1814	85	4.25
Wakefield/West Riding	1818	77	3.85
Northumberland, Durham, and Newcastle-upon-Tyne	1767	69	3.45
Stafford	1818	54	2.70
Bedfordshire county	1812	54	2.70
Nottingham	1811	48	2.40
Liverpool	1792	47	2.35
Devon	1801	47	2.35
Ticehurst	1792	40	2.00
St Peter's Bristol	1696	30	1.50
Guys	1791	20	1.00
Norwich Bethel	1713	17	0.85
Hereford	1797	15	0.75
Leicester	1794	12	0.60
Totals		1,355	69.10

Table 5.2 Private licensed madhouses in 1819

Location	Surname	Patients	Keepers (min)
Bethnal Green, Middlesex	Talbot	482	24.10
Hoxton, Middlesex	Miles	348	17.40
Bethnal Green, Middlesex	Rhodes	315	15.75
Hoxton, Middlesex	Burrow	118	5.90
Droitwich, Worcestershire	Rickets	102	5.10
Laverstock, Wiltshire	Finch	100	5.00
Hoxton, Middlesex	Warburton	78	3.90
Brislington, Somerset	Fox	73	3.65
Stapleton, Gloucester	Bompass	48	2.40
York, Yorkshire	Tuke	46	2.30
Clapton, Middlesex	Munro	41	2.05
Henley in Arden, Warwickshire	Burman	38	1.90
Kingsdown, Wiltshire	Langworthy	35	1.75
Alverstoke, Hampshire	Finch	32	1.60
Walton Lodge, Lancashire	Squires	32	1.60
Nursling, Hampshire	Middleton	29	1.45
Gatesheadfell, Durham	Nicholson	28	1.40
Chelsea, Middlesex	Bastable	25	1.25
Hackney, Middlesex	Fox	25	1.25
Bilston, Staffordshire	Proud	21	1.05
Islington, Middlesex	Annandale	20	1.00
Halstock, Dorset	Mercer	19	0.95
Hackney, Middlesex	Rees	19	0.95
Fivehead House, Somerset	Gillett	19	0.95
Lodden, Norfolk	Jollye	18	0.90
Thorpe, Surrey	Phillips and Summers	18	0.90

Table 5.2 (continued)

Location	Surname	Patients	Keepers (min)
Plaistow, Essex	Casey	17	0.85
Skillingthorpe, Lincolnshire	Willis	17	0.85
Fulham, Middlesex	Talfourd	17	0.85
Lakenham, Norfolk	Rigby and Wright	17	0.85
Spring Vale, Staffordshire	Bakewell	17	0.85
Fonthill Gifford, Wiltshire	Spencer	17	0.85
Kensington, Middlesex	Briand	16	0.80
Market Lavington, Wiltshire	Willett	15	0.75
Blakeley, Lancashire	Edwards	14	0.70
Newton, Lancashire	Hague	14	0.70
Horncastle, Lincolnshire	Fawcett	14	0.70
Newcastle-upon-Tyne, Northumberland	Paget	14	0.70
Hook Norton, Oxfordshire	Harris	14	0.70
Much Hadham, Hertfordshire	Jacob	13	0.65
Great Wigston, Leicestershire	Blunt	13	0.65
Billington, Lancashire	Chew	12	0.60
Cleve House, Somerset	Duck	12	0.60
West Malling, Kent	Perfect	11	0.55
Greatford, Lincolnshire	Willis	11	0.55
Chelsea, Middlesex	Jones	11	0.55
Tynemouth, Northumberland	Oxley	11	0.55
Chelsea, Middlesex	Burrows	10	0.50
Chelsea, Middlesex	Reedford	10	0.50
Pancras, Middlesex	Pell	10	0.50
Leicester, Leicestershire	Hill	9	0.45

Chelsea, Middlesex	Salmon	8	0.40
Lichfield, Staffordshire	Rowley	8	0.40
Blackheath, Kent	Holt	7	0.35
Hammersmith, Middlesex	Knight	7	0.35
Lower Tooting, Surrey	Sandiford	7	0.35
Habergham, Lancashire	Parkinson	6	0.30
Somerstown, Middlesex	[Pile]	6	0.30
York, Yorkshire	Backhouse	6	0.30
Hillingdon, Middlesex	Stilwell	5	0.25
Shrewsbury, Shropshire	Johnson	5	0.25
Chelsea, Middlesex	Bradbury	4	0.20
Winchmore Hill, Middlesex	Richardson	4	0.20
Henley in Arden, Warwickshire	Gibbs	4	0.20
York, Yorkshire	Mannering	4	0.20
York, Yorkshire	Skipwith	4	0.20
Chelsea, Middlesex	Press	3	0.15
Kingsland, Middlesex	Bignall	3	0.15
Turnham Green, Middlesex	Jackson	3	0.15
Paddington, Middlesex	Langdon	3	0.15
Chertsey, Surrey	Lucett	3	0.15
Frimley, Surrey	Irish	3	0.15
Henley in Arden, Warwickshire	Browne	3	0.15
Sutton Coldfield, Warwickshire	Terry	3	0.15
Long Bennington, Lincolnshire	Stafford	2	0.10
Guildford, Surrey	Hills	2	0.10
Total		2,576	128.80

The two hundred or more keepers in post in 1819 provided the subjects for close and even fierce scrutiny in the years immediately preceding parliamentary inquiries on the grounds of their alleged abuses of office. Institutions may have possessed stringent rules for the governance of patients and staff, but rules could be ignored. In the words of former patient Urbane Metcalf, 'the keepers do just as they please'.[85] Any absence of oversight by employers, either from complacency or carelessness, opened the way to 'flagrant abuses' of power.[86] At their most excessive, these abuses were said to have encompassed kidnapping, physical and sexual abuse, rape, and murder, reported at both public asylums and private madhouses, but not equally at all locations.[87] The larger institutions within or near the metropolis were identified with the abuses most frequently, while neutral reports, or quiet acknowledgement of a job well done in the provinces, did not achieve prominence.[88]

There is no substantial historiography about female keepers and their part in these allegations.[89] The women employed in asylums and madhouses became targets of opprobrium in the texts of former patients in similar ways to their male peers, albeit their evils are characterised in general terms – 'the scum of the earth' – rather than via detailed accounts of their iniquity.[90] This was perhaps a product of the authors of exposes typically being men, who were not subject to direct management by female staff. This means that, while both male and female anti-nurses were emerging among public understandings of the infrastructure of England's institutions for the insane, it was the men who dominated contemporary public inquiry and who are brought to the fore in histories.

Len Smith has written extensively on the male asylum keeper in the early nineteenth century, chiefly in terms of those who managed a madhouse but also in relation to the men employed to control or care for the patients (the latter being the focus of the discussion here).[91] He has countered the contemporary stereotype, the brutal keeper, by contextualising their de facto job description and their conditions of service. The work of a male keeper was physically taxing, emotionally draining, and conceptually complicated, qualities exacerbated by low wages, understaffing, and no appreciable training.[92] Like the female nurses in provincial infirmaries discussed in Chapter 3, keepers probably remained on duty at night in this period.[93] If men were recruited for their bodily strength yet urged to behave towards patients with gentleness, they were receiving 'mixed messages' about how best to perform their tasks and secure approval from employers.[94] At the same time, staff implemented management directions, and because the male staff were not gentlemen, they were scapegoated for institutional failures. In this way Smith renders the asylum anti-nurse comprehensible in context.

Some aspects of keepers' alleged rapacity were clearly material and related to their low levels of remuneration. If any resources were allocated to patients by physicians or family members, the keepers would routinely try to deprive the patients to their own advantage (such as by selling food not consumed, or requisitioning clothing). The men recruited as keepers were perhaps exhibiting the material behaviours and sensibilities associated with some sections of the labouring poor, among whom the desire for additional gain overcame sentiments of selflessness or generosity, yet were reproached for failing to have imbibed the ethos of a caring institution imagined (rather than realised) by the middling-sort medical men, the patients' families, or the charitable subscribers who observed them. 'The reform of working-class to middle-class standards' lay in the future.[95] In modern sociological terms, we might construe keepers who purloined patients' possessions as managing their emotions in pecuniary mode, perhaps suppressing other feelings in the pursuit of material gain, while avoiding the prescriptive and philanthropic modes of emotional labour which (if they were formalised within institutional rules) would have been the preferences of their critics.[96]

Other aspects of complaint against keepers were even more closely allied to working-class masculinity. Manhood was historically linked to physical strength, and the ability to deploy appropriate vigour to assert one's independence and honour: 'Refusal to fight could render a man open to mockery and insult' in the seventeenth century, and fighting or boasting about physical prowess 'could play an important part in a boy's transition to adulthood' throughout the eighteenth century.[97] Men relied on violence as 'a signifier of masculinity' in problematic ways in other contexts.[98] If patients hit out at their keepers, it would have gone severely against the cultural grain for men to have withheld return blows.[99] That said, the imposing physical presence of the keeper may have been deployed in other ways. There is assumed to be a long history to the distinction between the capacity for brute violence versus a version of manliness wherein violence is controlled.[100] In the twenty-first century, a strong attendant may be enough to calm a patient, and increase their sense of security on a ward.[101] This means that muscularity and energy were not necessarily at odds with any institutional delivery of disinterested care, but seem to have become so at this earlier date in reported instances of abuse. Coincidentally they were also qualities which later nursing leaders, for example, could not manipulate to fit with the reform agenda.[102]

At the same time, understandings of anger by the early nineteenth century were such that the emotion became particularly tied to men, making anger inherently masculine, but within a literature aimed at the instruction of ambitious middling youth and the desirability of controlling anger (which the domestic service, artisanal, and soldiering class from which most keepers were drawn could neither access nor appreciate).[103] Even the middling and elite might not take instruction in this regard. A contributor to the *Gentleman's Magazine* of 1804 regretted that 'most men [without qualification by status] still set a due value upon anger, and show by their practice that it is one of those passions which is in no danger of becoming paralytic for want of exercise'.[104]

Mark Neuendorf has characterised the exposés of asylum-keepers' brutality of the late eighteenth and early nineteenth century as aligning with an emotional register of forthright indignation among authors.[105] He sees this stance as newly freed from tropes of sensibility or the preservation of polite fictions, and no longer so prey to the risk that a patient's anger or accusations would be dismissed as a feature of their illness. The quantity and authentic detail of the abuse described by multiple former patients means that a measure of cruel handling was patently a feature of inpatient experience in at least some institutions. Yet this analysis can be pushed further in relation to the men who delivered the bodily care and control of asylum inmates: the stories told about male keepers clearly identified them as acting as conduits for the expression of other fears, specifically around loss of autonomy, the evaporation of family support, fear of other patients, and the stigma of mental illness.

Male employees held a candidly custodial role, in a sector that generally courted its patients rather than compelled them. Prosperous people suffering from physical illness or injury were treated consensually or not at all, whereas the mad from all social backgrounds were subjected to coercion (including by detention in an institution). This came as a shock to the middling and upper sort of patients who were deemed to be lunatics. Their deprivation of liberty, such as that experienced by Edward Goldney at the madhouse run by Joseph Mason, was ordered by house managers, perhaps with the best intentions.[106] Even so, confinement was applied by keepers, who were also responsible for managing any subsequent interventions in the form of close restraint or medicines. If violence was used by these men to guarantee that the prescribed drugs were taken, for example by ensuring that their patient was 'crammed with physic with a bullock's horn', they were breaching expected norms around both securing medical advice and following it at the same time that they obeyed their employer.[107]

Perceptions of behaviour by keepers were exacerbated by the fact that the families of those under confinement generally receded from their (the patient's) view. It may have been that a breakdown in family relations resulted in confinement in the first place, but institutional admission always entailed the departure of kin from patients' living spaces and feasibly involved neglect or active manipulation of patients once they had been placed in an asylum.[108] William Belcher inveighed against the risk of collusion between relatives, medical practitioners, and others in pursuit of material gain.[109] Quaker Edward Wakefield, who gave evidence to the Parliamentary Select Committee on Madhouses, repeated complaints in a similar vein at second hand, as when he described a female inmate of Bethlem who 'lamented that her friends who she stated to be respectable people, neither came to see her nor supplied her with little necessary comforts'.[110]

If keepers did their best to avoid their duties, and were frequently absent from their ward/gallery, they were therefore not on hand to assist their patients and protect them, specifically from physical exposure to the other patients.[111] Literate inmates complained after the fact about the lack of protection keepers offered from abuse or attack issuing from fellow residents. Urbane Metcalf observed that the keepers in Bethlem did nothing to prevent the patients from injuring each other or fighting, or might even promote physical abuse between patients (such as by delegating their own exercise of violence to a biddable patient).[112] Such protests aligned with (and were a substantial extension of) bitter complaints by both men and women about other patients on the grounds of the noise they made.[113] Keepers' lack of engagement with noise reduction marks them out, both in terms of the pre-professional nurse's role of regulation, and in relation to later strictures by Nightingale and others about the suppression of noise.[114]

Ultimately, keepers were feared to have a role in perpetuating and deepening the stigma of mental illness. They might have done this directly or indirectly. Direct denigration involved deriding patients, interpersonal threats, and violence.[115] Indirect abuse arose when keepers' behaviour had a target or an influence beyond the confines of the institution. Urbane Metcalf's narrative suggests that these included retailing hurtful anecdotes about patients' family members, while Select Committee evidence reports keepers delivering insults to patients' relations to prevent their future visits.[116]

At the same time that keepers became a focus for these wider fears, the cruelties they were said to have enacted can be seen as a spasmodic response to the personal perils of their occupation.[117] Men's employment experiences exposed them to institutional living and to 'dirty' work in ways that very probably impinged on their own sense of autonomy and self. Residential work in an asylum or madhouse deprived male employees of their own independent household, otherwise regarded as a cornerstone of male identity among middling and lower men.[118] Smith has characterised this as a 'relationship of dependency' akin to that of the patients.[119] Institutional living also had consequences for marriage, another of the components of adult maleness, as seen for the in-pensioners at Chelsea Hospital in Chapter 4. If the men were married before they took the job as a keeper, they were either required to break up their household or to siphon their wages to maintain it without their own physical presence.[120] If men married after they started work, their ability to maintain a relationship based on a typical combination of sex, affection, shared economic endeavour, and co-residence was reduced. Even where men married other institutional employees, they may not have had access to married quarters. This had implications for the getting of children and perceptions of virility, additional markers of manliness. Thus, their claims to masculinity were attenuated by the impact of asylum work on householding and family life.

In relation to dirty work, keepers first had to manage their own proximity to the mad. This was almost certainly problematic for men in post, but only perceptible among people of higher social standing than the keepers who reported their responses, such as at the York Asylum where 'there was a repugnance on the part of the Governors to enter the rooms where the patients were confined'.[121] The work which for other men was a source of pride (or at least aspirational access to personal pride) could not fill an identical function for keepers.[122]

Secondly, there was little scope for negotiation with their charges to mitigate their close contact. For Allen Ingram, the tone of Metcalf's publication underscores 'a denial of any possibility of dialogue or reciprocation between treaters and treated' while resident in Bethlem.[123] This barrier impinged on the keepers as well, across different institutions. 'W.J.', the only man to go into print to describe the work from the keeper's point of view, reported that the paramount feature of the role was that he got nothing back from patients owing to their 'insensibility to kindness'.[124] He elaborated with the specific example of a young male patient who seemed impervious to W.J.'s attention and became determined to misinterpret his efforts. The author concluded:

> To know that our kindnesses are not thrown away, but that they are felt, is a source of pleasurable feeling; but to find that our best efforts to please are given to the winds, and incapable of eliciting even an acknowledgement, is painful indeed, and hard to be endured.[125]

The nature of their charges' illness was such that keepers might have felt that meaningful communication was impossible, and therefore to attempt it was merely to invite failure.

Thirdly, the keeper as anti-nurse is someone whose need for social distance from patients became urgent on the grounds of their gender as men in a paid position of care. In many other occupational contexts, men were valued on the grounds of their physique and its productive capacity. Joanne Begiato has argued that blacksmiths, for example, were lionised as 'idealised virile workers' in this period as a symbol of appropriate muscularity.[126] Keepers did not use their muscles to manufacture anything and might have struggled to recognise the amelioration of mental illness as a suitable proxy. Furthermore, it had long been a question whether men could care, in the broadest sense, without incurring a charge of effeminacy. As one commentator of 1675 put it, 'Must we be guilty of effeminacy to perform Acts of Generosity? Can we not be charitable without being afflicted? And can we not relieve those that are in misery, unless we mingle our Sighs and their Sobs and Groans?'[127] Barker-Benfield acknowledges that 'The question persisted.'[128] The behaviour of keepers in the early nineteenth century is consonant with the idea that this remained a guilt to avoid at all costs. In modern professional terms, male keepers perhaps pursued 'internal demarcation' to differentiate their work from that of either women or effete men but took the practice to extremes, not merely avoiding effeminacy but resulting in violence and palpable harm.[129] This feature of men's experience may also help to explain the repeated allegation that madhouses were more likely to make their patients worse than to achieve cures, said to be the occasion of boasting by selected keepers.[130] In the reported instances of abuse, men were perhaps mulishly 'making' illness for their employer's benefit in a distorted version of productivity.

Fourthly, and as for female nurses, the handling and deployment of human ordure was a feature of the keepers' relationship with their charges. Dirtiness is to some extent a social construction, but there is little historical variation in the categorisation of excreta as dirt. The actor David Garrick, for example, cast 'beshit' as the opposite of clean in a letter of 1767.[131] The cause célèbre of James Norris, incarcerated under restraint in Bethlem, illustrates these continuities in context since in the run-up to Norris breaking his arm he was said to have 'made a dirt that he could not help'.[132] Lunatic patients were different to the cohorts of inpatients at either the ancient London hospitals or the provincial infirmaries because there was inevitably a subset of each asylum population that was incontinent, or in the terminology of the day 'wet and dirty' patients, with profound implications for asylum and madhouse employees. Behavioural symptoms aside, keepers were compelled to engage with the excreta of others if only by dint of handling the people concerned (i.e. even if the laundering of clothes and bedding, and the cleaning of rooms, was delegated to others).[133] At its most intense, cleaning the 'dirty' wards will have involved shovelling soiled straw, a combination of heavy and degrading work (and incidentally another cause of men's appointment for their muscularity).[134] The dangers of proximity to waste, and particularly plebeian human waste, have been examined by Kevin Siena across the same period covered by this book.[135] Siena was chiefly concerned with the risk of contagious disease but, as discussed in Chapter 3, Mark Jenner has extended the dangers to those involving social pollution. If Jenner's analysis of chamber-pot deployment held good within the walls of an asylum as well as without, then keepers may have felt themselves to be on the receiving end of weapons of the weak, even if the patients they kept had no intention to deploy their faeces and urine with this goal in mind.[136]

The behaviour of abusive keepers becomes more explicable if we assume that evidence of their aggressive attitude towards patients can be interpreted as the resistance of people who felt themselves to be targets in an unevenly weighted conflict. The necessity and continuity of keepers' exposure to human excreta were contained in a context that did not permit them explicitly to protest because refusal to work in this capacity would quickly have been brought to the attention of employers (if only by other keepers). I am arguing that the challenge this posed to men's status was such that keepers' violence (of word and action) was a form of resistance to the spoliation of self.[137] If this is correct, then keepers' conversion of patient ordure as a weapon against other (otherwise 'clean') patients (another way of exacerbating the stigma of mental illness) becomes rational. Urbane Metcalf claimed that use of the basement at 'new' Bethlem, the floor which housed incontinent patients, was employed by keepers as a place to punish patients who were initially/otherwise accommodated on other floors. He describes an instance where a keeper emptied the contents of a chamber pot into a man's shoes to ensure his transfer to the basement.[138]

This intentional and perhaps vengeful spoliation by keepers of patients was alleged on occasion to have become even more acute. An exposé of 1822 recounting historic abuses described one male patient having 'his mouth stuffed with HUMAN ORDURE' at Warburton's madhouse, to make him 'know good victuals' when they were offered.[139] Potential sensationalism aside, it seems likely that the conflicts arising from the delivery of care and control of waste by women in institutional nursing considered in Chapter 3 were amplified for men in the more high-stakes environment of an asylum into an existential threat to their masculine identity, such that their extreme response can be understood as a form of self-protection. Any cruelty betrayed by selected keepers is thus rendered comprehensible, if still inexcusable.

A further, more speculative, possibility is that the elevated status accorded to the patient from male nursing in other contexts – such as the possible advantage of being nursed by a male servant rather than a female servant, and the clear recognition of worth derived from being nursed by multiple men as was the case for Nelson – added another source of tension for male keepers in asylums and madhouses. If care by men conferred status on people who were otherwise acutely marginalised by dint of their diagnosis, by their proximity to others with the same diagnosis, and by reason of their divergent behaviour, and if the impact on the men themselves was in line with the 'dirty work' thesis of Hughes, Ashforth, and Kreiner (outlined in the Introduction to this book), what options were left to them to avoid their ceding all of their individual worth? Male keepers would have felt that their identities risked being spoiled beyond repair, if they somehow defrayed all of their own status in their delivery of male service to dirty patients. They would have been in a very difficult social position which, from their perspective, required urgent mitigation. We can see their brutality as their response to these challenges, a reassertion of status that looked inexplicable to outside observers but which was essential for some male insiders. The forms of restoration of manhood open to early modern men, for example via legal redress, were not available to keepers, leaving them only with violence.[140] The active pleasure reportedly expressed by male perpetrators of cruelty to patients can be interpreted as an attempt by men to repudiate the spoliation inherent in their workplace by asserting a cheerfully brutal persona.[141]

Fiction could hardly keep up with the horrors of the true-life depictions of keepers revealed by the revelatory publications by former patients. Nonetheless, at least one novel of the period captured aspects of the literal experience of madhouse confinement and combined them with the worst fears of the public. Radical author Thomas Holcroft, a man with a modicum of nursing experience himself, wrote the novel *Anna St Ives* in 1792.[142] The story follows Anna as she learns to distinguish between two suitors, the reckless and monied Coke Clifton versus the serious and deserving Frank Henley. She marries Henley, of course, but not before she and Frank have been subjected to a kidnapping plot where Clifton tries to force himself upon the virtuous Anna while holding Frank captive. In order to pursue his plans for abduction, Clifton employs an as-yet unopened private madhouse as the place to keep Frank, and employs the would-be madhouse keeper as his accomplice. Even Clifton's malignity is affronted by the 'foul-faced fellow' with whom he collaborates as merely one of a set of 'Satanic rascals ... I wonder by whom, where, and why such fellows are begotten!' In remarking that he seems 'more proper to make men mad than cure them', Clifton imitates a frequent refrain among madhouse survivors. This does not prevent him from employing both the methods of restraint typical of the institutional genre, a strait-waistcoat and gag, and displaying the perverse pleasure imputed to some keepers in their enjoyment of cruelty. In this way, Holcroft melodramatically conflates madhouse keeping with abduction, imprisonment, rape, and unmitigated evil as perpetrated upon the innocent and sane by men lacking any shred of humanity.[143] But Holcroft lacks the view of an insider. Neither Clifton nor his deputies are seen to have to cope with Frank's excreta.

Other literary models of masculinity were available, but they were muted, not directly about keepers, and very probably inaccessible to the men who were recruited to work in institutions for the mad. Henry Fielding's novel *Amelia* is generally concerned with the relationship between the titular heroine and her husband Captain William Booth.[144] In the early days of their marriage Booth proves feckless and unfaithful: but he is a good nurse. When Amelia is in labour, Booth 'lay behind her bolster, and supported her in my arms', a duty he finds emotionally painful.[145] Later when Amelia has a fever, Booth 'officiated as her nurse and never stirred from her'.[146] The couple both sit up with their child during illness. For his pains, Booth is dubbed by a female admirer 'an angel of a man'.[147] He is contrasted favourably with one of his senior military officers Major Bath, a man who undertakes nursing for his sister secretively with a fear of exposure as effeminate. Fielding satirises this position both at the time – Bath cries when his sister recovers, still apologising for the fact that 'nature will get the better of dignity' – and indirectly in retrospect when Bath dies in a duel defending his sensitive honour.[148] Fielding was an uxorious man in private life, and there are strong suggestions that he based Booth and Amelia on himself and his relationship with his wife. In the novel, love overcomes dignity without the need for either apology or fear, doing 'much to open up the issue of squaring manliness with male emotions and sympathy without incurring the charge of effeminacy'.[149] Furthermore, Fielding was a literary rival of Samuel Richardson, author of the quote at the start of this chapter, which raises the prospect that Grandison's denigration of male servants was composed as a strand of literary resistance to Fielding's depiction of a good male nurse two years earlier. Booth was not, however, a good predictor of the capacity for masculinity to accommodate his attitude wholesale or perhaps at all. If men were unwilling in private life to surrender their autonomy or dignity to their marital partner, the reluctance of men to take paid work to care for strangers becomes not only obvious, but obviously the potential motivator of anti-social behaviour.

Conclusion

Evidence of nursing by men can be found across all social groups and ages in this period, despite the paucity of commentary by men on their own actions. It was probably an inherent task for all male body servants, even if it was not a constant part of their employment: rather, the job was defined on other grounds, and nursing was a silent addition to their portfolio of labour. This ability to smuggle nursing into other roles may help to account for willing care of children by fathers, and to the care of each other in prison: the common interests of the family or among a community of inmates rendered male nursing both unavoidable and only a part of a wider identity. A lack of ability to disguise or excuse nursing introduced problems for men who were aware of the allegation that care by men was 'unnatural'. A wilful choice to care for others, particularly if unpaid for devoted attendance, posed a problem for men, whether as practically or conceptually irksome.

Not all male asylum keepers were violent towards their patients, yet the narratives that describe such violence in detail also offer clues as to why some men filling these roles may have felt obliged to behave brutally. In addition to the difficulties of the role described by Smith, this chapter has added the focus on keepers as a viable means to realise patients' wider concerns (including fears of abandonment by families). Most significantly, this discussion has linked aggressive behaviour by some keepers to the penalties of working with human waste. To see keepers' violence in the light of Ashforth and Kreiner's 'dirty work' thesis does not absolve it from judgement by contemporaries or successors: aggressive behaviour is, however, more comprehensible in this context. The next and final chapter studies nursing by men and women against a backdrop of international violence.

Notes

1 Sections from the first half of this chapter have previously been published as A. Tomkins, 'Male nurses in England and Europe before 1820: Beyond the madhouse', *Nursing History Review* 31 (2023), 150–70. I am grateful to the editor for permission to reproduce them here.
2 S. Richardson, *The History of Sir Charles Grandison* (London: the author, 1754), volume III, Letter XI.
3 M. Prosen, 'Nursing students' perception of gender-defined roles in nursing: A qualitative descriptive study', *BMC Nursing* 21: 104 (2022), 1–11.
4 'Madhouses' is a pejorative word, but was the term used by contemporaries into the early nineteenth century. Use of the word asylum began after the founding of the York asylum in 1772, and gradually

came to be used to denote public hospitals for the mad (as opposed to private licensed madhouses). The second part of this chapter will make use of this contemporary differentiation.

5 P.P. *A Return of the Number of Lunatics Confined in the different Gaols, Hospitals, and Lunatic Asylums* (1819), 1–3; P.P. *A Return of the Number of Houses Licensed for the Reception of Lunatics* (1819), 1–5; M. Arton, 'The rise and fall of the Asylum Worker's Association: The history of a "company union", *International History of Nursing Journal* 7: 3 (2003), 41–9.

6 For two notable exceptions ostensibly in this period see L. Smith, 'The relative duties of man: Domestic medicine in England and France, ca. 1685–1740', *Journal of Family History* 31: 3 (2006), 237–56, which focuses on men's medical decision-making about selves and families, and L. Culvert, '"A more careful tender nurse cannot be than my dear husband": Reassessing the role of men in pregnancy and childbirth in Ulster, 1780–1838', *Journal of Family History* 42: 1 (2017), 22–36 where the evidence of men's care generally falls after 1820.

7 For my definition of the anti-nurse, see the Introduction.

8 For the use of Samuel Bruckshaw's narrative of 1774 (for example) in institutional history, see L. Smith, *Private Madhouses in England, 1640–1815: Commercialised Care for the Insane* (London: Palgrave Macmillan, 2020), particularly chapter 8. For an exemplar history of the mad using the narratives of Urbane Metcalf and others, see R. Porter, *Mind-Forg'd Manacles: A History of Madness in England from the Restoration to the Regency* (London: Penguin, 1990).

9 C. Mackintosh, 'A historical study of men in nursing', *Journal of Advanced Nursing* 26: 2 (1997), 232–6; J. Evans, 'Men nurses: A historical and feminist perspective', *Journal of Advanced Nursing* 47: 3 (2004), 321–8. Alison Bashford finds that maleness was one of the 'insanitary' factors which had to be replaced by nursing reform: A. Bashford, *Purity and Pollution: Gender, Embodiment, and Victorian Medicine* (Basingstoke: Macmillan, 1998), p. 33.

10 C.J. Kauffman, *Tamers of Death: The History of the Alexian Brothers from 1300 to 1789* (New York: Seabury Press, 1976); C.J. Kauffman, *The Ministry of Healing: The History of the Alexian Brothers from 1789 to the Present* (New York: Seabury Press, 1978).

11 L.E. Sabin, 'Unheralded nurses. Male care givers in the nineteenth-century South', *Nursing History Review* 5: 1 (1997), 131–48.

12 For Sweden in this period, Maria Ågren finds men 'involved to a large extent' in caring, albeit under the broad heading of childcare, support for older people, and for the disabled – yet the more hands-on and

repetitive activities were more likely to be done by women. Men undertook more short-term activities such as treating wounds: M. Ågren, *Making a Living, Making a Difference: Gender and Work in Early Modern European Society* (Oxford: Oxford University Press, 2016), pp. 136–9.
13 P. Carter, *Men and the Emergence of Polite Society, Britain 1660–1800* (Harlow: Longman, 2001), pp. 209–11.
14 W. Van Reyk, 'Christian ideals of manliness in the eighteenth and early nineteenth centuries', *Historical Journal* 52: 4 (2009), 1053–73.
15 I. Mortimer, *The Dying and the Doctors: The Medical Revolution in Seventeenth-Century England* (Woodbridge: Royal Historical Society, Boydell Press, 2009), pp. 150–1.
16 Mortimer, *The Dying and the Doctors*, pp. 152, 164. There are few references in the probate accounts of other counties to male nursing, but this might be a factor of poor survivals; Mortimer, *The Dying and the Doctors*, p. 187.
17 S. Williams, 'Caring for the sick poor. Poor Law nurses in Bedfordshire, *c.*1770–1834', P. Lane, N. Raven, and K.D.M. Snell (eds), *Women, Work and Wages in England, 1600–1850* (Woodbridge: Boydell, 2004).
18 For many-to-many nursing by men see Chapter 6.
19 M. Pelling, *The Common Lot: Sickness, Medical Occupations, and the Urban Poor in Early Modern England* (London: Longman, 1998), p. 200; *Gentleman's Magazine* volume 87 part 1 (1817), p. 567.
20 Wedgwood Collection Barlaston, Wedgwood manuscripts, personal correspondence, letter of 21 November 1815 from Susannah Darwin to Josiah Wedgwood II.
21 H. Bradley, 'Across the Great Divide: The entry of men into "women's jobs"', C.L. Williams (ed.), *Doing 'Women's Work': Men in Nontraditional Occupations* (Newbury Park, CA: Sage, 1993), p. 23.
22 Gloucestershire Archives, HO 19/1/6 Gloucestershire Infirmary weekly board minutes 1786–95, 11–25 March 1790, 18 November–16 December 1790, 25 April 1793, 19 September 1793–22 May 1794; HO 19/1/7 Gloucestershire Infirmary weekly board minutes 1795–1804, 17 December 1795. In Worcester the infirmary employed Samuel Pirton for lodging and nursing female patients with smallpox, although Pirton seems to have been a cordwainer rather than an apothecary; Worcestershire Archives, BA5161/12 Worcester Royal Infirmary account book of general hospital expenses 1745–54, 17 June 1753 and 25 June 1754. It may of course have been Pirton's wife or daughter who did the actual nursing, or his female relations might

have inherited the role of delegated nurse; see Worcestershire Archives, BA5161/1 Worcester Royal Infirmary order books 1745–1800 and 1800–28, minute of 1 April 1785 and reference to 'nurse Purton's'.
23 H. Smith, *Letters to married women* (London: G. Kearsly, [1774]), p. 236.
24 S. Teedon, *The Diary of Samuel Teedon, 17 October 1791 to 2 February 1794* (London: [no details], 1902), p. 7 for Teedon attending his adult female cousin in company with Teedon's co-resident nephew 'doing what we could to relieve her'; S. Markham, *A Testimony of her Times: Based on Penelope Hind's Diaries and Correspondence 1787–1838* (Salisbury: Michael Russell, 1990), p. 22 for tender restraint offered by a gardener and neighbouring farmers to a minor clergyman during his final illness in 1796. W. Branch-Johnson (ed.), *The Carrington Diary (1797–1810)* (London: Christopher Johnson, 1956), p. 19 for a man nursing a former employee; R.C. Trench (ed.), *The Remains of the Late Mrs Richard Trench* (London: Parker, Son, and Bourn, 1862), pp. 385–6 for an unnamed clergyman sharing the nursing of his brother-in-law who was dying at Madeira, reported 1818; R.M. James, 'Health care in the Georgian household of Sir William and Lady Hannah East', *Historical Research* 82: 218 (2009), 694–714, on p. 711 for nursing Sir William East during gout by his son Augustus.
25 J. Malcolm, *Reminiscences of a Campaign in the Pyrenees and South of France in 1814* (Cambridge: Ken Trotman, 1999), p. 305.
26 M. Storey (ed.), *Two East Anglian Diaries* (Woodbridge: Boydell for the Suffolk Record Society, 1994), p. 160.
27 T. Lobb, *A Treatise of the Smallpox* (London: T. Woodward and C. Davis, 1731) p. xxxiv.
28 A. Sutton (ed.), *An Edinburgh Diary 1793–1798* (Stroud: Sutton, 2016), p. 101.
29 H. Newton, *The Sick Child in Early Modern England, 1580–1720* (Oxford: Oxford University Press, 2012), see conclusion to chapter 3. See also the website Orlando: Women's Writing in the British Isles from the Beginnings to the Present, John Fenwick, husband of author Eliza Fenwick, for a nine-year-old son being deputised to nurse his father: https://orlando.cambridge.org/index.php/profiles/fenwel (accessed 16 January 2023).
30 J. Ayres (ed.), *Paupers and Pig-Killers: The Diary of William Holland, a Somerset Parson, 1799–1818* (Stroud: Sutton, 2000), pp. 66–7 for 2 February 1802.
31 E.M. Forster (ed.), *Original Letters from India: 1779–1815* (London: Hogarth Press, 1925), p. 126.

32 Huntington Library Stutterd Letters, SFP 143 John to Thomas 22 February 1787. I am indebted to Karen Harvey for this reference.
33 J. Beresford (ed.), *John MacDonald: Memoirs of an XVIII Century Footman* (New York: Harper and Brothers, 1927), p. 134.
34 K. Straub, *Domestic Affairs: Intimacy, Eroticism and Violence between Servants and Masters in Eighteenth-Century Britain* (Baltimore, MD: Johns Hopkins University Press, 2009), chapters 5 and 6.
35 S.E. Brown, 'Assessing men and maids: The female servant tax and meanings of productive labour in late eighteenth-century Britain', *Left History* 12: 2 (2007), 11–32, on pp. 12–13; T. Meldrum, *Domestic Service and Gender 1660–1750: Life and Work in the London Household* (Harlow: Longman, 2000), pp. 173–4.
36 M. Bundock, *The Fortunes of Frances Barber* (New Haven, CT: Yale University Press, 2015), pp. 169–71.
37 J. Boswell, *The Life of Samuel Johnson* (London: J.M. Dent and Sons, 1951), volume II, p. 606.
38 For a concise treatment of the long relationship between the two men, see G. Gerzina, *Black England: Life before Emancipation* (London: Allison and Busby, 1995), pp. 45–54.
39 M. Cappe (ed.), *Memoirs of the Life of the Late Mrs Catherine Cappe* (London: Longman, Hurst, Rees, Orme, and Brown, 1822), chapter 40 for all quotes and details relating to John Hacket.
40 There is a baptism for John Malloney Hackett on 26 November 1781 in Barbados, son of Philip Hackett and Eliza Ann: www.findmypast.co.uk (accessed 15 September 2022).
41 O. Equiano, *The Interesting Narrative of the Life of Olaudah Equiano or Gustavus Vassa, the African* (New York: Modern Library, 2004), pp. 108 and 126 relating to events in 1763–65.
42 T. Holcroft, *Memoirs of the Late Thomas Holcroft Written by Himself* (London: Longman, Hurst, Rees, Orme, and Brown, 1816), volume I, p. 160.
43 K. Everest, 'Keats, John', *Oxford Dictionary of National Biography*, https://doi.org/10.1093/ref:odnb/15229 (accessed 17 August 2021).
44 Everest, 'Keats'.
45 The full text of the letters written by John Keats are available online: see *The Project Gutenberg eBook, Letters of John Keats to his Family and Friends*, https://www.gutenberg.org/files/35698/35698-h/35698-h.htm (accessed 24 November 2021); for quote, see letter from John Keats to George and Georgiana Keats, 13 or 14 October 1818.
46 Letter from John Keats to Charles Wentworth Dilke, 21 September 1818.

47 The full text of letters written by Joseph Severn are available online; see *Joseph Severn's Letters from Rome – John Keats* on English History, https://englishhistory.net/keats/joseph-severns-letters-from-rome/ (accessed 24 November 2021).
48 Letter from Joseph Severn to John Brown, 14–17 December 1820.
49 Letter from Joseph Severn to William Haslam, 15 January 1821.
50 Letter from Joseph Severn to Mrs Brawne, 11 January 1821.
51 Letter from Joseph Severn to John Brown, 14–17 December 1820.
52 F. Nightingale, *Notes on Nursing – What It Is and What It Is Not* (London: Harrison, 1859), p. 13 for the 'true nurse calling' requiring what is good for the patient first, and only then the nurse's consideration of self or 'what it was their place to do'.
53 E.K. Abel, *Hearts of Wisdom: American Women Caring for King 1850–1940* (Cambridge, MA: Harvard University Press, 2000), p. 4.
54 J. Alleine, T. Alleine, et al., *Life and Death of the Rev Joseph Alleine* (New York: Robert Carter, 1840), p. 91 for an example of many-to-one nursing carried out by women mentioned in Chapter 1.
55 W. Beatty, *Authentic Narrative of the Death of Lord Nelson* (London: T. Davison, 1807), full text available online at https://www.gutenberg.org/files/15233/15233-h/15233-h.htm (accessed 3 September 2021).
56 L. Brockliss, J. Cardwell, and M. Moss, *Nelson's Surgeon: William Beatty, Naval Medicine, and the Battle of Trafalgar* (Oxford: Oxford University Press, 2005), p. 156.
57 Chevalier was mentioned only once by Beatty, as helping to turn Nelson onto his right side.
58 Benjamin West is quoted in P. Paret, *Imagined Battles: Reflections of War in European Art* (Chapel Hill, NC: University of North Carolina Press, 1997), pp. 50–1.
59 Bonham's Auction House website, manuscript list of Lord Nelson's servants, sold in 2005, with auction house commentary, https://www.bonhams.com/auctions/11430/lot/209/ (accessed 26 August 2021).
60 K. Williams, 'Ideologies of nursing: Their meanings and implications', R. Dingwall and J. McIntosh (eds), *Readings in the Sociology of Nursing* (Edinburgh: Churchill Livingstone, 1978), p. 40.
61 Pelling, *Common Lot*, p. 181; C. Beck, 'Cared for by his messmates', paper delivered at the European Social Science History Conference 2021.
62 P. McRorie Higgins, *Punish or Treat?: Medical Care in English Prisons 1770–1850* (Victoria, British Columbia: Trafford, 2007), pp. 56–61; P.P. *Report from the Commissioners on the Cold Bath Fields Prison* (1809), p. 23 for a turnkey acting as doctor's mate and nurse of the men's infirmary.

63 The apothecary of New Prison and Bridewell, Clerkenwell, reported in February 1791 that 'John Yall is in the Sick Ward as Nurse, John Smith Has been ill but remains in the Ward as an Assistant'; Middlesex Sessions papers, Justices' working documents, see London Lives LMSMPS508610010, www.londonlives.org (accessed 5 December 2022).
64 P.P. *Report from the Committee on the Prisons within the City of London and Borough of Southwark 1. Newgate* (1818), p. 103.
65 *Some Account of St Bartholomew's Hospital London* (London: J. Smeeton, 1800), p. 12 claims there was one sister, one nurse, and one night nurse for each ward of around fourteen patients at Barts; London Metropolitan Archives, H9/GY/T/01/019 Guy's Hospital archive memorandum book of John Hollister 1738–65.
66 P.P. *Report from the Committee on the State of the Gaols of the City of London* (1814), p. 55.
67 P.P. *Second Report from the Committee on the Prisons within the City of London and Borough of Southwark 2. Giltspur-Street Prison. 3. Whitecross-Street Prison. 4. Borough Compter. 5. Bridewell* (1818), p. 250.
68 P.P. *Report from the Committee on the King's Bench, Fleet, and Marshalsea Prisons* (1815), p. 234; J. Neild, *State of the Prisons in England, Scotland and Wales* (London: J. Nichols and Son, 1812), p. 137.
69 A. Tomkins, 'Stafford Infirmary and the "unreformed" nurse, 1765–1820', I. Atherton, M. Blake, A. Sargent, and A. Tomkins (eds), *Local Histories: Essays in Honour of Nigel Tringham* (Stafford: Staffordshire Record Society, 2022).
70 L.D. Smith, 'Behind closed doors; Lunatic asylum keepers, 1800–60', *Social History of Medicine* 1: 3 (1988), 301–27, on p. 306.
71 P.P. *Select Committee on State of Gaols, and Best Method of Providing for Reformation of Offenders* (1819), p. 371.
72 P.P. *Report from the Committee on the King's Bench, Fleet, and Marshalsea Prisons* (1815), pp. 189, 197.
73 P.P. *Royal Commission on State, Conduct, and Management of Fleet, Westminster and Marshalsea Prisons* (1819), p. 71.
74 J. Caulfield, *Portraits, Memoirs, and Characters of Remarkable Persons* (London: T.H. Whiteley, 1820), volume III, pp. 168–75.
75 See Chapter 1.
76 Stereotyping male nurses as gay is an observed phenomenon of the early twenty-first century and may have long roots: T. Harding, 'The construction of men who are nurses as gay', *Journal of Advanced*

Nursing 60: 6 (2007), 636–44. However, S. O'Driscoll, 'The molly and the fop: Disentangling effeminacy in the eighteenth century', C. Mounsey (ed.), *Developments in the Histories of Sexualities: In Search of the Normal, 1600–1800* (Lewisburg, PA: Bucknell University Press, 2013) argues that the conflation of effeminacy and sodomy in this period cannot be assumed. For some of the norms of men sharing accommodation which took place without necessarily incurring assumptions of their effeminacy, see G. Williamson, *Lodgers, Landlords, and Landladies in Georgian London* (London: Bloomsbury Academic, 2021).

77 Smith, *Private Madhouses*, p. 2.
78 W. Battie, *A Treatise on Madness* (London: J. Whiston and B. White, 1758); Porter, *Mind-Forg'd Manacles*, pp. 150–5.
79 A. Cruden, *The Adventures of Alexander the Corrector* (London: the author, 1754); The Madhouses Act 1774, 14 Geo. 3 c. 49; P.P. *Report from the Committee on Madhouses in England* (1814–15).
80 P.P. *Return ... Lunatic Asylums* (1819) and P.P. *Return ... Houses* (1819).
81 For 6.2 see P.P. *Return ... Lunatic Asylums* (1819), which includes the data for the Ticehurst and Hereford asylums, despite their being private, and the information for St Peter's in Bristol which were contained within a workhouse; patient figures for St Lukes are taken from P.P. *Report from the Select Committee appointed to Enquire into the State of Lunatics* (1807), p. 21; patient figures for Guys are taken from London Metropolitan Archives, H9/GY/A/161/001 Guy's Hospital memorandum book of Thomas Callaway 1807–09; dates of founding are taken from either C. Chalklin, *English Counties and Public Building 1650–1830* (London: Hambledon, 1998), p. 201 or L.D. Smith, '"The keeper must himself be kept": Visitation and the lunatic asylum in England, 1750–1850', G. Mooney and J. Reinarz (eds), *Permeable Walls: Historical Perspectives on Hospital and Asylum Visiting* (Amsterdam: Rodopi, 2009). This table omits all patients held in gaols, houses of correction, or coincidental returns from infirmaries that lacked dedicated wards for the insane, on the grounds that specialist staff were not notably recruited to cater for mad patients. For 6.3 see P.P. *Return ... Houses* (1819); The Retreat has been added using details from S. Tuke, *Description of the Retreat, an Institution near York for Insane Persons of the Society of Friends* (York: W. Alexander, 1813), p. 220; Pile's name at Somerstown was excluded from the report of 1819 but is taken here from P.P. *Report ... Lunatics* (1807), p. 25; the patients column aggregates the patients in

multiple houses owned and run by the same licensee, i.e. by Burrow, Miles, Rhodes, and Talbot.
82 P.P. *Report* ... *Madhouses* (1814–15), evidence of Richard Powell p. 78 and Lucas Pepys p. 107.
83 Tuke, *Description*, p. 99.
84 H.C. Cameron, *Mr Guy's Hospital 1726–1948* (London: Longman, Green & Co., 1954), pp. 71–2.
85 U. Metcalf, *The Interior of Bethlem Hospital* (London: the author, 1818), partially reproduced in A. Ingram, *Patterns of Madness in the Eighteenth Century: A Reader* (Liverpool: Liverpool University Press, 1998), pp. 256–64, on p. 257.
86 Smith, '"The keeper"', p. 206.
87 Felonies committed within madhouses could be concealed in ways that were not possible outside, bringing some of the same personnel into view: see the prosecution for murder in 1759 of William Tipton, formerly a keeper for Michael Duffield's madhouse in Chelsea 1741–58, case t17591205-34, www.oldbaileyonline.org (accessed 22 November 2022). He was acquitted, partly on the evidence of multiple other keepers.
88 Poet William Cowper was so attached to his keeper at the St Albans madhouse where he was a patient in 1764–65 that he employed him as a servant (to the chagrin of the madhouse proprietor): W. Cowper, *Memoir of the Early Life of William Cowper Esq* (London: R. Edwards, 1816), pp. 64, 73–4; I am indebted to Len Smith for this reference. Even a patient in Lancashire who thought himself wrongly confined admitted 'that he has been well treated in the house'; Lancashire Archives, QSP/2585/6 relating to Dr Chew's asylum in Billington, 1809. Smith argues that favourable conclusions by asylum visitors are given credibility by the appearance of critical reports at other times or for other places; Smith, *Private Madhouses*, p. 241.
89 Although see L.D. Smith, *Lunatic Hospitals in Georgian England, 1750–1830* (New York: Routledge, 2007), p. 63 for some failings by female managers.
90 J. Mitford, *A Description of the Crimes and Horrors in the Interior of Warburton's Private Mad-House* (London: Benbow, 1825), volume I, p. 25.
91 Smith, '"The keeper"'; Smith, 'Behind closed doors'.
92 Smith, 'Behind closed doors', p. 312; L.D. Smith, *'Cure, Comfort and Safe Custody': Public Lunatic Asylums in Early Nineteenth-Century England* (London: Leicester University Press, 1999), p. 138. An account by a patient who struggled with his male keepers in the 1650s,

and who credited his recovery partly to 'hard keeping', can be found in [G. Trosse], *The Life of the Reverend Mr George Trosse* (Exeter: Joseph Bliss and Richard White, 1714), pp. 53–76. A very detailed account by a patient of the multiple challenges he posed to his keepers in the years up to 1821 are included in P.S. Knight, *Observations on the Causes, Symptoms and Treatment of Derangement* (London: Longman, Rees, Orme, Brown, and Green, 1827), pp. 151–2.
93 Smith, *Cure, Comfort and Safe Custody*, p. 140.
94 Smith, 'Behind closed doors', p. 326.
95 Bashford, *Purity and Pollution*, p. 30.
96 S.C. Bolton and C. Boyd, 'Trolley dolly or skilled emotion manager? Moving on from Hochschild's Managed Heart', *Work, Employment, and Society* 17: 2 (2003), 289–308.
97 E. Foyster, *Manhood in Early Modern England: Honour, Sex and Marriage* (London: Longman, 1999), p. 178; E. Foyster, 'Boys will be boys? Manhood and aggression, 1660–1800', T. Hitchcock and M. Cohen (eds), *English Masculinities 1660–1800* (London: Longman, 1999), p. 151.
98 J. McEwan, 'Attitudes towards male authority and domestic violence in eighteenth-century London courts', J. Van Gent and S. Broomhall (eds), *Governing Masculinities in the Early Modern Period: Regulating Selves and Others* (London: Routledge, 2011), p. 262.
99 Recourse to physical force remained a valued working-class masculine trait well beyond 1820; see for example A. Clark, 'The rhetoric of Chartist domesticity', *Journal of British Studies* 31: 1 (1992), 62–88, on p. 71 for its political deployment in the 1840s.
100 K. Thomas, *The Ends of Life: Roads to Fulfilment in Early Modern England* (Oxford: Oxford University Press, 2009), p. 72; D. Morgan, 'Theater of war. Combat, the military, and masculinities', H. Brod and M. Kaufman (eds), *Theorising Masculinities* (London: Sage, 1994), p. 177.
101 Personal communication with Len Smith, November 2022.
102 Bashford, *Purity and Pollution*, p. 33.
103 Foyster, 'Boys', pp. 157–9; Smith, *Cure, Comfort and Safe Custody*, p. 135.
104 *Gentleman's Magazine*, volume 74 (1804), p. 301, quoted in Foyster 'Boys', p. 166.
105 M. Neuendorf, *Emotions and the Making of Psychiatric Reform in Britain, c.1770–1820* (Cham: Springer Nature Switzerland, 2021), p. 217.
106 L.D. Smith, '"God grant it may do good two all": The madhouse practice of Joseph Mason, 1738–79', *History of Psychiatry* 27: 2 (2016), 208–19, on p. 210.

107 W. Belcher, *Address to Humanity* (London: Allen and West, 1796), p. 5.
108 Some of the earliest complaints about private madhouses, if not about keepers per se, related to the collusion of families with madhouse keepers; P.P. *Journal of the House of Commons for 22 February 1763*, pp. 486–9.
109 Belcher, *Address to Humanity*, p. 15.
110 P.P. *Select Committee on Provisions for better Regulation of Madhouses in England Report, Minutes of Evidence, Appendix* (1814–15), p. 11, quoted in Ingram, *Patterns*, p. 248.
111 Metcalf, *Bethlem Hospital*, in Ingram, *Patterns*, p. 260.
112 Metcalf, *Bethlem Hospital*, in Ingram, *Patterns*, pp. 262–3.
113 Belcher, *Address to Humanity*, p. 4; A.M. Crowe, *A Letter to Dr Robert Darling Willis* (London: the author, 1811), p. 14.
114 Nightingale, *Notes on Nursing*, chapter 4: 'Noise'.
115 Knight, *Observations*, p. 150 for keepers who made their patient the butt of their jokes. NB this patient's reason returned in May 1821, so the experiences he describes in his memoir date to 1820 or earlier.
116 Metcalf, *Bethlem Hospital*, in Ingram, *Patterns*, p. 259; P.P. *Report ... Madhouses* (1814–15), p. 3, evidence of Godfrey Higgins.
117 There are explicit modern parallels. In the twentieth century, 'defensive working practices are developed in order to help staff cope with situations that might cause them distress'; I. Eyers and T. Adams, 'Dementia care nursing, emotional labour and clinical supervision', T. Adams (ed.), *Dementia Nursing Care: Promoting Well-being in People with Dementia and their Families* (Basingstoke: Palgrave Macmillan, 2007), p. 188 citing T. Kitwood, *Dementia Reconsidered* (Buckingham: Open University Press, 1997).
118 J. Tosh, 'The old Adam and the new man: Emerging themes in the history of English masculinities, 1750–1850', T. Hitchcock and M. Cohen (eds), *English Masculinities 1660–1800* (London: Longman, 1999), p. 223; H. Barker, 'Soul, purse, and family: Middling and lower-class masculinity in eighteenth-century Manchester', *Social History* 33: 1 (2008), 12–35, on p. 17 and *passim*.
119 Smith, *Cure, Comfort and Safe Custody*, p. 146.
120 The maintenance of household as evidence of personal male self-mastery had long roots; A. Shepard, *Meanings of Manhood in Early Modern England* (Oxford: Oxford University Press, 2003), p. 70.
121 Smith, '"The keeper"', p. 204 quoting P.P. *Report ... Madhouses* (1814–15), p. 144. Stigmatising attitudes among health professionals including nurses remains a problem in the twenty-first century;

B.S. Carrara, C.A.A. Ventura, S.J. Bobbili, O.M.P. Jacobina, A. Khenti, and I.A. Costa Mendes, 'Stigma in health professionals towards people with mental illness: An integrative review', *Archives of Psychiatric Nursing* 33: 4 (2019), 311–18.

122 It seems highly unlikely that keepers were at all influenced by evangelical moralising of work: Tosh, 'Old Adam', pp. 234–6.

123 Metcalf, *Bethlem Hospital*, in Ingram, *Patterns*, p. 256.

124 W.J., *Practical Observations on Insanity* (London: J. Anderson et al., 1828) but also alluding to the years before 1820. L. Parry Jones, *The Trade in Lunacy: A Study of Private Madhouses in England in the Eighteenth and Nineteenth Centuries* (London: Routledge & Kegan Paul, 1972), p. 185 tentatively identifies the author as William Jones, an employee at the Whitmore House madhouse in 1808.

125 W.J., *Observations*, pp. 55–6.

126 J. Begiato, *Manliness in Britain, 1760–1900* (Manchester: Manchester University Press, 2020), pp. 169–70.

127 A. Le Grand, *Man without Passion, or, The wife stoick* (London: Harper and Amery, 1675), p. 278.

128 G.J. Barker-Benfield, *The Culture of Sensibility: Sex and Society in Eighteenth-Century Britain* (Chicago, IL: University of Chicago Press, 1996), p. 104.

129 Bradley, 'Across the Great Divide', p. 23.

130 Mitford, *Crimes and Horrors*, volume I, pp. 1–2.

131 D.S. Sechelski, 'Garrick's body and the labor of art in eighteenth-century theater', *Eighteenth-Century Studies* 29: 4 (1996), 369–89, on p. 383.

132 B.E. Ashforth and G.E. Kreiner, '"How can you do it?": Dirty work and the challenge of constructing a positive identity', *Academy of Management Review* 24: 3 (1999), 413–34, on p. 415: P.P. Select Committee on Provisions for the Better Regulation of Madhouses in England: First Report (1815–16), p. 41.

133 W.J. suggested a staffing structure where a 'superior' staff member responsible for moral superintendence directed a lowlier member of staff to conduct the hands-on 'personal care'; W.J., *Observations*, pp. 49–50. This sounds rather like the Sister/nurse/helper structure observed in Chapter 2 at St Bartholomew's Hospital.

134 For the use of straw among dirty patients see Metcalf, *Bethlem Hospital*, in Ingram, *Patterns*, p. 260.

135 K. Siena, *Rotten Bodies: Class and Contagion in 18th-Century Britain* (New Haven, CT: Yale University Press, 2019).

136 M. Jenner, 'Chamberpots at Dawn', seminar paper, Keele University, 6 March 2019.

137 For a similar response by men forced into close contact with waste produced by others, under even more challenging circumstances for the charges themselves, see E. Christopher, *Slave Ship Sailors and Their Captive Cargoes, 1730–1807* (Cambridge: Cambridge University Press, 2006), pp. 171–3.
138 Metcalf, *Bethlem Hospital*, in Ingram, *Patterns*, pp. 258, 260–1.
139 Mitford, *Crimes and Horrors*, volume I, p. 6.
140 Foyster, *Manhood*, chapter 5.
141 Mitford, *Crimes and Horrors*, volume I, p. 15 for Warburton's keeper who allegedly gloried in his inhumanity. For a discussion of the potential for trauma to explain abusive behaviours by male and female nurses, see Chapter 6.
142 All quotes are taken from T. Holcroft, *Anna St Ives* (London: Oxford University Press, 1970), a modern edition of the original 1792 text, pp. 376–9.
143 The trope of madhouse incarceration was continued by other authors, but only after 1820, and in relation to the dubious or wrongful admission of patients rather than the outright criminality of staff; see, most prominently, W. Collins, *The Woman in White* (London: Sampson Low, Son, & Co., 1860) and C. Reade, *Hard Cash* (London: Sampson Low, Son, & Marston, 1863).
144 H. Fielding, *Amelia* (London: A. Millar, 1752).
145 Fielding, *Amelia*, volume I, p. 237.
146 Fielding, *Amelia*, volume II, p. 61.
147 Fielding, *Amelia*, volume I, p. 237.
148 Fielding, *Amelia*, volume I, p. 242.
149 A. Fletcher, *Gender, Sex and Subordination in England 1500–1800* (New Haven, CT: Yale University Press, 1995) p. 338.

6

Nursing in wartime 1793–1815

You never hear any of those grumblers say a word about the comforts provided for the sick and wounded, their favourite talk is of evils for which there could be no remedy.[1]

War imposed demands on the resources of the nations engaged in combat and on those whose lands were the scene of fighting. The resource issues raised by maintenance of a standing army and its deployment in the field have given rise to a weighty historiography, including in relation to the significance of conflict for the development of medicine and medical careers.[2] The history of nursing in wartime before the 1850s, in contrast, has thus far been written with the grumblers in mind. The many-to-many nursing requirements of the sick and injured were characterised by nurse reformers as inadequate and squalid. Work by Paul Kopperman has attempted to recalibrate responses to care for the army in the pre-reform period making some impact on military history but less difference to histories of nursing. Very recent work by Erin Spinney starts to reset our expectations.

Admittedly the analysis of Private William Wheeler, the author of the quote above, pointed entirely the other way from the grumblers. Despite seeing active service from 1809 onwards, and being wounded and hospitalised in Spain during 1814, he advanced a rosy view of care facilities for the private solider. His was perhaps the perspective of an ordinary labouring man whose expectations of life and social support either within or beyond the army were slim, despite his inadvertent skill as a writer and his passion for books.[3] When he became unfit for service, Wheeler's optimism was well-founded in his own case because he was able to return home to Walcot near Bath as a Chelsea out-pensioner.[4]

This chapter first provides a brief survey of the state of emergency nursing and medicine *c*.1793–1815, and then a short outline of the conflicts and theatres of war which engaged English personnel in this period plus the personal narratives they generated. It goes on to consider the spontaneous or inadvertent nursing by men and women on the battlefield or in its vicinity during these years and compares their endeavours with accounts of salaried care by nurses and orderlies. As in earlier chapters, the application of context to wartime nursing illuminates the achievements of individuals against the constraints of gender and status. Just as medical history has overwritten accounts of military surgeons as 'ill-educated butchers', so this chapter re-evaluates female army followers and orderlies as filling roles other than as self-serving exploiters of the vulnerable.[5] It surveys, too, the scope for twenty-first century understandings of trauma to inform perceptions of wartime carers as fellow victims. At the same time the chapter illustrates the contemporary value of the stereotypical anti-nurse in consolidating racial, status, and gender prejudice against foes and even allies. Finally, the chapter focuses on the aftermath of the Battle of Waterloo, and nursing in Brussels, to find cultural precursors of the reformed 'lady' nurse.

The chapters in this book so far have been tied closely to English nurses and their patients. This chapter broadens the field to include British voices, in acknowledgement of the diversity of backgrounds among wartime writers. A small number of German authors are also included here as the allies of British soldiers and simultaneously as sometime patients or carers.

Emergency nursing and medicine: first aid before the phrase

Immediate responses to illness and particularly to injury or acute threat to life were ubiquitous long before the formalisation of *premier secours*, or first aid, and could prove essential.[6] As one eighteenth-century military physician put it, 'The art of being timely is almost a medicine.'[7] History's first responders were inevitably a heterogeneous mix of family, friends, employees, employers, or strangers dependent on whether the sudden condition was revealed at home, at work, or elsewhere. Alice Thornton, as a conscientious employer, good housewife, and humane woman, for example, gave de facto first aid to her servants, including when she removed a piece of goose from her maid's throat when it was choking the maid in 1661.[8] The unplanned assistance of others could be critical in securing good outcomes for patients, as when bystanders staunched the flow of blood arising from Samuel Wood's drastic industrial injuries in 1737 using loaf sugar.[9]

There were some types of emergency for which there was no precedent, but wherever crises could be typified there was a value in making knowledge widespread. Printed advice was available for those dealing with accidents well before 1660 and grew by fits and starts thereafter.[10] Interventions and techniques gained ground. Sudden loss of blood from a limb might be stemmed by the swift application of a tourniquet.[11] Similarly burns and scalds were treated more comfortably and efficiently if attendants knew that fluids were advantageous and were wary of adhesions between burned skin and clothing, bedding, or dressings.[12] An increasing awareness of the need for quick action was institutionalised in the founding of the Royal Humane Society, designed to rescue from death (and premature burial) the victims of drowning. This British charity of 1774 was modelled on one founded in Amsterdam in 1767 for the resuscitation of people apparently drowned in one of that city's many canals. The Humane Society offered an active spur to the development of resuscitation techniques because it offered prizes for essays in life-saving and medals to some of those who used them successfully.[13]

Allied to swift attention was the development of triage, credited to French surgeon Dominique Larrey (1766–1842), to deal with overwhelming demands on the many-to-many care and treatment model imposed by wartime. This involved dividing potential patients into three groups according to their injuries, a technique with both 'ruthless and philanthropic aspects' if utilised chiefly to restore the wounded men to fighting fitness as quickly as possible.[14] It was implemented first for French soldiers between 1806 and 1808 and, along with other developments in transporting the wounded, made a significant impact in reducing mortality among ordinary servicemen. The impact of triage on care as opposed to on medicine would theoretically have required withholding support for some patients on the basis of a systematic requirement to attend others first. It may be impossible to determine what impact this had on carers and their charges in terms of their understanding of nursing, but it seems plausible that consciously to refrain from caring according to rote would have been regarded with a similar scepticism to that directed at care only in exchange for payment. The ideal of care throughout the period was to react spontaneously and compassionately without regard to either remuneration or system.

British involvement in European wars 1793–1815: nursing, infrastructure, and evidence

The delivery of nursing to soldiers in early modern Europe has been little discussed until very recently.[15] The quality of care given during the English Civil War and Interregnum has been assessed as much better than expected if only calibrating by nineteenth-century preconceptions: conflicts subsequent to the 1640s have attracted a moiety of interest in wartime nursing on the basis of a regrettably slim source base.[16] What distinguishes the events between 1793 and 1815 is the combination of long periods of action with a proliferation of relevant texts.

France declared war on Britain, Holland, and Spain in February 1793 and began a period of conflict which only ended decisively with the defeat of Napoleon at Waterloo in June 1815. Hostilities saw no enemy action in mainland Britain but required British soldiers to fight on the continent alongside Dutch, German, Spanish, and Portuguese allies. The memoirs of men who wrote about their experiences are concentrated to a lesser extent on military action in the Low Countries in the later 1790s and to a greater degree on the pitched battles and military life of the Iberian Peninsula between 1808 and 1814. The Battle of Waterloo in 1815 developed a literature all of its own.

The issue of care for soldiers was not of course a new problem from 1793 onwards. In the broadest sense the need to foster manpower, including by disease prevention, formed a part of contemporary narratives around, for example, the Seven Years War from 1756 to 1763.[17] Yet despite the frequency with which England was engaged in continental warfare throughout the eighteenth century, there were no large, permanent army hospitals constructed or run within the country before 1780. Small-scale regimental hospitals were augmented by temporary arrangements near to the sites of conflict, accommodated in tents or in buildings which were rented or requisitioned for the purpose.[18] The American War of Independence, spanning 1775 to 1783, apparently prompted the creation of general military hospitals on the south coast of England, although little is known about them, while the wars with France from 1793 to 1815 spurred the building of establishments at Gosport, Plymouth, and Walmer. The architecture of the Plymouth hospital featured blocks linked by a common arcade, where each floor in every block had its own nurse's room.[19] Female nurses and male orderlies were established features of the official provision for sick and wounded soldiers by the mid-eighteenth century and assumptions about the women's activities were akin to those for their equivalents in provincial infirmaries.[20] In this sense they fit with wider historiographical assessments of the relationship between military and hospital medicine.[21]

The Army Medical Board was established in 1793 and, among other tasks, specified the proper features of regimental and army hospitals and the necessary resources for medical attention. The published versions of the *Regulations* are much better at acknowledging the desirable existence of nurses and orderly men than they are at detailing their duties. In the light of this 'lackluster regulatory apparatus', more attentive to inventory than to care, the practical dimensions of army nursing must be gleaned from elsewhere.[22]

Testimony can be secured from the multiple memoirs of the events written between 1793 and 1815, or from letters and diaries written concurrently with or shortly after the action. Many such works have been published since 1815. Writings used for the analysis below have been selected for their attention to human as well as military matters and form a subset of published work calendared by Robert Burnham.[23] My intention here is to examine small sections of numerous accounts to contribute to the historiography of nursing, in distinct contrast to their typical use by military historians to study aspects of fighting.[24]

Conflicts prior to the wars of 1793 to 1815 generated relatively few, or truncated first person accounts, by combatants. Aspiring military writers may indeed have been 'confronted with a paucity of suitable precedents' when it came to life-writing before the 1790s, but their successors overcame their reticence in style, because a profusion of publications from the start of the first war with France up to the mid-1830s signalled the increasing popularity of the format.[25] Clusters of memoirs have been used to examine both the literary and historical potential of the field.[26] A key feature of the memoir for my purposes is the lapse of time between historical events and the act of writing. Time gives the author the space and opportunity to tell and retell the story to themselves and to others, to check facts, rewrite and forget, a process which facilitates the introduction of a specific agenda. Memoirs could even be disguised as something else: the modern editor of James Hope's 'letters', for example, raises questions about whether the material was fashioned into letters in accordance with literary tradition rather than copied from letters literally sent through the post.[27] The memoir-as-travelogue was already well established among men who travelled to fight, and strove to write, among foreign scenes.[28] Serjeant William Clarke's account was neglected for two hundred years in the belief that it was the text of a novel, rather than a memoir.[29] Even at the simplest level, the writer's agenda will have differed between those who wrote lifelong autobiographies and others recalling only phases of life (such as military service). Participation in or proximity to one of the most notable battles of any conflict is likely to have influenced writers in other ways, too, as they strove to position themselves in relation to historic events.[30] This context does not inevitably mean that they were writing fiction, but that they were shaping memory for specific stated, tacit, or unconscious ends.[31] These ambitions could include the recasting of war as an individual adventure, with a concomitant loss of information about quotidian domestic matters.[32]

Letters and diaries make up the remainder of the narratives used here. In contrast to memoirs, these are diurnal writings with an immediacy that is less susceptible to the expression of subsequent agendas by the original writers.[33] They are eminently open to shaping, however, particularly by non-authorial editors who can cut, interpolate, gloss, and otherwise control the release of the material for publishers' and/or ideological ends.[34] At the same time, the determination to keep diaries or write letters by people under stress can be seen retrospectively as an act of defiance in the face of authority or (during wartime) the threat of sudden death.[35] These competing motivations among authors and editors can make interpretation complicated. Most usefully for the purposes of this chapter, though, letters and diaries illustrate the emergence of the mundane account of wartime experience, as it is only the writer who notes the daily, repetitious events in life that notices the minutiae of care.[36] Coincidentally in giving details about wounding and care, writers were avoiding studied expressions of stoicism and the 'ideology of sacrifice' preferred by the state.[37]

The analysis below of spontaneous and organised nursing arises from the study of over a hundred published memoirs, diaries, and collections of letters.[38] Most such sources from soldiers make little or no mention of the physical consequences of war on men's bodies and their need for nursing, a form of suppression already noticed in the literature.[39] The majority of the writing which does give notice to nursing activity comes from rank-and-file soldiers, non-commissioned, and junior officers. The more senior the author in the army's hierarchy at the time of the need for nursing, the less likely they were to give sustained attention to care, whether on the battlefield or elsewhere. Some memoirists even refer to prolonged stays in hospital without giving any detail of their experience of treatment or recuperation.[40] Nonetheless among those who did describe nursing work, there are forms of coalescence between writers and across genres about the features of this work. One or two writers might not be thought authoritative on their own: an array of writers, publishing at different times for different audiences, represents a form of unforced consensus.

Spontaneous care: nursing by wives, comrades, lodging hosts, and the anti-nurse as racial stereotype

Armies in the late eighteenth and early nineteenth centuries were ostensibly male-only environments. In fact, women were routinely present as 'on the strength', being permitted to accompany male combatants for their provision of cooking, laundry, and care, or tolerated as camp followers. In both capacities they were generally depicted as of doubtful virtue, a 'disruptive influence', or as likely to strip the dead for spoils as to tear up rags for dressing wounds, descriptive abuse which spoke to gender and status difference as much as to lived experience.[41] Most histories of nursing during wartime thus far have been drawn to the development of official services rather than to their prehistory, doubtless owing to the survival of coherent archives for discrete organisations.[42]

The personal narratives analysed here demonstrate that women, chiefly regimental wives, had the theoretical capacity to supply a patchwork of immediate nursing attention.[43] It was routine for six wives to accompany every hundred men, with the women at least notionally receiving pay and victuals from the army in exchange for their services, sometimes necessitating a ballot of those women who were willing to travel as adjuncts to the army.[44] A failed ballot did not necessarily prevent women from following their spouses without official recognition. Therefore, the women who followed the army might do so in ways which made a difference to their status in the eyes of the military authorities (and to the cost of campaigns) but made no appreciable impact on their travelling alongside the 'baggage' or on their attentions to the men. These women were at less risk of violent injury than their combatant husbands, but they were not safe even when performing supportive or nursing work.[45] The very fact of their marching with soldiers over problematic terrain exposed them to drowning, for example, in rivers and bogs.[46]

Yet there are almost no detailed accounts of ordinary women's actions as carers in this wartime context.[47] Instead the women were critiqued for their marital practices – women who were widowed while on campaign frequently made a swift remarriage, suggesting to contemporaries that their affections were shallow at best – or for their plundering the dead in the aftermath of a battle.[48] Similar allegations directed at plague nurses, that were surveyed in the Introduction to this book, have been mitigated by historians' reference to the women's paucity of alternatives for economic survival. The continued relevance of economic pressure on women in this later period has been confirmed by Catriona Kennedy, and John Lynn makes the case for 'pillage as fundamental to the campaign economy'.[49] Contemporaries, though, were content to live with the paradox involved in making use of scavenged materials, such as 'Waterloo teeth' converted into dentures, at the same time as damning the resource-gatherers.[50]

The easy stereotypes of the common soldier's female camp follower were contrasted at the time with women of higher social standing, such as the wife of Colonel Dalbiac, described in 1811 while in Portugal as 'a complete soldier's wife, rain or no rain, sun or no sun, it is equally the same to her, her whole thought is her husband'.[51] Susanna Dalbiac was the daughter of a military family who married in 1804 and thereafter followed her husband everywhere, always sleeping in her husband's tent.[52] During the Battle of Salamanca in 1812 she watched the colonel from within the range of French artillery fire, and after the battle sought him among the dead and wounded on the battlefield. Colonel Dalbiac survived, so his wife turned her attention to others among the wounded until the 'final retreat'.[53] In anticipation of the nurse reformers, Mrs Dalbiac was a lady who contemporaries hesitated to label decisively as a nurse.[54]

Lowlier women were occasionally directed into nursing as a means to remain honourably widowed rather than becoming dishonourably remarried. The wife of Corporal Cunningham of the 42nd Regiment, her husband having been killed during the Battle of Toulouse, displayed the wifely devotion of right feeling despite her lowly background. She insisted on accompanying the corporal's corpse to its burying place with every mark of grief, such that the esteem for her husband and for her own status as a widow ensured favourable attention. She was recruited to nurse the company's commanding officer 'and under his protection was restored in decent respectability to her home.'[55] The status of women's would-be protectors was highly relevant to their life chances. The author of this anecdote was at some pains to point out that 'The only protection a poor solider can offer to a woman suddenly bereft of her husband ... would, under more favourable circumstances, be considered as an insult' and to exonerate women from a charge of callous remarriage by presenting it as her 'only alternative'.[56]

The most concentrated focus for retrospective popular attention to an ordinary woman was provided by the 'Heroine of Matagorda'. Agnes Reston (née Harkness) (1773–1856) accompanied her husband to war and took a small child with her (a son of approximately 4 years old). At the fort of Matagorda near Cadiz in 1810 she assisted the doctor in dressing wounds by tearing up her own and her husband's clothes, earning her attribution as a nurse, and participated in general aspects of defence such as carrying sandbags, but it was her distinguished bravery that secured her lasting fame. While under bombardment by French cannon, Reston volunteered to fetch water from the well despite being exposed to constant fire. The rope of the bucket was even detached by shot at her first attempt to fill it, but with the help of a sailor she retrieved the pail and returned with water for the wounded.[57] Reston was a woman whose bodily courage and diffused compassion – she took the task of fetching water from a drummer boy who was afraid to go – represented the kind of selflessness that was otherwise associated only with women who nursed their relations to the detriment of their own strength.[58]

Joseph Donaldson, whose volumes of memoirs helped to advertise Reston's work, regretted her lack of official material reward.[59] The Secretary at War apparently had no funds or other means for the formal recognition of such exemplary women.[60] Agnes Reston lacked the social cachet of being a colonel's wife (in the manner of Susanna Dalbiac) being the wife of a serjeant in the 94th Regiment. She did not fit the stereotype of the camp follower, so contemporaries did not know what to make of her, until she was championed by Donaldson. By the time his work attracted widespread notice, Reston had lived out the majority of life. After her husband's death she continued to work as a nurse, including in the Glasgow Hospital, but also seemingly undertook domestic nursing since it was her attention to a single fever patient in Glasgow 1843 that helped to revive her fame.[61] Public recognition, when it came, generated a subscription in the manner (but not the magnitude) of the funds raised for Florence Nightingale while the latter was in the Crimea, and an annuity was purchased to give Reston an income of £30 a year.[62] Yet Reston was selfless to the last, donating money to other local charities from her own small funds.[63] In contrast with responses to Susanna Dalbiac, Agnes Reston was in essence a lady nurse without reaching the social status of a lady.

The immediate demands of those wounded in battle were not always met by either female or male attendants, since multiple accounts by soldiers include reference to the men trampled underfoot, or left on the field, as a consequence of attack or retreat.[64] Nonetheless the men whose memoirs of army service during the period 1793 to 1815 described their own or others' calls for help characterised a variety of ways that *other men* offered first aid or rudimentary nursing to each other.[65] They shared water, wine, and brandy (including with the enemy), applied tourniquets or dressings, fabricated slings, offered companionship as comfort, and carried or dragged one another to places of greater safety.[66] As Holly Furneaux has established, the gentle soldier was not wholly an invention of the mid-nineteenth century.[67]

Similarly memoirs of military hospitals mention spontaneous 'kindnesses' between men who were not technically employed to care which, like those in the field, involved the enemy as well as allies across different types of narrative.[68] Moyle Sherer's recollections of the hospital at Elvas included a report of English and French soldiers 'performing little kind offices for each other' which is poignant if unspecific.[69] There was an explicit acknowledgement of the femininity that was entailed by at least one writer who claimed, 'you will often see a rough but kind-hearted soldier, seated for hours by the bedside of a wounded comrade, administering to his wants, smoothing his pillow, and tending him with all the gentleness and affection of a woman'.[70]

The outbreak of war in 1793 saw householders across the European continent accommodate, feed, and care for strangers who fell at their door or were billeted upon them. Numerous memoirs of English military men recall the attention given by landlords and landladies to the wounded in Belgium, Holland, Portugal, Spain, and even France, as well as in England.[71] This might reasonably be termed 'second aid', since lodgings were usually located some distance from battles or skirmishing.

Writers were likely to recall instances of particularly good attention, more frequently and in more detail than was the case with care from regimental wives.[72] Charles Leslie was billeted with his friend, and benefitted from a nurse who was both the daughter of the householder and a nun of the Order of St Clare (who had returned home on the destruction of her convent). This woman procured bandages, applied poultices, made drinking chocolate, and kept up the spirits of her patients with 'cheerful conversation'.[73] Similarly a wounded colonel was attended before, during, and after the operation to remove his leg by the daughter of his Spanish host.[74] Kind treatment was not dependent on the high social status of the landlord or landlady.[75] A bricklayer's daughter supplied the roasted apples for Thomas Bunbury's 'low' diet following his thigh wound in 1813; he summarised 'nothing could exceed the kindness of this poor creature'.[76] In recuperation, Charles Kinloch was billeted upon a Portuguese family who 'paid me as much attention as if I had been their own son'.[77] A supposition of fictive kinship was presumably important to the men who, in extremis, called out to their mothers for aid.[78] This literature lionised the voluntary care of one person for another. Whether it was a 'Portuguese gentleman' who brought drinking chocolate and biscuits to the wounded in the streets, Dutch villagers who scraped together a few provisions for the wounded in transit, or the Spanish landlady who loosened bandages when called in the night, the patients were touched by and grateful for the expression of unforced compassion.[79]

All such spontaneous assistance contrasted with stories of off-the-cuff exaction of wilful harm upon the wounded and dying, considered at length by Gavin Daly.[80] 'Anti-nurse' narratives in this vein were used by British writers to expand their existing racial stereotyping of the Spanish and Portuguese allies as unmanly and cowardly in battle, and generally uncommitted to the cause of their own liberation, to encompass brutality as well.[81] The Spanish soldiers, guerrilla fighters, and observing civilians were all noted for their cruelty to the French after any military engagements, including their butchering of the wounded.[82] These were actions that British authors were generally keen to deprecate. Captain George Bowles felt himself obliged to save wounded Frenchmen after the Battle of Talavera from the risk of being murdered by the Spanish who proved 'beyond measure astonished at being prevented'.[83] The Spanish people who acted in this way were supposedly reacting to the French invasion of 1808, and to the imposition of Napoleon's brother Joseph in substitution for their own monarch, and were not open to dissuasion. John Mills found himself in conversation with a Spanish soldier who had allegedly assisted in the murder of sixteen cartloads of wounded Frenchmen after the Battle of Fuentes d'Onoro: 'Instead of being ashamed of it, he considered it as a great feat; nor could I persuade him that the situation of a wounded man differed materially from another.'[84] It seems that the Spanish periodically assumed the anti-nurse position by design, for the purpose of revenge.

Portuguese people were presumed to be similarly motivated by their experience of French occupation from late 1807 to 1808 and by their opposition to the French military annexation of Spain, such that they too were reported as committing brutal reprisals including stoning to death.[85] Consequently, French soldiers feared murder at the hands of Portuguese brigands, and preferred to place confidence in their English opponents for care, although any accounts in this strain by English memoirists may well have been inflated by a desire to promote an image of English graciousness in victory.[86] These depredations sometimes had specific reference to masculine identity. A German ally of the British reported a form of torture enacted by the Portuguese on the French, which involved nailing them alive to barn doors, emasculating them, and placing the severed penises in the victims' mouths.[87]

In contrast to these perceptions of allies as extravagantly violent, the French were pretty uniformly described by British authors as brave in combat and generous to their defeated opponents.[88] When wounded, the French and English soldiers might well be attended in the same premises by the same personnel, apparently without rancour and with generosity or even friendship.[89] Consequently English soldiers were reticent about their own behaviour in the anti-nurse mould, although some do exist.[90] Instead their accounts underline the spontaneous compassion that they delivered or witnessed from their comrades, to draw lines of distinction between rapacious foes and the humane British.[91] William Wheeler's account is unusual in deriving from military action in the Netherlands as late as 1809, but was prolix (rather than otherwise out of line with parallel narratives) in his patriotic admiration about care for the enemy's wounded:

> Amidst all this pain and misery, it is delightful to see the very same soldiers, who an hour before were dealing destruction about them, tendering all the assistance in their power to a fallen enemy. What a boast to belong to such a country.[92]

This pattern of commentary on anti-nursing, or its repudiation, cannot be explained by crude allegiance to congregationalism, as the French, Spanish, and Portuguese were all Catholic while the English, German, and other allied forces were chiefly Protestant. Instead there was a British discourse of national difference that expressed preconceptions of the 'superstitious, dirty, and backward Portuguese national character', and a perception of Spain as a much-diminished power 'some century's behind England in everything' in contrast to France as a 'civilised' nation.[93] British critiques contained a classist element in relation to armies' leadership, with the assumption that Spanish officers were little above the country's peasantry in terms of education and culture.[94] This suggests that, to move beyond the rationales for responses to violence offered by Gavin Daly, and aligning with analyses by Catriona Kennedy, the anti-nurse was an additional device for the consolidation of British masculinity by dint of horrified observation of cruelty carried out by others.

Organised care by nurses and orderlies

The earliest regulations for English military nursing were probably devised in 1644 in relation to the Parliamentary forces of the English Civil War. These prioritised soldiers' wives, which von Arni optimistically interprets to mean that the women recruited for nursing purposes were accustomed to discipline and used to taking the initiative.[95] Army nurses were urged to be kindly adherents of Christian morality, and were subject to penalties for inadequate attention or displays of bad temper, yet were given latitude over their areas of presumed expertise including over cooking equipment.[96] The concentrated and distinctive nature of military nursing during the 1640s, whereby men might have fought quite close to home and where the presence of wives was not limited by the difficulties of overseas travel, means that nurses' service was probably quite different in the civil wars when compared with later continental European experiences.

Army nurses in the eighteenth century were not necessarily subject to any finer formal regulations, but they were recruited according to local arrangements. In the hospital at Oosterhout established to meet military needs in the War of the Austrian Succession, the nurses were given clear, written instructions (which coincidentally strongly suggests they were selected for literacy). The accompanying 'rules' for nurses did not have the status of regulations: they did make clear the timetable for serving meals and the importance of following orders.[97] Nurses accustomed to such a routine would have been an asset. During the Seven Years War, for example, Colonel John Cosnan in Portugal gave tacit confirmation to the idea that the army valued women with experience of nursing in its hospitals, over and above the generic skills of a soldier's wife.[98] This means that when army physician Donald Monro published his *Observations on the Means of Preserving the Health of Soldiers* in 1780 his topic was not without precedent but clearly required elaboration in relation to care. Even so, Monro's ambitious list of requirements for nurse behaviour and activity in military hospitals was not adopted.[99]

British army regulations relating to nursing by women issued from the 1790s onwards were very limited as well.[100] In regimental hospitals women were to cook, administer medicines, and assist with the laundry, but were somewhat interchangeable with male orderlies.[101] In the regulations governing general hospitals their work was barely described, although both nurses and orderlies were asked 'to take care to have always in the respective Wards, gruel and panado, with such other drinks as may be ordered for the Patients, ready during both night and day'.[102] The intake of nourishing fluids was clearly a priority, no matter who was doing the caring. Consequently, Erin Spinney judges female nursing as 'important but not essential' to the army's conception of care.[103]

Regulations relating to orderly men were a little more precise than the equivalents for women, if only because they specified, for example, the need to recruit one orderly to every eight hospital patients.[104] Orderly men were supposed to empty bedpans immediately after use, and sweep/scrape the floors every morning in an echo of the discussions of dirty work in Chapters 3 and 5 above.[105] Also in line with the rules for provincial infirmaries, military patients were supposed to assist the nurses and orderlies if able to do so in the same ways as their non-combatant peers, namely in making beds, cleaning wards, and helping fellow patients.[106]

General hospitals were established by the British in Portugal between 1807 and 1814 at major centres of population such as Abrantes or (more usually) on or near the coast for convenience of access to transport such as in Oporto, Coimbra, and Lisbon. Hospital capacity at Coimbra in February 1812 included space in the Convent of Francisco (holding four hundred wounded) and the College of Arts (holding one thousand).[107] Smaller, temporary hospitals were opened in response to the locations covered by troops and near to the sites of battle.

As was the case for spontaneous nursing, there is scant information about the women who were paid to nurse in military hospitals in the works of male writers.[108] Those accounts that survive observe the stereotypes for domestic nurses as either ideal, or conversely as morally dubious. John Malcolm, a prisoner of the French while in hospital in Toulouse in 1814, reported two different experiences of female attention which illustrate these polarities: first he was stripped and put to bed by two nurses 'without any coy delays, or the slightest attempt at a blush'.[109] He clearly interpreted the women's business-like approach to his nakedness as brazen rather than as evidence of nursing experience. Second he was embraced by a hospital visitor who he remembered years later as a 'ministering angel'.[110] One moment of compassion proved more memorable than the two nurses' physical service (service moreover rendered suspect for Malcolm by the women's lack of embarrassment). John Cooper, in contrast, only remembered being neglected by a woman in a temporary hospital at Villa Vicosa, even though he had given her some small loaves.[111]

Paul Kopperman has assumed that during the American Revolutionary War nursing duty was disliked by soldiers' wives if it separated them from their husbands, and when it exposed them to contagion or injury.[112] Such exposure was a genuine risk in this later period: a wife to a serjeant in the 82nd Regiment who was a nurse on William Wheeler's ward in the hospital at Fontarabia in 1814 reputedly pricked her finger on a bandage pin, suffered amputation of her hand, and even then died.[113] The reluctance of women who were officially present with the army 'on the strength' to volunteer as hospital nurses was palpable in 1809, towards the conclusion of the disastrous Walcheren campaign, when they were apparently threatened with loss of rations if they refused to take on nursing duty.[114]

A much more detailed appreciation of the nurses' lives (if not of their nursing work) is supplied by Catherine Exley of Batley in Yorkshire.[115] She was the wife of Joshua Exley, a foot soldier in the 34th Regiment, who was given permission to accompany her husband to Portugal during the summer of either 1809 or 1810. Hers was the life of an ordinary working woman who possessed no resource in adversity. When left on her own for example – in the early years of their marriage Joshua was sent to Madeira without his wife – she returned to Batley and gave birth to her first child in the parish workhouse. It is interesting to note that she used no synonyms for stigma about her need for Poor Law assistance, nor did she identify any meanness on the part of the parish authorities, reporting instead that 'every comfort was afforded me'.[116]

Her life in Portugal was similarly impoverished but more distressing. Her little boy sickened, so she sewed together some clothes and stuffed them with straw to serve as a mattress for him. The child died (the first of three Exley infants to expire overseas) and it was only owing to the kindness of other soldiers that she was able to afford a burial (her husband Joshua being on manoeuvres). At her second experience of childbirth she relied again on the charity of fighting men for accommodation, food, textiles, and resources for the midwife. A subsequent fit of illness occasioned a collapse, when the wife of a corporal ensured she was 'attended night and day until

I could move about', while a further medical crisis (catching fever from her husband) entailed her being taken to 'the house set apart for the women' near to the general hospital at Abrantes.[117] She was thus known to have been the recipient of care, in both spontaneous and organised ways, which was perhaps a factor influencing the manner of her later delivery of nursing. This is also a lone shred of evidence that the army's temporary hospital arrangements could accommodate wives as well as soldiers.[118]

The fact of Catherine Exley's working as a nurse is mentioned in just a few short lines. She was a nurse under her husband who had been appointed as a hospital ward master, apparently in a temporary hospital a little before (and in close proximity to) the Battle of Albuera in May 1811. In this post she took care of the sick and managed the provisions, until maternity and illness again deprived her of the ability to work. She was then employed one-to-one as the nurse of an adjutant's wife until she caught the same illness as her patient. Thereafter her life following the regiment in Spain proved one of near constant mobility, requiring the giving and receiving of assistance to prevent or ameliorate injury. In this way the detail of Exley's account suggests that the line between female English nurses and female English patients in Portugal and Spain was non-existent. To be an ordinary woman in the train of the army was to be both a carer and an object of care, in formal and informal ways.

The male orderlies appointed to hospitals were stereotyped as neglectful, self-serving, or actively cruel.[119] William Brown's experience of the hospital at Coimbra in 1809 and/or 1810 therefore followed this pattern in describing the orderlies as inattentive to the medical superintendent's orders 'so that the sick were often left to shift from themselves … they whose duty it was to administer to our comfort, were as callous to our sufferings as if they had been enemies'.[120] Worse was reported by the men who suffered specific loses to orderlies, as when clothes and haversacks were stolen, or where orderlies were reported as the perpetrators or colluders of murder.[121] Close inspection of multiple memoirs, however, offers a more variegated picture of competence and kindness.[122] When recovering from a wound in 1794, John Stevenson of the Guards fell ill while in hospital in France. He was removed to a fever ward where he thought himself 'well attended to ... I had nothing to complain of in that respect' at the hands of male nurses who had chiefly been recruited from among German prisoners of war.[123] John Douglas took the view that the Irishman who attended him in the hospital at Celorico 'behaved like a brother'.[124] A Spanish orderly at a hospital at Valladolid was singled out by Johann Maempel for specific praise, since he 'nursed me with the greatest care ... he often made my bed five times in a day'.[125] Painstaking attention could be contingent on shared history. An anonymous Scotsman treated at the hospital in Deal in 1809 discovered that his hospital orderly was a fellow Glaswegian. The orderly went on to display 'the utmost kindness and solicitude ... because I drew my breath first among a certain heap of stones'.[126]

There were never enough men to treat the high numbers of wounded after each major battle, and some of the injured were sufficiently objective to attribute the slow attention paid to them to the number of men who were in a worse condition.[127] William Swabey estimated that there were 'two hundred probably having only one hospital mate to dress their wounds or minister to their diseases'.[128] Orderlies were equally thin on the ground, and unlike medical men their duties did not cease when patients died: at Celorico in the summer of 1811 'The hospital orderlies were exhausted by attending, burying, and clearing away the dead.'[129]

Such men as there were suffered additional negative stereotyping, since there was a widespread assumption that hospital orderlies recruited from among the lightly wounded soldiers on campaign were 'shirkers' who took hospital posts to avoid battle.[130] This presumption of cowardice is problematic because service as an orderly was not a guarantee that a man would not come under fire, and the conditions of service in a hospital were grim.[131] Memoirists and diarists referred with horror to the pile of limbs which built up outside a hospital, and to the cries of the patients waiting for amputation, which they characterised as worse than the sights and sounds of mutilation encountered during the heat of battle.[132] The smell of infected wounds was reputedly revolting.[133] Furthermore, the work was emotionally draining. Friedrich Lindau worked in the hospital at Hamelin alongside his father and mother following their town's surrender to the French in November 1806. They attended

Prussians and French wounded alike. Lindau's self-approval for attentive care is not to be relied upon, but his narrative is notable for the authenticity of detail by which he characterised 'the horrors of the hospital'.[134] He worked among the dying, who gasped, prayed, and screamed while he tried to dispense medicine, tea, and restraint for the feverish.

Against these immediate penalties of hospital service were the longer-term risks of constant exposure to illness and injury. Colour Serjeant George Calladine was made an orderly to a hospital in in 1817 (coincidentally in Ceylon rather than any of the European theatres of war: his writing is included here for the rarity value of an orderly's diary). Calladine found the situation quite profitable in financial terms but it took its toll on his health: 'I was getting completely wearied of my situation ... I found my health continually declining by being so much among the sick and having such bad sores to dress. I began to lose my appetite.'[135] Yet he found he could not simply declare an intention to resign the duty. He had to be caught doing something categorically wrong so, after a ten-month stint in the hospital, he intentionally got drunk and refused to attend when the doctor summoned him.[136] This earned his discharge to guard duty and suggests that the 'bad' behaviour of other orderlies or in different hospitals might be attributed to their desire to get away from the hospital environment and to return to active service.

The final group of people who were effectively paid to care were the male servants of army officers. These men were generally viewed favourably. George Simmons' servant Henry Short 'took great care of me', making Simmons 'as easy and comfortable as a forlorn bedridden person could be in a strange land'.[137] Charles Crowe's 'man' Barney Bradley assisted Crowe to staunch haemorrhaging.[138] This sort of caring service was no sinecure, though, since servants could also fall ill and require hospitalisation.[139] George Wood's servant, the evocatively named Thomas Standfast, died.[140]

In sum, paid nursing by women was ubiquitous and largely unnoticed, while attitudes to paid nursing by men were differentiated somewhat by the status and expectations of the commentator. There was an undercurrent in all of these narratives of the role of emotion work which was desired by patients yet apparently missing from any care which was not spontaneous or freely given. John Cooper, incidentally a gloomy commentator throughout, wrote that having 'no one to care a straw for me' was 'worst of all'.[141] At this time, medical voices started to intimate that perhaps female attention to the wounded soldier was superior to male, and that women should be charged with the 'chief care' of the sick.[142] Such opinions seem to have had little impact before 1820, but their presence shows that thinking along these lines predated conflict in the Crimea.

Women, men, and trauma

Earlier chapters in this book have discussed the risks to those who nursed. In the context of domestic nursing in Chapter 1, these were characterised as including exhaustion from sleeplessness, revulsion, and guilt. For the institutional nurses of provincial infirmaries, Chapter 3 considered challenges to the five senses and the contribution of 'dirty work' to their vexed social position, while men who nursed in Chapter 5 left infrequent but telling clues about the ways that care impinged on their sense of self. These all have their parallels for the women and men who nursed in wartime, with the additional palpable risk of their care work inducing a form of trauma in them.[143]

There is historiographical contest over the detection of trauma in people before the word and its associated experiences were codified by psychology professionals.[144] Even so, Donna Trembinski has argued that the words which were available to historical actors in the medieval and early modern periods to signify mental distress, namely mania and melancholia, contain sufficient similarities with the modern diagnosis to justify the periodic identification of trauma victims in the distant past.[145] Subsequent work has emphasised that is not necessary or wise to attempt retrodiagnoses on the basis of criteria devised by twentieth-century psychology; at the same time it is patronising to assume that pervasive exposure to violence in the past inured people to mental injury.[146] It is possible, nonetheless, to consider people's exposure to war in terms of 'how they experienced it and how they dealt with it' without falling into either of these ontological traps.[147] The psychological distress arising from participation in the Seven Years War (1756–63) has been characterised as 'emotional turmoil ... without a framework' in a context where personal emotional expression was discouraged.[148] Wartime trauma in an era before diagnostic sophistication is perhaps best defined as 'war-induced mental impairment' or, in the words of one sufferer during the English Civil War, 'distraction'.[149]

There is literary evidence that 'contemporary perceptions of war trauma ... were present within the publications of the period', and authors of wartime narratives were certainly not oblivious to the risk of something akin to trauma, if only to others.[150] William Lawrence's memoir, for instance, wondered whether recovery from the consequences of war was possible, saying in relation to the Portuguese civilians 'It must have taken years to get over the misery and grief, if they ever did.'[151] The sources used in this chapter do not tend, however, to contain direct evidence of the authors' own severe distress. They do not report that they wept or gave other physical signs of mental disturbance, and sometimes claimed that their feelings had hardened in response to scenes of battle, dismemberment, and decapitation.[152] They did invoke synonyms that might flag psychological pain when they expressed horror at the physical carnage of war or profound pity for the loss of life. Some of their feelings, akin to alienation from others rather than self, were perhaps channelled into rejection of any anti-nurse behaviour (noticed above).

Philip Shaw has detailed the use of 'nostalgia' to indicated soldiers' mental suffering.[153] Aside from such substitutions, Catriona Kennedy has also observed the wilful excision of detail from wartime narratives that she labels the 'inexpressibility motif'.[154] This is a good fit for Haddy James, for example, a surgeon treating the wounded in a house at the rear of a battle, who felt 'it was all too horrible to commit to paper'.[155] Trauma by its modern definition is a blanket term for something that 'cannot be expressed adequately in language'.[156] This is naturally unhelpful for historians who depend on texts, and is at odds with a supposed use of written correspondence, for example, to process psychological suffering.[157] Any supposition of trauma experienced by the women and men who cared for the sick and wounded during the years 1793 to

1815 must therefore remain speculative, albeit within a suggestive context and based on an extensive roster of reading.

In particular, a reconsideration of the stereotypes for camp-followers and hospital orderlies respectively through an awareness of the potential for trauma-like distress is valuable. If we assume that exposure to extreme violence and suffering, as either a perpetrator, a witness, or a victim, could feasibly cause something akin to (or a precursor of) modern 'trauma', then we might expect to find symptoms of it in outliers of behaviour or expression. These are categorised for modern analyses under the headings of intrusion (including unwanted thoughts), avoidance (such as evasion of responsibilities), and arousal (meaning a form of over-stimulation).[158] Under the heading of arousal, for example, not everyone who is irritable or who behaves compulsively has previously been traumatised, but irritation out of place, or addictive patterns of consumption, may still be important markers. Similarly callous behaviour could arise either as a habitual personality trait or as the side effect of numbed emotions in a way that might reasonably predate the modern labelling of compassion fatigue. For context, exposure to traumatised patients in the twentieth and twenty-first centuries had mental health impacts on healthcare workers: even if they did not undergo the same experiences, empathy risked 'vicarious traumatization' or 'secondary traumatic stress'.[159]

Numerous commentators for the period 1793 to 1815 reported that the aftermath or evidence of battle was shocking, much worse than engagement in fighting, providing scenes of horror without parallel, beyond description, and even beyond imagining.[160] The knowledge that some of the wounded could not be helped other than by murder meant that ordinary soldiers who were not capable of committing acts of euthanasia fled because 'We could not bear it.'[161] Yet this was the human context of labour for those dealing with the wounded, requiring 'incessant attendance of the most painful nature' whether in the 'loathsome wards of a hospital' or elsewhere.[162] Lieutenant William Hay summed up the difference between fighting and its aftermath as witnessed at a convent-turned-hospital: 'Seeing suffering on the field of battle, where all are alike exposed and actively engaged, is nothing compared with this, which made me feel quite sick.'[163] If these events had taken place in the twentieth century, researchers might have sought to confirm the presence of psychological distress among care workers by reference to nightmares or flashbacks, work avoidance, numbed emotions, compulsive behaviour, symptoms of arousal such as hypervigilance, or impairment of functioning. Research by survey is not open to historians: observation of indicative behaviour is the closest alternative. A tiny cohort of the writers described nightmares or other forms of intrusive thought in themselves at the time or subsequently to their military service.[164] This does not mean that others definitively did not experience such things, or that their accounts lack reference to any of the relevant indicators. Indeed, in the light of modern understandings of trauma, women's apparent display of hard-hearted and self-centred actions in, for example, plundering the dead, is possibly a symptom of their distress. Similarly for male orderlies 'skulking' and displays of neglect or cruelty to the wounded are congruent with a heightened sense of vulnerability, emotional distance, and aggression, a sense of being victimised by clients, and such behaviours are directly indicative of work avoidance, all the symptoms of modern 'burnout'.[165] Under these circumstances the drunken orderly potentially becomes an exemplar of trauma-inspired compulsive behaviour.[166] Edward Costello offers a brief vignette of the alcoholic hospital orderly, incidentally in years before alcohol addiction was medically recognised. After the Battle of Salamanca in 1812 Michael Connelly, who was slightly wounded, was appointed as a hospital serjeant. According to Costello he was, unusually, 'exceedingly attentive to the sick' but 'drank like a whale'.[167] Connelly consumed wine rations of any dying or dead patients until he 'drank himself out of the world', dying 'like a beast'. Historians of nursing would so far have written off Connelly as an inadequate carer owing to frequent intoxication: he might better be characterised as another type of combat victim.

Given the uncertainties involved, this narrative survey does not conclusively 'find' trauma in this period, much less diagnose anyone retrospectively, but does offer trauma as one component of an explanation for negative nurse stereotypes. If this line of thinking is right, historians possess a new way to incorporate evidence of callous or harmful actions of nurses and orderlies into a reappraisal of their work.

Waterloo, Brussels, and the pre-reform 'lady' nurse[168]

The inhabitants of Brussels were demonstrably not the first in the wars of 1793 to 1815 to nurse people to whom they were not related, and without recompense. What was novel about the days after the battles of Quatre Bras on 16 June and Waterloo on 18 June in 1815 was the concentration of medical and nursing effort within a relatively small geographical compass, the vast numbers of men wounded, and the pervasive eagerness of civilians to offer help. This did not mean that the wounded of Waterloo received sufficient attention to their wants: commentators confirm that it took five days to clear the battlefield, and that lives were certainly lost as a result.[169] The wounded lay unattended, or were the further victims of 'cruel handling' as plunderers stripped the dead and wounded alike of their clothes and other belongings; Prussian patrols (but allegedly not British) shot both their own men and French soldiers who were deemed so badly injured as to be irrecoverable.[170] Once in Brussels, however, the wounded were treated with as much care and effectual humanitarianism as was possible, by townspeople rapidly swamped by injured soldiers.

Official 'hospital' style accommodation in hastily requisitioned churches and other large structures ran out immediately. Inhabitants therefore took both officers and rank-and-file soldiers into their own homes; 'the people opened their houses, which literally became hospitals'.[171] 'There was hardly a door without a number, showing how many were lodged within.'[172] 'In the greater number there were not fewer than four, six, or eight'.[173] A family in the Place de Louvain were said to have 'received and tended no less than fifty wounded Englishmen'.[174] Elizabeth Ord, an English woman in Brussels, wrote her own account in addition to the more famous one by her stepfather Thomas Creevey.[175] She described how 'we had five badly wounded Prussian common soldiers billeted upon us at 12 o'clock that night [18 June] and as we have no outbuildings we were obliged to lay them on the floor of our dining room, it was so late we could get no straw for them or could do anything but feed them.'[176] The recipients of this attention were aware of the generous spirit in which house-room was offered. Friedrich Lindau, a rifleman in the King's German Legion who had suffered a bullet wound to the back of the head, recalled 'I was treated in a very friendly way by my hosts', even though he remembered being in a lot of pain at the time.[177] Eventually even household accommodation was exhausted, and hundreds of men were laid in the streets on straw, whether under canvas or in the open, on every spare patch of ground.[178]

Most notable in this chaotic environment was the gender and social standing of the people offering practical and comfort or emotion work reported by multiple observers.[179] Captain Thomas Hobbs noticed largesse from 'People of the first rank' while Frances D' Arblay pointed out that 'M. de Beaufort, being far the richest of my friends at this place ... had officers and others quartered upon him without mercy.'[180] Lieutenant James Hope recalled 'Many of the most respectable ladies in Brussels stood all day at the gate by which the wounded entered, and to each soldier, as they arrived, distributed wine, tea, coffee, soup, bread, and cordials of various kinds.'[181] John Davy reported 'The most delicately brought up women, and persons of all ranks were occupied in this way.'[182] The houses of the 'best' families were open, and the ladies busy 'attending and dressing their wounds and nursing them like their own children'.[183] Ladies also left their homes to deliver succour: 'ladies of the highest rank were not ashamed to traverse from hospital to hospital in the dead hour of night and employ their persons and property in this work of humanity'.[184] Richard Henegan, an army commissary, claimed that ladies 'took upon themselves to assist the surgeons in their painful duties'.[185] A young female member 'of one of the first families in Brussels' dressed the wound of a serjeant-major despite having a cut on her finger, and 'her life very nearly paid the forfeit of her humanity' owing to infection.[186]

Some authors moved from general praise to specific examples. Rifleman Lieutenant George Simmons was quartered on the 'very respectable' Mr Overman, a German merchant and banker, in May 1815, and returned to the Overman house on the Rue de l' Etoile after Waterloo apparently with a fatal wound; he had been shot through the liver and was told he could not survive.[187] It is not clear whether Simmons was nursed by a daughter or a servant of the house, but whoever the young woman was she won sentimental gratitude from Simmons. He wrote just a month later: 'My dear little nurse has never been ten minutes from me since I came to the house ... For ten nights together she never went to bed, but laid her head on my pillow.'[188] The ladies of the house supported him definitively and apparently physically in September, when he was sufficiently recovered to go out with them for a walk 'which amused the people that passed'.[189] Years later, in an additional memoir written for the benefit of his son, Simmons claimed that before Waterloo, Overman had instructed him to return to the house if wounded '& my wife & daughter will be proud to nurse you'. Here he confirmed that 'one or other of the family never left me, night or day, until I was out of danger', suggesting that the 'dear little nurse' had in fact been one of Overman's daughters Julia, Harriett, or Eulalie.[190] Simmons provides a rare instance of a writer with a double voice, who both experiences and remembers their experience.[191]

Among the memoirists, if not always the letter and journal writers, there was clearly some retrospective idealisation of the women who offered assistance, in both the short and the long term: 'the softest hands in each house smoothed the couch of the agonised warrior' wrote literary editor John Scott sentimentally, as early as 1816.[192] William Pitt Lennox, who was a young cornet at the time of the battle, later rhapsodised 'Beautiful as woman is in all the charities of life, never does she appear so pre-eminently beautiful as in the chamber of sickness or death', but forbore to reveal the identity of any of the Brussels 'ministering angels' for fear of their blushes.[193] It is important to position Lennox's comments in particular in the wider chronology of the nineteenth century, given that his memoir was first published in 1864, during the high period of nursing reform 1855–85: he may have been writing in the knowledge of Florence Nightingale's reputation and her recommendations for nurse activity, thereby allowing his later understanding of nursing to infiltrate his memory of earlier lady nurses.

Furthermore, the broader view of activity in Brussels somewhat qualifies the picture of 'humane and indefatigable exertions' to admit that generosity was not *entirely* unstinting.[194] The Ord-Creevey household, for example, perceived limits to what the inhabitants could offer its temporary military guests. As soon as their billeted soldiers had been fed, an additional servant was hired to wash the men and make them comfortable until both men and mattresses could be removed to space in a church.[195] Author Charlotte Waldie confessed that she purposefully did not act the nurse, when she might readily have done so. She excused herself on the grounds that she did not think it safe for 'ladies' to bind wounds, and thereby planted a seed in the imaginations of her very many British readers: tacitly, lady nurses would have been even more prevalent if they had been competent or, in other words, trained.[196]

But the consistency of accounts across different genres of personal writing confirms that, rosy retrospectives aside, the attention paid to the wounded was largely indiscriminate, delivered by ordinary women and ladies alike, and carried with it elements of what would come to be seen, fifty years later, as a Nightingale-style ideal of nursing.[197] For example: a young woman of approximately 18 was allegedly observed dispensing hot and cold refreshments. 'She moved along with an eye of lightening, glancing about for those whom she thought most in need of her assistance'. On encountering a Highlander with an injured thigh

> she knelt at his side, and gently moving aside his blood-stained kilt, commenced washing the wounded part; the Scotchman seemed uneasy at her importunity. But with the sweetest voice imaginable, she addressed him in English with 'Me no ashamed of you – indeed I will not hurt you! And the wounded man, ere he could recover his rough serenity, found his wound bandaged, and at ease, under the operations of this fair attendant.[198]

The unnamed woman combined the keen observational skill, lack of fuss or embarrassment, and clear soothing voice, recommended by Nightingale a generation or two later, but without the author writing in full knowledge of the nursing reform movement, since his memoirs were first published in 1841.[199]

This near ubiquity of nursing activity among the inhabitants of Brussels was not explicitly inspired by any role models, such as the Sisters of Charity, although it probably owed some debt to the different social context for nursing on the continent: Catholic nursing Sisterhoods were common there, and ensured that nursing did not carry the same association with women's proximity to material (and spiritual) poverty as was the case in Britain. Similarly, it is possible that the nursing energies displayed in Brussels had some origins in the customary largesse of wealthy women towards the poor. Part of the explanation certainly lies in the sheer number of wounded and the relatively short distance between the battlefield and the amenities of Brussels. One estimate of 23 June 1815 put the number of wounded in Brussels at 22,000.[200] Additional factors include the localised collapse of social barriers: Waldie describes such uncertainty and trepidation in Brussels until the decisive announcement of the Allies' victory that all ranks spoke to each other regardless of former social divisions in order to obtain news. Furthermore, 18 June 1815 was a 'day of horror' for the inhabitants of Brussels, so their gratitude that their defenceless city had been spared, and not overrun by either of the opposing armies, was made concrete.[201] Combine these high-stakes emotions with a recent history of relatively light or comparatively amiable experience of housing billeted soldiers in the months preceding the Battle of Waterloo and the humane, sometimes emotional, Belgian reaction to what was in front of their eyes becomes more readily comprehensible. Military men had grown 'from lodgers to be acquaintances, from acquaintances companions, and from companions friends'.[202] The former hosts of Thomas Hobbs wept when he was returned to them wounded after Quatre Bras, suggesting that they were engaged in emotional work as well as physical care (or perhaps they were just overwrought, as Waterloo had not then been fought).[203] Basil Jackson ascribed this to Christian charity (among the Catholic Belgians), and as a tribute to the character of the soldiers who had earned the good opinions of city folk before Napoleon's final period of military activity.[204] Contemporary George Walton detected a scintilla of friendly competition when he recalled 'it seemed as if the inhabitants vied with each other in their zeal and activity to administer to the wants of the sufferers'.[205] Doubtless Elaine Scarry would add that the function of soldiers' suffering – to confer reality and authority on state conflict – had the auxiliary effect of drawing in Belgian observers as spontaneous participants in the memorialisation of the battle.[206] The scale of injury precluded a recourse to mass stoicism, which so often proved the alleged choice of the individual soldier, so the next best response to such widespread distress, loss, grief, and bewilderment was generous sympathy: tending to specific wounds contributed to the healing of the body politic.[207]

The humanitarian response *avant la lettre* to the wounded of Waterloo was referenced throughout the first half of the nineteenth century. This was achieved at first in piecemeal form, with the sporadic publication of military memoirs or documents, and of eyewitness accounts, rather than retrospective histories. *The Battle of Waterloo, containing the accounts published by authority, British and Foreign, and other relative documents, with circumstantial details, previous and after the battle* ran to at least seven editions in 1815 alone.[208] The quantity of material made available was such that, by 1830, the *Monthly Review* 'suggested that the British reading public must be in possession of everything there could be to know' about the wars after 1808.[209] The quality of wartime memoirs improved too, particularly from the mid-1820s, when some volumes took on novelistic qualities.[210]

Two of the most significant publications in terms of the Waterloo literature, and emphatic in their capacity for memorialisation, were those written by women. Charlotte Eaton (née Waldie) first published a description of her days in Brussels in 1817, and her volume was reissued in the early 1850s. Waldie's account is written in elegiac mode, where all participants were blessed with retrospective glory: 'every private soldier acted like a hero'.[211] She was therefore inclined to idealise the whole affair, but this does not make her claims about Belgian generosity and humanity any less significant in terms of their cultural purchase.[212] Another literary heroine's perspective was revealed when Frances Burney's diaries were released in successive volumes from 1841 onwards, with the entries dealing with 1815 published in 1846. Burney dwelled on the same events as Waldie at less length, but with more personal investment in the scenes around her.[213]

Therefore when William Makepeace Thackeray published his novel *Vanity Fair* in 1847–48, depicting incidents in the final conflict with Napoleon, the literary landscape was already well populated with contextual material.[214] Furthermore, as Catriona Kennedy has pointed out, in the novel 'the entire campaign is filtered through the experiences of the women left behind in Brussels'.[215] The actions of Amelia Osborne and Mrs O'Dowd in caring for Tom Stubble at their hotel in Brussels consolidated the images of genteel and prosperous women tending to the wounded. The two woman 'watched incessantly by the wounded lad' who had received a spear in the leg at Quatre Bras on 16 June, and in doing so proved their bravery when 'the cannon of Waterloo began to roar'.[216] Amelia's brother Jos Sedley leaves the city to a commentary of sarcasm from Mrs O'Dowd, and Mrs Becky Crawley makes a calculated decision to stay for her own potential advancement; but the two self-appointed nurses (both staunch for their combatant husbands, as well as attending the hapless Stubble) are selflessly immovable. Thackeray reminded his readers 'All of us have read of what occurred' at Waterloo, 'never tired of hearing and recounting the history of that famous action'.[217] The battle was additionally replete with famous consequences, including the response in Brussels. *Vanity Fair* drew together the existing narratives of Waterloo and assembled them in fictional form, and in doing so underscored both the emblematic significance of the battle for a generation and the scope for women as nurses at all social levels. In this way the events in Brussels in 1815 provided an early model for the lady nurse through the canon of literature they generated.

Conclusion

The presence and nursing actions of women who accompanied their soldier husbands overseas were typically glossed or omitted by the men who wrote memoirs, letters, and diaries about their wartime experiences. The women themselves did not have the capacity or inclination to match their male relatives in setting biographical accounts down on paper. Even Catherine Exley only wrote years later and described her life as a camp follower as a prefix to her spiritual awakening. Therefore, any evidence relating to female nurses in this context is hard won and difficult to verify. Only a woman notable for bravery first and nursing second, the Heroine of Matagorda, can have her career mapped sketchily from a patchwork of sources. This does not mean, however, that easy assumptions about women's inadequacy can be accepted. Thousands of women delivered nursing care without being singled out for bravery.

Women and men have been stereotyped for their faults as carers when it is necessary to ask, if not confirm, whether their exploitative behaviours were driven by trauma. The connection between trauma and alcohol suggested above provides a useful analogy for finding harm before the development of diagnostic terminology. Human bodies were clearly susceptible to inebriation before the word was coined: it is entirely possible for damage to have been caused by exposure to visual rather than oral intake. The hardhearted, hard-drinking nurses or orderlies were perhaps protecting or soothing themselves, a practice which we might now understand if not exonerate but which nurse reformers of the later nineteenth century (intent on the patient being put first) would be bound to abhor.

Most such criticisms are missing from accounts of Brussels after the Battle of Waterloo. Instead, the fighting men and observers alike depict a city temporarily oriented almost exclusively to care, regardless of gender, social, or national barriers. In this crisis, prosperous and high-status women found a time-limited calling to nursing, a vocation in miniature, that both preceded Florence Nightingale's insistence on the elevated motivations of lady nurses and laid down expectations for the emergence of that persistent ideal.

Notes

1 B.H. Liddell-Hart, *The Letters of Private Wheeler 1809–1828* (Moreton-in-Marsh: Windrush Press, 1999), p. 196.
2 For the military-fiscal state, see for example J. Brewer, *The Sinews of Power: War, Money and the English State, 1688–1783* (New York: Alfred A. Knopf, 1989); in relation to medical professionalisation see M. Ackroyd, *Advancing with the Army: Medicines, the Professions, and Social Mobility in the British Isles, 1790–1850* (Oxford: Oxford University Press, 2006).
3 The National Archives (hereafter NA), WO 97/652/53 Royal Hospital Chelsea soldiers' discharge papers for William Wheeler 1828; Liddell-Hart, *Wheeler*, p. 9. Before recruitment to the militia Wheeler was a mason's labourer: WO 96/277/372 Militia Attestation Papers for William Wheeler 1809.
4 NA HO 107 for the 1851 census of Walcot.

5 C. Kelly, *War and the Militarisation of British Army Medicine, 1793–1830* (London: Pickering and Chatto, 2011), p. 4.
6 For the first use of premier secours, see F.X. Becq, *Moyens Salutaires d'Administrer, en cas d'asphyxie, les premier secours que cet état exige* (Brussels: M.E. Ramplebergh, 1821).
7 P. Kopperman, *'Regimental Practice' by John Buchannan, MD: An Eighteenth-Century Medical Diary and Manual* (London: Routledge, 2016), p. 84.
8 L.M. Beier, *Sufferers and Healers: The Experience of Illness in Seventeenth-Century England* (London: Routledge & Kegan Paul, 1987), p. 238.
9 C. Spence, *Accidents and Violent Death in Early Modern London 1650–1750* (Woodbridge: Boydell, 2016), pp. 173–5.
10 S. Bradwell, *Helps for Suddain Accidents* (London: Thomas Purfoot, 1633).
11 For the application of a 'common' tourniquet see 'Particulars of the fate of Thomas Dowley', *Morning Post*, 30 June 1791; for the workings of a more complex 'screw' tourniquet see [A.], 'New patents lately enrolled', *Whitehall Evening Post*, 3–5 June 1800.
12 'Burns and scalds', *Oracle*, 27 October 1797.
13 B. Rodgers, *Cloak of Charity: studies in eighteenth-century philanthropy* (London: Methuen, 1949), pp. 10–11.
14 H. Nakao et al., 'A review of the history of the origin of triage from a disaster medicine perspective', *Acute Medicine and Surgery* 4: 4 (2017), 379–84, on p. 379.
15 J.A. Lynn II, *Women, Armies, and Warfare in Early Modern Europe* (Cambridge: Cambridge University Press, 2008), pp. 122–4 notices nursing briefly. E. Spinney, 'Women's work: Nurses, orderlies and the gendered division of care in Revolutionary and Napoleonic era British army hospitals', *Nursing History Review* 31 (2023), 127–49 is a welcome addition to the field.
16 E.G. von Arni, 'Who cared? Military nursing during the English Civil Wars and Interregnum, 1642–60', G. Hudson (ed.), *British Military and Naval Medicine* (Amsterdam: Rodopi, 2007).
17 E. Charters, 'The caring fiscal-military state during the Seven Years War, 1756–1763', *Historical Journal* 52: 4 (2009), 921–41.
18 P. Kopperman, 'Medical services in the British Army 1742–1783', *Journal of the History of Medicine* 34: 4 (1979), 428–55, on pp. 429–30.
19 H. Richardson, *English Hospitals 1660–1948: A Survey of their Architecture and Design* (Swindon: Royal Commission on the Historical Monuments of England, 1998), pp. 87–8.

20 Kopperman, 'Medical services', p. 436: D. Monro, *Observations on the Means of Preserving the Health of Soldiers; and of conducting Military Hospitals* (London: J. Murray and G. Robinson, 1780), volume I, pp. 121–4.
21 Kelly, *British Army Medicine*, p. 2.
22 Spinney, 'Women's work', p. 138.
23 R. Burnham and G. Glover, 'British memoirs of the Napoleonic Wars', http://www.napoleon-series.org/research/bibliographic/British Memoirs/c_british.html (accessed 5 November 2019).
24 Among a vast literature, see particularly P. Griffith (ed.), *Modern Studies of the War in Spain and Portugal, 1808–1814* (London: Greenhill, 1999), which comprises the supplementary volume IX of a modern edition of C. Oman, *History of the Peninsular War* (Oxford: Clarendon, 1902–30).
25 R. Lawson-Peebles, 'Style wars. The problems of writing military autobiography in the eighteenth century', A. Vernon (ed.), *Arms and the Self: War, the Military, and Autobiographical Writing* (Kent, OH: Kent State University Press, 2006), p. 65.
26 N. Ramsey, *The Military Memoir and Romantic Literary Culture, 1780–1835* (Abingdon: Routledge, 2016); C. Kennedy, *Narratives of the Revolutionary and Napoleonic Wars: Military and Civilian Experience* (Basingstoke: Palgrave Macmillan, 2013).
27 S. Monick (ed.), *The Iberian and Waterloo Campaigns: The letters of Lt James Hope (92nd (Highland) Regiment) 1811–1815* (Dallington: Naval & Military Press, 2000), pp. viii, xxiv.
28 S.D. Broughton, *Letters from Portugal, Spain & France 1812–1814* (Stroud: Nonsuch, 2005).
29 G. Glover (ed.), *A Scots Grey at Waterloo: The Remarkable Story of Sergeant William Clarke* (Barnsley: Frontline, 2017).
30 Ramsey, *Military Memoir*, p. 36.
31 Kennedy, *Narratives*, chapter 1, first section on 'writing and fighting'.
32 Ramsey, *Military Memoir*, pp. 176–7.
33 Vernon (ed.), *Arms and the Self: War, the Military, and Autobiographical Writing* (Kent, OH: Kent State University Press, 2006), p. 23.
34 M. Jolly, 'Myths of unity: Remembering the Second World War through letters and their editing', A. Vernon (ed.), *Arms and the Self: War, the Military, and Autobiographical Writing* (Kent, OH: Kent State University Press, 2006).
35 L. Bloom, 'Women's confinement as women's liberation: World War II civilian internees in South Pacific camps', A. Vernon (ed.), *Arms and*

the Self: War, the Military, and Autobiographical Writing (Kent, OH: Kent State University Press, 2006).
36 Lawson-Peebles, 'Style wars', p. 71.
37 Ramsey, *Military Memoir*, p. 18.
38 The list of works used is given as the 'Printed primary sources' section of the bibliography for this book.
39 Kennedy, *Narratives*, p. 75.
40 C. O'Neil, *The Military Adventures of Charles O'Neil* (Worcester, MA: Edward Livermore, 1851), p. 255; G. Glover (ed.), *The Diary of William Gavin Ensign and Quarter-Master of the 71st Highland Regiment, 1806–1815* (Godmanchester: Ken Trotman, 2013), p. 83.
41 P.E. Kopperman, 'The British high command and soldiers' wives in America, 1755–1783', *Journal of the Society for Army Historical Research* 60: 241 (1982), 14–34, on pp. 17–21; K. Wilson, *The Island Race* (London: Routledge, 2002), pp. 97–8, 104–5.
42 J. Brooks and C. Hallett (eds), *One Hundred Years of Wartime Nursing Practices, 1854–1953* (Manchester: Manchester University Press, 2015), p. 2; A. Summers, *Angels and Citizens: British Women as Military Nurses, 1854–1914* (London: Routledge, 1988).
43 A. Venning, *Following the Drum: The Lives of Army Wives and Daughters* (London: Headline, 2006), p. 195; N. St John Williams, *Judy O'Grady and the Colonel's Lady: The Army Wife and Camp Follower since 1660* (London: Brassey's Defence Publishers, 1988), p. 55.
44 *General Regulations and Orders for the Army* (London: W. Clowes, 1811) p. 255; G.R. Gleig, *The Subaltern* (Edinburgh: W. Blackwood and Sons, 1845) pp. 10–11 for a sentimental depiction of a woman balloted to remain behind.
45 Liddell-Hart, *Wheeler*, p. 99; J.S. Cooper, *Rough Notes of Seven Campaigns: 1809–1815* (Staplehurst: Spellmount, 1996), p. 117.
46 A.L.F. Schaumann, *On the Road with Wellington* (London: Greenhill, 1999), p. 130; J. Anton, *Retrospect of a Military Life* (Cambridge: Ken Trotman, 1991), pp. 116–17.
47 See [C. Leslie], *Military Journal of Colonel Leslie* (Aberdeen: Aberdeen University Press, 1887), p. 155 for women finding straw and a blanket, an unusual reference to ordinary women.
48 W.F.K. Thompson (ed.), *An Ensign in the Peninsular War: The Letters of John Aitchison* (London: Michael Joseph, 1994), p. 212; G. Glover (ed.), *John Westcott's Journal of the Campaign in Portugal* (Godmanchester: Ken Trotman, 2018), p. 39; J. Harley, *The Veteran, or 40 Years' Service in the British Army: The Scurrilous Recollections*

of *Paymaster John Harley 47th foot – 1798–1838* (Solihull: Helion, 2018), p. 215.
49 Kennedy, *Narratives*, p. 80; Lynn, *Women*, pp. 145–50.
50 British Dental Association Museum holdings include sets of 'Waterloo' teeth: www.bda.org/museum (accessed 15 December 2022).
51 G. Glover (ed.), *Campaigning in Spain and Belgium: The Letters of Captain Thomas Charles Fenton, 4th Dragoons & the Scots Greys 1809–15* (Huntingdon: Ken Trotman, 2010), pp. 34–5.
52 W. Tomkinson, *The Diary of a Cavalry Officer in the Peninsula and Waterloo Campaign 1809–1815* (London: S. Sonnenschein, 1894), p. 188.
53 Thompson, *John Aitchison*, p. 212.
54 For one very detailed account of nursing by a high-status wife, albeit following Waterloo, see M. De Lancey, *A Week at Waterloo* (London: Reportage Press, 2008). I discuss this text in some detail in A. Tomkins, 'Waterloo, Brussels, and developments in humanitarian nursing', *UK Association for the History of Nursing Bulletin* 8: 1 (2020).
55 Anton, *Retrospect*, p. 142.
56 Anton, *Retrospect*, p. 142.
57 J. Donaldson, *Scenes and Sketches of a Soldier's Life in Ireland* (Edinburgh: William Tait, 1826), pp. 186–7; T. Garretty, *Memoirs of a Sergeant Late in the Forty-Third Light Infantry Regiment Previously to and During the Peninsular War* (Cambridge: Ken Trotman; 1998), p. 79.
58 See Chapter 1.
59 J. Donaldson, *Recollections in the Eventful Life of a Soldier* (Philadelphia, PA: G.B. Zieber and Co., 1845), p. 79.
60 Donaldson, *Scenes and Sketches*, p. 189. She had sought the continuation of her husband's army pension, which was denied; 'Mrs Reston', *Chambers Miscellany* (1845), 17–26, on p. 24. For the efforts of other widows of ordinary soldiers to secure pensions, see J. Hurl-Eamon, *Marriage and the British Army in the Long Eighteenth Century* (Oxford: Oxford University Press, 2014), pp. 54–5.
61 'The heroine of Matagorda', *The Times*, 5 September 1843.
62 'Mrs Reston', p. 25.
63 See for example *Glasgow Herald*, 30 June 1854 and 19 November 1855.
64 Cooper, *Seven Campaigns*, p. 25.
65 This was also a feature of earlier conflicts; see Kopperman, *'Regimental Practice'*, p. 158.
66 Garretty, *Memoirs*, p. 159; S. Morley, *Memoirs of a Sergeant of the 5th Regiment of Foot* (Godmanchester: Ken Trotman, 1999), pp. 67, 75;

G. Glover (ed.), *Adventurous Pursuits of a Peninsular War & Waterloo Veteran: The Story of Private James Smithies 1st (Royal) Dragoons, 1807-15* (Godmanchester: Ken Trotman, 2011), p. 60; R.N. Buckley (ed.), *The Napoleonic War Journal of Captain Thomas Henry Browne, 1807-1816* (London: Bodley Head, 1987), p. 161; Schaumann, *On the Road*, pp. 191, 329; *Memoirs of a Sergeant Late in the 43rd Light Infantry Regiment* (London: John Mason, 1835), pp. 93, 159; C. Hibbert (ed.), *The Wheatley Diary: A Journal and Sketchbook kept during the Peninsular War and the Waterloo Campaign* (Moreton-in-Marsh: Windrush Press, 1997), p. 79; G. Simmons, *A British Rifle Man* (London: A.C. Black, 1899), pp. 78, 82, 93, 292-3; Glover, *William Gavin*, p. 97; E. Hathaway (ed.), *A Dorset Soldier: The Autobiography of Sgt William Lawrence 1790-1869* (Staplehurst: Spellmount, 1993), p. 67.

67 H. Furneaux, *Military Men of Feeling: Emotion, Touch, and Masculinity in the Crimean War* (Oxford: Oxford University Press, 2016), pp. 2, 16-18.

68 Simmons, *British Rifle Man*, p. 80; H. Jones, 'Seven Weeks Captivity in ST. Sebastian, in 1813', W. Maxwell, *Peninsular Sketches; by Actors on the Scene* (Cambridge: Ken Trotman, 1998), volume II, p. 307; S. Monick (ed.), *Douglas's Tale of the Peninsula and Waterloo 1808-15* (London: Leo Cooper, 1997), p. 87.

69 M. Sherer, *Recollections of the Peninsula* (London: Longman, 1824), p. 168.

70 W. Maxwell, *Peninsular Sketches; by Actors on the Scene* (Cambridge: Ken Trotman, 1998), volume II, p. 356.

71 J. Blakiston, *Twelve Years' Military Adventure in Three Quarters of the Globe* (London: Henry Colburn, 1840), volume II, pp. 257-8; R. Eadie, *On Campaign with the 79th (Cameron Highlanders) Through Portugal and Spain* (Darlington: Napoleonic Archive, 2006), p. 45; P. Hawker, *Journal of a Regimental Officer during the Recent Campaign in Portugal and Spain under Lord Viscount Wellington* (London: Ken Trotman, 1981), p. 127; A. Bamford (ed.), *Triumphs and Disasters: Eyewitness Accounts from the Netherlands Campaign, 1813-1814* (Barnsley: Frontline, 2016), p. 168; Simmons, *British Rifle Man*, p. 343.

72 Simmons, *British Rifle Man*, pp. 48, 120; E. Hathaway (ed.), *A True Soldier Gentleman: The Memoirs of Lt. John Cooke 1791-1813* (Swanage: Shinglepicker, 2000), p. 113.

73 [Leslie], *Military Journal*, p. 157.

74 R. Henegan, *Seven Years Campaigning in the Peninsula and the Netherlands, from 1808 to 1815* (London: Henry Colburn, 1846) volume I, p. 360.

75 G. Wood, *The Subaltern Officer: a narrative* (Godmanchester: Ken Trotman, 1986), p. 130 for a bed prepared by a 'very poor' Spanish widow.
76 T. Bunbury, *Reminiscences of a Veteran* (London: C.J. Skeet, 1861), volume I, p. 228.
77 G. Glover (ed.), *A Hellish Business: From the Letters of Captain Charles Kinloch 52nd Foot 1806–16* (Godmanchester: Ken Trotman, 2007), p. 98.
78 Simmons, *British Rifle Man*, p. 126.
79 W. Brown, *The Autobiography or Narrative of a Soldier: The Peninsular War Memoirs of William Brown of the 45th Foot* (Solihull: Helion, 2017), p. 57; E. O'Keeffe (ed.), *Narrative of the Eventful Life of Thomas Jackson, Militiaman and Coldstream Sergeant, 1803–15* (Solihull: Helion, 2018), p. 82; Blakiston, *Twelve Years*, volume II, pp. 257–8.
80 G. Daly, '"Barbarity more suited to savages": British soldiers' views of Spanish and Portuguese violence', *War & Society* 35: 4 (2016), 242–58.
81 C. Kennedy, 'John Bull into battle: Military masculinity and the British army officer during the Napoleonic wars', K. Hagemann and G. Mettele (eds), *Gender, War and Politics: Transatlantic Perspectives, 1775–1830* (Basingstoke: Palgrave Macmillan, 2010), pp. 139–40.
82 Simmons, *British Rifle Man*, p. 32; Garretty, *Memoirs*, p. 73.
83 G. Glover (ed.), *A Guards Officer in the Peninsula and at Waterloo: The Letters of Captain George Bowles, Coldstream Guards 1807–1819* (Godmanchester: Ken Trotman, 2008), p. 19.
84 I. Fletcher (ed.), *For God and Country: The Letters and Diaries of John Mills, Coldstream Guards, 1811–14* (Staplehurst: Spellmount, 1995), p. 61.
85 A.H. Haley (ed.), *The Soldier who Walked Away: Autobiography of Andrew Pearson, a Peninsular War Veteran* (Woolton: Bullfinch, 1987), p. 79.
86 Glover, *Smithies*, p. 60.
87 Schaumann, *On the Road*, p. 156.
88 For example, Simmons, *British Rifle Man*, p. 33.
89 Glover, *William Gavin*, p. 95; Buckley, *Thomas Henry Browne*, p. 245; Simmons, *British Rifle Man*, pp. 102–3; Hathaway, *Lawrence*, p. 61; Liddell-Hart, *Wheeler*, p. 150; A. Brett-James (ed.), *Edward Costello: The Peninsular and Waterloo Campaigns* (London: Longman, 1967), p. 109.

90 Hathaway, *Lawrence*, p. 76 for an admission of thefts from a mortally wounded French soldier.
91 Brett-James, *Edward Costello*, p. 59; J. Anderson, *Recollections of a Peninsular Veteran* (Uckfield: Naval & Military Press, 2010), p. 14.
92 Liddell-Hart, *Wheeler*, p. 32.
93 Kelly, *British Army Medicine*, p. 95; Kennedy, 'John Bull', p. 139; G. Glover (ed.), *From Corunna to Waterloo: The Letters and Journals of Two Napoleonic Hussars* (London: Greenhill, 2007), p. 53; Daly, 'Barbarity', pp. 255–6.
94 Kennedy, 'John Bull', p. 140.
95 Von Arni, 'Who cared?', p. 126.
96 Von Arni, 'Who cared?', pp. 127–9.
97 Kopperman, 'Medical services', p. 440.
98 Kopperman, 'Medical services', pp. 438–9.
99 Monro, *Observations*, pp. 121–3.
100 For fuller consideration of this topic, see Spinney, 'Women's work'.
101 *Regulations to Regimental Surgeons &c for the Better Management of the Sick in Regimental Hospitals* (London: J. Jones, 1799), p. 37; *Instructions for the Regulation of Regimental Hospitals and the Concerns of the Sick* (London: W. Clowes and Co., 1812), p. 12.
102 *Regulations for the Management of the General Hospitals in Great Britain* (London: W. Clowes and Co., 1813), pp. 29–36 relates to the hospital servants, but with no entries dedicated to nurses and orderlies; quote given on p. 42.
103 E. Spinney, 'Naval and military nursing in the British Empire c.1763–1830' (PhD thesis, University of Saskatchewan, 2018), pp. 232, 236.
104 *Regulations* (1813), p. 49.
105 *Regulations* (1798), p. 31.
106 *Regulations* (1813), p. 42.
107 Glover, *John Westcott*, pp. 90–1.
108 NB Broughton, *Letters*, p. 134 and Harley, *Veteran*, pp. 193–4 for brief but favourable reports of nursing by the French Sisters of Charity.
109 J. Malcolm, 'Reminiscences of a campaign in the Pyrenees and the South of France in 1814', *Memorials of the Late War* (Edinburgh: Constable, 1828), volume I, p. 301.
110 Malcolm, 'Reminiscences', p. 303.
111 Cooper, *Seven Campaigns*, p. 33.
112 Kopperman, 'Medical services', p. 439.

113 Liddell-Hart, *Wheeler*, p. 153.
114 Staffordshire Record Office, D 661/9/6/2/4/3 orderly books of Major General William Dyott, order no. 6 14 October 1809. I am grateful to Dr Ian Atherton for this reference.
115 R. Probert (ed.), *Catherine Exley's Diary: The Life and Times of an Army Wife in the Peninsular War* (Kenilworth: Brandrum, 2014).
116 Probert, *Diary*, p. 24; baptism of 24 January 1808, see www.findmypast.co.uk (accessed 24 January 2023); Hurl-Eamon, *Marriage*, p. 56.
117 Probert, *Diary*, pp. 26–7.
118 This detail expands on regulations that gave women and children access to army medical attention; *Regulations* (1813), p. 45.
119 S. Reid (ed.), *A Soldier of the Seventy-First from De la Plata to Waterloo 1806–1815 by Joseph Sinclair* (London: Frontline, 2010), p. 67; Cooper, *Seven Campaigns*, p. 34; J.C. Maempel, *Adventures of a Young Rifleman, in the French and English Armies, during the War in Spain and Portugal, from 1806 to 1816* (Leonaur, 2008), p. 128; R. Brown, *An Impartial Journal of a Detachment from the Brigade of Foot Guards, Commencing 25th February 1793 and Ending 9th May 1795* (London: John Stockdale, 1795), p. 225. These characterisations persisted into the nineteenth century and histories of the Crimean War; Furneaux, *Military Men*, pp. 210–11.
120 Brown, *Autobiography*, pp. 42–3. He served as a ward orderly in his turn at Moimenta da Beira (p. 119).
121 Garretty, *Memoirs*, pp. 172–3; E. Buckham, *Personal Narrative of Adventures in the Peninsula during the War in 1812–13* (Cambridge: Ken Trotman, 1995), pp. 81–2. This was a feature of orderlies' behaviour in earlier conflicts, and among the lower grades of medical men; Kopperman, 'Medical services', p. 432; F. Hall, *Recollections in Portugal and Spain during 1811 and 1812* (Godmanchester: Ken Trotman, 2002), pp. 35–6.
122 Hathaway, *Lawrence*, p. 72.
123 G. Glover (ed.), *The 3rd (Scots) Guards in Time of War: The Memoirs of Sergeant John Stevenson, 1793–1814* (Godmanchester: Ken Trotman, 2018).
124 Monick, *Douglas's Tale*, p. 67.
125 Maempel, *Adventures*, pp. 87–8.
126 *Vicissitudes in the life of a Scottish Soldier* (London: Henry Colburn, 1827), p. 103.
127 Simmons, *British Rifle Man*, p. 36; *Memoirs of a Sergeant*, p. 170.
128 W. Swabey, *Diary of Campaigns in the Peninsula for the Years 1811, 12 and 13* (London: Ken Trotman, 1984), p. 151.

129 Hathaway, *Cooke*, p. 94.
130 Fletcher, *John Mills*, p. 252; Monick, *Douglas's Tale*, pp. 66, 75; Brett-James, *Edward Costello*, p. 91. This was an assumption voiced earlier; see Kopperman, 'Regimental Practice', p. 118.
131 W. Surtees, *Twenty-Five Years in the Rifle Brigade* (Edinburgh: Ballantyne and Company, 1833), pp. 255–6.
132 Schaumann, *On the Road*, p. 193; G. Glover (ed.), *An Eloquent Soldier: The Peninsular War Journals of Lieutenant Charles Crowe of the Inniskillings, 1812–1824* (Barnsley: Frontline, 2011), p. 264; Glover, *William Clarke*, p. 208.
133 Maempel, *Adventures*, p. 127; Cooper, *Seven Campaigns*, p. 14.
134 J. Bogle and A. Uffindell (eds), *A Waterloo Hero: The Reminiscences of Freidrich Lindau* (London: Frontline, 2009), p. 21; J.E. Daniel, *Journal of an Officer in the Commissariat Department of the Army* (London: the author, 1820), p. 325 for the horror of a temporary hospital.
135 M.L. Ferrar (ed.), *The Diary of Colour-Serjeant George Calladine 19th Foot 1793–1837* (London: Eden Fisher & Co., 1922), p. 60.
136 *Regulations* (1798), p. 35 stated that 'Orderly Men acting in the Hospital, should be considered as being in a permanent situation, and not liable to be removed except in case of Misdemeanour'; quoted by Spinney, 'Naval and military nursing', p. 239.
137 Simmons, *British Rifle Man*, pp. 82, 89.
138 Glover, *Eloquent Soldier*, pp. 200–5.
139 Fletcher, *John Mills*, pp. 64, 78.
140 Wood, *Subaltern Officer*, pp. 151–2.
141 Cooper, *Seven Campaigns*, p. 33.
142 R. Jackson, A *System of Arrangement and Discipline for the Medical Department of Armies* (London: John Murray, 1805), pp. 252–60.
143 For wartime reference to human excrement and the scope for dirty work, see Cooper, *Seven Campaigns*, p. 37; Schaumann, *On the Road*, p. 40.
144 P.J. Bracken, 'Post-modernity and post-traumatic stress disorder', *Social Science and Medicine* 53: 6 (2001), 733–43.
145 D. Trembinski, 'Comparing premodern melancholy/mania and modern trauma: An argument in favor of historical experiences of trauma', *History of Psychology* 14: 1 (2011), 80–99.
146 W.J. Turner and C. Lee (eds), *Trauma in Medieval Society* (Leiden: Brill, 2018), introduction.

147 C. Lee, 'Healing words: St Guthlac and the trauma of war', W.J. Turner and C. Lee (eds), *Trauma in Medieval Society* (Leiden: Brill, 2018), p. 273.
148 D. Taylor, 'Trauma and emotion in the battlefield correspondence of Andrew Mitchell (1708–1771)', *Emotions: History, Culture, Society* 2: 2 (2018), 292–311, on p. 292.
149 E. Peters, 'Trauma narratives of the English Civil War', *Journal for Early Modern Cultural Studies* 16: 1 (2016), 78–94, on p. 78; www.civilwarpetitions.ac.uk (accessed 1 February 2023).
150 E. Butcher, 'War trauma and alcoholism in the early writings of Charlotte and Branwell Bronte', *Journal of Victorian Culture* 22: 4 (2017), 465–81, on p. 465.
151 Hathaway, *Lawrence*, p. 58.
152 Hathaway, *Lawrence*, p. 67. Simmons, *British Rifle Man*, p. 293 confesses metaphorically to 'a tear'.
153 P. Shaw, 'Longing for home: Robert Hamilton, nostalgia and the emotional life of the eighteenth-century soldier', *Journal for Eighteenth-Century Studies* 39: 1 (2016), 25–40.
154 Kennedy, *Narratives*, p. 19.
155 J. Vansittart (ed.), *Surgeon James's Journal 1815* (London: Cassell 1964), p. 37; see also P. Coleman (ed.), George *Walton 1796–1874: The Journal and Diary of a Rifleman of the 95th who Fought at Waterloo* (Studley: Brewin Books, 2016), p. 32 for a hospital scene judged impossible to describe.
156 Trembinski, 'Comparing', p. 83.
157 Taylor, 'Trauma'.
158 E. Domingues-Gomez, 'Prevalence of secondary traumatic stress among emergency nurses', *Journal of Emergency Nursing* 35: 3 (2009), 199–204, on p. 199.
159 S. Collins, 'Working with the psychological effects of trauma: Consequences for mental health-care workers – a literature review', *Journal of Psychiatric and Mental Health Nursing* 10: 4 (2003), 417–24; Domingues-Gomez, 'Prevalence'; Butcher, 'War trauma'.
160 Simmons, *British Rifle Man*, p. 32; Monick, *Douglas's Tale*, pp. 82–3; Liddell-Hart, *Wheeler*, p. 153; Hathaway, *Cooke*, pp. 183, 204; Brett-James, *Edward Costello*, p. 108; Monick, *James Hope*, pp. 66, 267.
161 Reid, *Joseph Sinclair*, p. 115; see also Glover, *William Clarke*, p. 206.
162 Hall, *Recollections*, pp. 36–7. The quote relates to hospital mates, but there is every reason to extend the reflection to orderlies.

306   Nursing the English from plague to Peterloo

163 A. Bamford (ed.), *Reminiscences 1808–1815 under Wellington: The Peninsular and Waterloo Memoirs of William Hay* (Solihull: Helion, 2017), p. 116.
164 O'Keeffe, *Jackson*, p. 85; for a discussion of George Gleig in this context, see Butcher, 'War trauma', pp. 272–4.
165 Collins, 'Working with the psychological effects'; for general 'avoidance' see Bogle and Uffindell, *Friedrich Lindau*, pp. 142, 150.
166 Butcher, 'War trauma', pp. 475–80.
167 Brett-James, *Edward Costello*, p. 109.
168 An extended version of this section of the chapter has previously been published as Tomkins, 'Waterloo'. I am grateful to the editor for permission to reproduce some of the content here.
169 G. Glover (ed.), *The Waterloo Archive, volume III: British Sources* (Barnsley: Frontline, 2011), narrative of Donald Finlayson, pp. 217–18; O'Neil, *Military Adventures*, p. 253.
170 Glover, *William Clarke*, p. 218; Bamford, *William Hay*, p. 118.
171 W. Verner, *Reminiscences of William Verner (1782–1871) 7th Hussars* (London: Society for Army Historical Research, 1965), p. 48.
172 G. Glover (ed.), *The Waterloo Archive, volume I: British Sources* (Barnsley: Frontline, 2010), p. 221.
173 Monick, *James Hope*, p. 271.
174 B. Jackson, *With Wellington's Staff at Waterloo: The Reminiscences of a Staff Officer During the Campaign of 1815 and with Napoleon on St Helena* (Leonaur, 2010), chapter 5.
175 H. Maxwell (ed.), *The Creevey Papers* (London: John Murray, 1903), volume 1, pp. 224–39.
176 Glover, *Waterloo Archive, volume I*, p. 229.
177 Bogle and Uffindell, *Friedrich Lindau*, p. 179.
178 Brett-James, *Edward Costello*, p. 154; W. Pitt Lennox, *Fifty Years' Biographical Reminiscences*, 2 volumes (London: Hurst and Blackett, 1863), volume I, p. 248.
179 There was at least one Spanish precedent for this; Thompson, *John Aitchison*, p. 177.
180 I am indebted to Gareth Glover for his personal communication regarding Captain Thomas Hobbs's experience in Brussels; W.C. Ward (ed.), *Diaries and Letters of Madame D'Arblay* (London: Frederick Warne and Co., 1892), volume III, p. 364.
181 Monick, *James Hope*, p. 269.
182 Glover, *Waterloo Archive: volume I*, p. 219 for the testimony of hospital assistant John Davy.
183 Bamford, *William Hay*, p. 117.

184 Glover, *William Clarke*, p. 201.
185 Henegan, *Seven Years*, pp. 336–7.
186 J. Scott, *Paris Revisited in 1815, by way of Brussels* (London: Longman, Hurst, Rees, Orme, and Brown, 1816), pp. 168–9.
187 Simmons, *British Rifle Man*, p. 368.
188 Simmons, *British Rifle Man*, p. 371.
189 Simmons, *British Rifle Man*, p. 373.
190 G. Glover (ed.), *The Waterloo Archive, volume IV: British Sources* (Barnsley: Frontline, 2012), pp. 203, 208, 222 for the account by George Simmons. See also Scott, *Paris Revisited*, p. 87 for confirmation of the involvement of wives and daughters.
191 Vernon, *Arms and the Self*, pp. 24–5.
192 Scott, *Paris Revisited*, p. 87.
193 Lennox, *Reminiscences*, pp. 248–9.
194 Lennox, *Reminiscences*, pp. 248–9.
195 Glover, *Waterloo Archive, volume I*, p. 229.
196 C. Eaton [neé Waldie], *Waterloo Days; the narrative of an Englishwoman resident at Brussels in June, 1815* (London: George Bell, 1888), p. 78.
197 Coleman, *George Walton*, p. 3; F. Nightingale, *Notes on Nursing – What It Is and What It Is Not* (London: Harrison, 1859).
198 Brett-James, *Edward Costello*, p. 155.
199 Nightingale, *Notes on Nursing*, throughout but particularly the chapters on 'Noise' and 'Observation of the Sick'.
200 Glover, personal communication, relating to Captain Thomas Hobbs.
201 Monick, *James Hope*, p. 268.
202 Scott, *Paris Revisited*, p. 86.
203 Glover, personal communication, relating to Captain Thomas Hobbs.
204 Jackson, *Waterloo*, chapter 5.
205 Coleman, *George Walton*, p. 34.
206 E. Scarry, *The Body in Pain: The Making and Unmaking of the World* (Oxford: Oxford University Press, 1985), pp. 114–15.
207 For stoicism see Ramsey, *Military Memoir*, pp. 17–19.
208 *The Battle of Waterloo, containing the accounts published by authority, British and Foreign, and other relative documents, with circumstantial details, previous and after the battle*, 7th edition (London: J. Booth; T. Egerton, 1815).
209 Ramsey, *Military Memoir*, p. 51.
210 Ramsey, *Military Memoir*, pp. 63–5.
211 Eaton [neé Waldie], *Waterloo Days*, p. 156.
212 Eaton [neé Waldie], *Waterloo Days*, pp. 78, 99, 117, 154.

213 Ward, *Madame D'Arblay*, volume III.
214 Stendahl, *The Charterhouse of Parma* (1st edition 1839; World Classics edition Oxford: Oxford University Press, 1997), chapter 3.
215 Kennedy, *Narratives*, p. 188.
216 W.M. Thackeray, *Vanity Fair* (London: Bradbury and Evans, 1848), chapter 32.
217 Thackeray, *Vanity Fair*.

Conclusion

On 16 August 1819, England witnessed a severe demand for emergency nursing in Manchester. The events at St Peter's Field, described variously as a riot or massacre, occasioned sixty-one admissions to the Manchester Infirmary of whom half were treated as inpatients. Victims bore a variety of wounds arising from sabre cuts, blows, crushing, and trampling. Beyond the immediate institutional response there were uncounted hundreds of injured, such that multiple households in the wider Manchester region accommodated those able to walk away, and Poor Law institutions were meeting the care needs of those affected even years afterwards. Thomas Buckley died of his injuries in November 1819, while his son died in Chadderton Workhouse six years later.[1] No direct records of the resulting nursing have survived, as the Manchester Infirmary minutes are opaque on the finer detail of its unprecedented influx of patients and memoirs like those of Samuel Bamford skirt over the mundane aftermath in recognition of the overwhelming horror of the event.[2] The women and men who assisted others with first aid *avant la lettre* and personal care are imperceptible.[3]

There can be strong grounds to suppose, though, that the response in Manchester after Peterloo in no way matched the humanitarian outpouring of assistance across social boundaries seen in Brussels following Waterloo; Peterloo's victims were treated by their social equals rather than their social superiors. We can also assume that whatever the failings of nurses for the Peterloo wounded, any nascent critique of carers would have been smothered by the larger and much tougher project of bringing the authorities (including the Manchester Magistracy, Yeomanry, and the Home Office) to account.

Beyond these drastic events, where any sins of nurses were perhaps dwarfed by the egregious misuse of power, these chapters have demonstrated that there were multiple grounds on which goodwill might be withdrawn from nurses in the pre-reform period. The stereotypical older, poor woman, working in close quarters with disease, decay, and human waste, could feasibly deliver her service in line with expectations. Any discrepancy between what clients wanted and what nurses could achieve, however, offered a variety of ways to denigrate the nurse simply for being herself.

Domestic nurses had to manage physical risk and the scope for emotional bruising. Exhaustion from unalleviated night nursing was merely the most obvious physical risk (aside, of course, from contracting their patient's illness), yet one which unpaid nurses repudiated. Revulsion and even potentially trauma were suppressed.[4] Vulnerable patients required kindness, so nurses tended to subordinate their own needs – up to a point. Once they became vulnerable carers, they protected themselves by withholding kindness, or at least by allowing patients to perceive the nurses' own competing requirements. This was the criteria on which domestic paid nurses were deprecated. Women's failure to establish entitlement to their own wants could induce feelings of illness (as was the case for Sarah Harriet Burney) or mental collapse (most dramatically experienced by Mary Lamb).

The demands of nursing could pose a threat to identity. This form of exposure occurred wherever women and men felt effaced by the needs of their patients. In the absence of a vocation or spiritual calling to nurse, as was promoted for nurses under mid-nineteenth-century reforms, people's sense of self was undermined by the combination of physical exertion and by the patient dominating all of their thoughts. John Keats and Joseph Severn expressed this most explicitly, and Chapter 5 argues that this male prominence among the testimony by individual literary nurses was a consequence of the shortfall between normative expectations of masculinity and the nursing role. Women were less likely to perceive an entire loss of self, because normative femininity required a measure of subordination. The early emergence of the lady nurse in Brussels, among women who accepted nursing duties spontaneously as an act of social condescension and pressing duty, provides an otherwise missing link between the pre-reform nursing experience, women's identities, and the emergence of an aspiration to recruit nurses from among gentlewomen.

The constraints on care went beyond the personal. The anti-nurse was, throughout the period, a useful ideological tool for expressing differences in priorities between patients and carers or between nations. In domestic settings, commentators generally stopped short of identifying female anti-nurses in practice, but scrutiny of men in asylums found clear evidence of male brutality. The perpetrators were presumed to be motivated by the prospect of material gain: it is perhaps more just to assume that their violence sprang from a form of self-protection, given their requirement to undertake dirty work on behalf of stigmatised patients. Similarly, the extravagant anti-nurse violence reported during the wars of 1793 to 1815 was possibly a reflection of lived experience, but definitely a way for British combatants to define their masculinity against an opprobrious 'other'. The anti-nurse template arguably resurfaced in England in the 1840s in the persons of Betsy Prig and especially Sarah Gamp, Charles Dickens's fictional nurses, bringing the dangers of acquisitive and potentially death-dealing nursing much closer to home.[5] The unreformed female nurse was, I would suggest, recast as an anti-nurse to underline the urgency of the arguments for women's training and social uplift. For the nurse to place 'her own comfort above patient needs' had transitioned from an individual's survival strategy to a deplorable failing that demanded 'severe discipline' by the 1850s.[6]

Institutional female nurses were no more aberrant from 1660 to 1820 than their domestic counterparts. They may occasionally have drunk alcohol, and been reproached or dismissed as a result, but their missteps on the wards of St Bartholomew's Hospital are seen most often in their handling of petty textiles. This, too, must be seen in a context where nurses were widely regarded as specialised servants, and domestic servants enjoyed access to textile perquisites as a routine component of their material reward. The wider experience of hospital and infirmary nurses speaks more reliably to the esteem of employers, and rewards for work well done. Provincial infirmaries found ways to acknowledge their debt to good nurses in the form of policed gratuities and in offering nurses a bed when they were, themselves, unwell. Relationships between the women generated support from fellow female ward staff. At St Bartholomew's Hospital and Chelsea Royal Hospital, this was expressed in the ways that nurses found fictive kin among their colleagues. Chelsea Hospital was unique in two additional respects: first, it routinely afforded women access to actual kin when it acted as an effectual marriage broker, and sometimes paid women to care for a group of men that included their own husbands. Second, it was only at Chelsea that a generous hospital context aligned with the continuity and confidence of nursing staff to produce a microclimate of care from which both the residents and the female ward staff benefitted.

The 'dirty' work inherent to the nursing role in all locations found little or no mitigation in this period, meaning that both women and men had to find their own ways to avoid personal spoliation. Female nurses in provincial infirmaries used the levying of small fees, against the rules, to demarcate themselves from patients while simultaneously making their contact with ordure a matter of financial reward rather than solely a source of taint. Male nurses were in a different but no less precarious position, but (if the argument levied here is correct) managed their anxieties rather differently, by lashing out at patients.

This research indicates important pathways for the development of the historiography of nursing in future. First, naval nursing requires detailed coverage. The Royal Naval Hospital Haslar was the largest hospital for the sick or wounded in England, from the time of its opening in around 1753 until well into the nineteenth century. Its capacity was augmented by a smaller institution at Stonehouse, Plymouth (which was nonetheless very large in comparison to other, civilian hospitals), and on hospital ships. This specialised variety of military nursing deserves full treatment owing to its scale and to the rich texture of women's lives offered by a close reading of its archives, and will secure its due in work planned by Erin Spinney and Geoff Hudson.[7] Second, the London hospitals which were newly opened in this period also generated data about nurses. The scale of institutional provision in the metropolis, combined with the numbers of nursing employees across all venues, may at best offer the opportunity to witness nursing careers across different institutions. Third, historians of nursing and the Poor Law should be alert to the possibilities of using workhouse records to retrieve aspects of institutional nursing. There may of course be an ideal such source for workhouse nursing currently lying unused in a county or other archive, but beyond a fortunate discovery it may be necessary to adopt a tangential approach. This topic may feasibly be accessible via inquests following deaths in workhouses, in the form of detailed coroners' papers and witness statements. There is reason for optimism around this technique, not least because Charmian Mansell has very recently been able to demonstrate how the features of care can be unpicked from legal inquiries, in her example a case brought before provincial church courts.[8] These three options are the most obvious for an extension of the experiences of nursing in England and Britain more widely. The most exciting and expansive widening of the field, however, would comprise a global adoption of the remit to see nurses before 1820 as more than simply unreformed. This could be attempted wherever textual archives survive for either institutional or domestic nurses, whether they were male or female, paid or unpaid, perhaps by using or adapting the sociological analyses attempted here. There is much work to be done about the historical delivery of care, interwoven with recovery of evidence giving opinions about carers, before we can lay claim to a comprehensive appreciation of nursing before either nurse training or professional organisation developed. I look forward to my own provisional conclusions being adjusted and refined as future researchers join the task of investigating the women and men who worked as nurses before the 1850s.

On the basis of the chapters above, the women and men who nursed the English before 1821 were stereotyped on the grounds of gender expectations, social status, and an unwillingness among all but the most acute observers to allow for the nurse's own point of view. This created the grounds of tension for multiple individuals and groups. In addition to these burdens the pre-reform nurses had no identifiable economic sector, knowledge base, or nascent representation. William Buchan's attempt to make medicine, for example, available to lay people while still drawing clear lines of authority and responsibility between practitioners and patients points up the central problem for nurses in this period: nurses were lay people with less social or intellectual credit than their male peers at any social level who lacked access to boundary-keepers like Buchan for their own practice.[9] The need for nurse reform, when it was perceived in the early nineteenth century, can be reconstrued as the need for nurses to consolidate and express untainted authority.

Notes

1. R. Poole, *Peterloo: The English Uprising* (Oxford: Oxford University Press, 2019), p. 351.
2. Manchester Royal Infirmary, MRI/4/1/1316 weekly board minutes 1816–1819; S. Bamford, *Passages in the Life of a Radical* (London: T. Fisher Unwin, 1843), chapter 25.
3. As was common with cases of riot, studied for patterns of prosecution: injuries were dealt with beyond formal institutions to avoid identification of participants. I am grateful to Dr Ian Atherton for raising the issue of riots earlier than 1819 for their relevance to nursing.
4. This was the ideal for the reformed nurse and her successors; K. Roberts, 'An ambiguous presence: Wartime constructions of the body of the nurse', *UK Association for the History of Nursing Bulletin* 10: 1 (2022), www.bulletin.ukahn.org (accessed 12 June 2024).
5. C. Dickens, *The Life and Adventures of Martin Chuzzlewit* (London: Chapman and Hall, 1844); A. Summers, 'The mysterious demise of Sarah Gamp: The domiciliary nurse and her detractors, *c.*1830–1860', *Victorian Studies* 32: 3 (1989), 365–86.
6. C. Helmstadter, 'A third look at Sarah Gamp', *Canadian Bulletin of Medical History* 30: 2 (2013), 141–59.
7. E. Spinney, *Carers for the Sick and Hurt: British Naval Nursing 1763–1820* (forthcoming); G. Hudson, *Canadian Journal of Health History* (forthcoming).
8. C. Mansell, 'Reconstructing the labour of care in early modern England', *Historical Journal* 67: 1 (2023), 1–21.
9. W. Buchan, *Domestic Medicine*, [16th edition] (London: A. Strahan, T. Cadell jun., and W. Davies, 1798); C.E. Rosenberg, 'Medical text and social context: Explaining William Buchan's *Domestic Medicine*', *Bulletin of the History of Medicine* 57: 1 (1983), 22–42.

Select bibliography

Archival sources

Barts Health Archives

SBHB/HA/1/5, St Bartholomew's Hospital minutes of the board of governors 1647–65/6; SBHB/HA/1/6, 1665/6–75; SBHB/HA/1/7, 1675–89; SBHB/HA/1/8, 1689–1708; SBHB/HA/1/9, 1708–19; SBHB/HA/1/10, 1719–34; SBHB/HA/1/11, 1734–48; SBHB/HA/1/12, 1748–57; SBHB/HA/1/13, 1757–70; SBHB/HA/1/14, 1770–86; SBHB/HA/1/15, 1786–1801; SBHB/HA/1/16, 1801–15; SBHB/HA/1/17, 1815–26.

SBHB/HA/4/1, St Bartholomew's Hospital board of governors' order book 1653–1739.

SBHB/HB/12, St Bartholomew's Hospital salary account and receipt books 1645–1716.

SBHB/SA/20/1, St Bartholomew's Hospital indemnity for Sarah Mansell's employment by surgeon Percival Pott, 1757.

SHBSBL/CW/3/1, St Bartholomew the Less churchwardens' correspondence, letter from Sister Elizabeth Russell 1747.

Birmingham Archives

MS 1423/2, Birmingham General Hospital trustees' minutes 1766–84; MS 1423/3, 1784–93; MS 1423/4, 1794–1803; MS 1423/5, 1803–15; MS 1423/6, 1815–23.

Cheshire Record Office

ZH1/1/1, Chester Infirmary Board minutes 1755–58; ZH1/1/2, 1763–68; ZH1/1/3, 1768–73; ZH1/1/4, 1773–78; ZH1/1/5, 1778–82; ZH1/1/6, 1783–87; ZH1/1/7, 1787–94; ZH1/1/8, 1794–99; ZH1/1/9, 1799–1804; ZH1/1/10, 1805–08; ZH1/1/11, 1808–15; ZH1/1/12, 1815–22.

ZH1/24, Chester Infirmary minutes of the board of economy 1801–06, including statistics of other infirmaries 1787–1817.
ZH1/88-89, Chester Infirmary visitors' books 1802–14, 1814–57.

Gloucestershire Archives

HO 19/1/1, Gloucester Infirmary weekly board minutes 1744–55; HO 19/1/2, 1755–62; HO 19/1/3, 1762–70; HO 19/1/4, 1770–77; HO 19/1/5, 1778–86; HO 19/1/6, 1786–95; HO 19/1/7, 1795–1804; HO 19/1/8, 1804–13; HO 19/1/9, 1814–21.

Liverpool Archives

614 INF/1/1, Liverpool Royal Infirmary quarterly board minute book 1749–96; 614 INF/1/2, 1796–1823.

London Metropolitan Archives and Guildhall Library Manuscripts

DL/AL/C/003/9052/039/071, DL/AM/PW/1754/055, DL/AM/PW/1763/005, DL/C/0366/0426/024, wills of Royal Hospital Chelsea nurses and inmates 1719–78.

Manchester Royal Infirmary

MRI/4/1/1316, weekly board minutes 1816–19.

The National Archives

HO 17/97/8, criminal petition of Lydia Weston 1822.
PROB 11/455/181, PROB 11/480/115, PROB 11/486/47, PROB 11/529/406, PROB 11/552/219, PROB 11/554/12, PROB 11/559/149, PROB 11/565/99, PROB 11/566/18, PROB 11571/88, PROB 11/584/72, PROB 11/589/320, PROB 11/590/288, PROB 11/590/365, PROB 11/591/447, PROB 11/595/51, PROB 11/597/255, PROB 11/615/183, PROB 11/623/304, PROB 11/625/346, PROB 11/626/410, PROB 11/630/154, PROB 11/657/86, PROB 11/657/263, PROB 11/662/393, PROB 11/692/266, PROB 11/700/261, PROB 11/710/132, PROB 11/717/319, PROB 11/719/350, PROB 11/721/100, PROB 11/722/443, PROB 11/752/496, PROB 11/760/65, PROB 11/762/195, PROB 11/784/75, PROB 11/798/250, PROB 11/813/128, PROB/11/813/302, PROB 11/817/62, PROB 11/833/142, PROB 11/839/175, PROB 11/852/370,

PROB 11/862/18, PROB 11/872/387, PROB 11/892/112, PROB 11/892/204, PROB 11/896/365, PROB 11/898/95, PROB 11/924/83, PROB 11/925/356, PROB 11/927/10, PROB 11/959/172, PROB 11/973/277, PROB 11/975/371, PROB 11/990/321, PROB 11/1108/276, PROB 11/1149/246, PROB 11/1188/138, PROB 11/1205/128, PROB 11/1290/102, PROB 11/1367/180, PROB 11/1390/133, PROB 11/1412/227, PROB 11/1450/168, PROB 11/1544/541, PROB 11/1559/213, PROB 11/1579/146, PROB 11/1590/174, PROB 11/1596/253, PROB 11/1610/411, PROB 11/1636/13, PROB 11/2202/125, wills of Royal Hospital Chelsea nurses and inmates 1700–1854.

PROB 18/33/33, probate dispute Walker versus Kay concerning nurse Mary Whitton 1714.

RG 4/4330, register of marriages (1691–1765), baptisms (1691–1796), and burials (1692–1797) at Royal Hospital Chelsea.

RG 4/4387, baptisms (1797–1812) and burials (1797–1813) at Royal Hospital Chelsea.

SP 32/4/6, a list of soldiers disabled by their wounds now in the Royal Hospital Chelsea 1692.

WO 12/11589-91, Royal Hospital Chelsea musters 1788–94, 1795–1808, and 1809–20.

WO 23/124-31, Royal Hospital Chelsea musters 1702–12, 1714, 1717, 1728–59, 1763–69, 1770–76, 1777–82, and 1783–89.

WO 23/134, Royal Hospital Chelsea list of in-pensioners and staff 1794–1813, recording deaths 1795–1816.

WO 245/4, 5, 6, 7, Royal Hospital Chelsea salary books 1743–53, 1764–73, 1773–84, and 1782–89.

WO 247/6, 7, 8, 9, Royal Hospital Chelsea inventories 1754–60, 1761–65, 1775–76, and 1780–82.

WO 248/30, Royal Hospital Chelsea warrants to William Cheselden 1739–44.

WO 250/459–467, Royal Hospital Chelsea journals 1715–49, 1750–71, 1771–75, 1778–82, 1783–87, 1787–93, 1793–98, 1799–1805, 1806–06.

WO 250/469, Royal Hospital Chelsea index to journals 1703–55.

WO 250/475, Royal Hospital Chelsea board minutes 1783.

Shropshire Archives

3909/1/1, Salop Infirmary weekly board minutes 1745–56; 3909/1/2, 1756–70; 3909/1/3, 1770–84; 3909/1/4, 1784–99; 3909/1/5, 1799–1814; 3909/1/6, 1814–27.

3909/5/4, Salop Infirmary matron's incident book 1747–53.

Staffordshire Record Office

D685/1/1, Stafford General Infirmary general board minutes 1765–1820.
D685/2/1, Stafford General Infirmary weekly board minutes 1766–69; D685/2/2, 1769–75; D685/2/3, 1775–82; D685/2/4, 1782–89; D685/2/5, 1789–95; D685/2/6, 1795–1803; D685/2/7, 1803–12; D685/2/8, 1812–22.
D 685/18, Stafford Infirmary visitors' book 1766–1811.

Worcestershire Archives

BA5161/1, Worcester Royal Infirmary order books 1745–1800 and 1800–28.
BA5161/12, Worcester Royal Infirmary account book of general hospital expenses 1745–54.

Printed primary sources (exclusively relating to chapter six)

Anderson, J., *Recollections of a Peninsular Veteran* (Uckfield: Naval & Military Press, 2010) *Vicissitudes in the Life of a Scottish Soldier* (London: Henry Colburn, 1827).
Anton, J., *Retrospect of a Military Life* (Cambridge: Ken Trotman, 1991).
Bamford, A. (ed.), *With Wellington's Outposts: The Peninsular and Waterloo Letters of John Vandeleur* (Barnsley: Frontline, 2015).
Bamford, A. (ed.), *Triumphs and Disasters: Eyewitness Accounts from the Netherlands Campaign, 1813–1814* (Barnsley: Frontline, 2016).
Bamford, A. (ed.), *Reminiscences 1808–1815 under Wellington: The Peninsular and Waterloo Memoirs of William Hay* (Solihull: Helion, 2017).
Blakiston, J., *Twelve Years' Military Adventure in Three Quarters of the Globe*, volume II (London: Henry Colburn, 1840).
Blathwayt, G., *Recollections of My Life including Military Service at Waterloo* (Cambridge: Ken Trotman, 2004).
Bogle, J. and A. Uffindell (eds), *A Waterloo Hero: The Reminiscences of Freidrich Lindau* (London: Frontline, 2009).
Brett-James, A. (ed.), *Edward Costello: The Peninsular and Waterloo Campaigns* (London: Longman, 1967).
Broughton, S.D., *Letters from Portugal, Spain & France 1812–1814* (Stroud: Nonsuch, 2005).
Brown, R., *An Impartial Journal of a Detachment from the Brigade of Foot Guards, Commencing 25th February 1793 and Ending 9th May 1795* (London: John Stockdale, 1795).

Select bibliography 319

Brown, W., *The Autobiography or Narrative of a Soldier: The Peninsular War Memoirs of William Brown of the 45th Foot* (Solihull: Helion, 2017).

Buckham, E., *Personal Narrative of Adventures in the Peninsula during the War in 1812–13* (Cambridge: Ken Trotman, 1995).

Buckley, R.N. (ed.), *The Napoleonic War Journal of Captain Thomas Henry Browne, 1807–1816* (London: Bodley Head, 1987).

Bunbury, T., *Reminiscences of a Veteran*, volume I (London: C.J. Skeet, 1861).

Cadell, C., *Narrative of the Campaigns of the Twenty-eighth Regiment, since Their Return from Egypt in 1802* (London: Whittaker, 1835).

Chesterton, G.L., *Peace, War, and Adventure: An Autobiographical Memoir of George Laval Chesterton* (London: Longman, Brown, Green & Longmans, 1853).

Coleman, P. (ed.), *George Walton 1796–1874: The Journal and Diary of a Rifleman of the 95th who Fought at Waterloo* (Studley: Brewin Books, 2016).

Cooper, J.S., *Rough Notes of Seven Campaigns: 1809–1815* (Staplehurst: Spellmount, 1996).

Daniel, J.E., *Journal of an Officer in the Commissariat Department of the Army* (London: the author, 1820).

Dansey, C.C., *The Peninsular Letters of 2nd Captain Charles Dansey Royal Artillery* (Godmanchester: Ken Trotman, 2006).

De Lancey, M., *A Week at Waterloo* (London: Reportage Press, 2008).

Dent, W., *A Young Surgeon in Wellington's Army: The Letters of William Dent* (Old Woking: Unwin Brothers, 1976).

Dobbs, J., *Recollections of an Old 52nd Man* (Staplehurst: Spellmount, 2000).

Donaldson, J., *Scenes and Sketches of a Soldier's Life in Ireland* (Edinburgh: William Tait, 1826).

Donaldson, J., *Recollections in the Eventful Life of a Soldier* (Philadelphia, PA: G.B. Zieber and Co., 1845).

Eadie, R., *On Campaign with the 79th (Cameron Highlanders) Through Portugal and Spain* (Darlington: Napoleonic Archive, 2006).

Eaton, C. [neé Waldie], *Waterloo Days; The Narrative of an Englishwoman Resident at Brussels in June, 1815* (London: George Bell, 1888).

Ferrar, M.L. (ed.), *The Diary of Colour-Serjeant George Calladine 19th Foot 1793–1837* (London: Eden Fisher & Co., 1922).

Fletcher, I. (ed.), *For God and Country: The Letters and Diaries of John Mills, Coldstream Guards, 1811–14* (Staplehurst: Spellmount, 1995).

Fletcher, I. (ed.), *In the Service of the King: The Letters of William Thornton Keep* (Staplehurst: Spellmount, 1997).

Garretty, T., *Memoirs of a Sergeant Late in the Forty-Third Light Infantry Regiment Previously to and During the Peninsular War* (Cambridge: Ken Trotman, 1998).

Gleig, G.R., *The Subaltern* (Edinburgh: W. Blackwood and Sons, 1845).
Glover, G. (ed.), *The 1812 Diary of Ensign Carter 30th Foot* (Godmanchester: Ken Trotman, 2006).
Glover, G. (ed.), *A Hellish Business: From the Letters of Captain Charles Kinloch 52nd Foot 1806–16* (Godmanchester: Ken Trotman, 2007).
Glover, G. (ed.), *From Corunna to Waterloo: The Letters and Journals of Two Napoleonic Hussars* (London: Greenhill, 2007).
Glover, G. (ed.), *The Diary of a Veteran: The Diary of Sergeant Peter Facey, 28th (North Gloucester) Regiment of Foot 1803–19* (Godmanchester: Ken Trotman, 2007).
Glover, G. (ed.), *A Staff Officer in the Peninsula and at Waterloo: The Letters of the Honourable Lieutenant Colonel James Stanhope 1st Foot Guards 1809–15* (Godmanchester: Ken Trotman, 2007).
Glover, G. (ed.), *A Guards Officer in the Peninsula and at Waterloo: The Letters of Captain George Bowles, Coldstream Guards 1807–1819* (Godmanchester: Ken Trotman, 2008).
Glover, G. (ed.), *The Waterloo Diary of Captain James Naylor, 1st King's Dragoon Guards* (Godmanchester: Ken Trotman, 2008).
Glover, G. (ed.), *At Wellington's Headquarters: The Letters of Robert Duffield Cooke Army Pay Corps 1811–14* (Godmanchester: Ken Trotman, 2009).
Glover, G. (ed.), *Campaigning in Spain and Belgium: The Letters of Captain Thomas Charles Fenton, 4th Dragoons & the Scots Greys 1809–15* (Huntingdon: Ken Trotman, 2010).
Glover, G. (ed.), *The Waterloo Archive, volume I: British Sources* (Barnsley: Frontline, 2010).
Glover, G. (ed.), *Adventurous Pursuits of a Peninsular War & Waterloo Veteran: The Story of Private James Smithies 1st (Royal) Dragoons, 1807–15* (Godmanchester: Ken Trotman, 2011).
Glover, G. (ed.), *An Eloquent Soldier: The Peninsular War Journals of Lieutenant Charles Crowe of the Inniskillings, 1812–1824* (Barnsley: Frontline, 2011).
Glover, G. (ed.), *Captain Thomas Edwardes-Tuckers Peninsular Diary, 23rd (Royal Welch Fusiliers) Regiment of Foot, 1813–14 A.D.C to Sir Thomas Picton* (Godmanchester: Ken Trotman, 2011).
Glover, G. (ed.), *The Waterloo Archive, volume III: British Sources* (Barnsley: Frontline, 2011).
Glover, G. (ed.), *The Waterloo Archive, volume IV: British Sources* (Barnsley: Frontline, 2012).
Glover, G. (ed.), *The Diary of William Gavin Ensign and Quarter-Master of the 71st Highland Regiment, 1806–1815* (Godmanchester: Ken Trotman, 2013).

Glover, G. (ed.), *A Hussar Sergeant in the King's German Legion: The Memoirs of Cavalry Sergeant Ebbecke, 2nd Hussar Regiment King's German Legion, 1803–1815* (Godmanchester: Ken Trotman, 2017).
Glover, G. (ed.), *A Scots Grey at Waterloo: The Remarkable Story of Sergeant William Clarke* (Barnsley: Frontline, 2017).
Glover, G. (ed.), *The American Sharpe: The Adventures of an American Officer of the 95th Rifles in the Peninsula & Waterloo Campaigns* (Barnsley: Frontline, 2017).
Glover, G. (ed.), *John Westcott's Journal of the Campaign in Portugal* (Godmanchester: Ken Trotman, 2018).
Glover, G. (ed.), *The 3rd (Scots) Guards in Time of War: The Memoirs of Sergeant John Stevenson, 1793–1814* (Godmanchester: Ken Trotman, 2018).
Haley, A.H. (ed.), *The Soldier who Walked Away: Autobiography of Andrew Pearson, a Peninsular War Veteran* (Woolton: Bullfinch, 1987).
Hall, F., *Recollections in Portugal and Spain during 1811 and 1812* (Godmanchester: Ken Trotman, 2002).
Harley, J., *The Veteran, or 40 Years' Service in the British Army: The Scurrilous Recollections of Paymaster John Harley 47th Foot – 1798–1838* (Solihull: Helion, 2018).
Hathaway, E. (ed.), *A Dorset Soldier: The Autobiography of Sgt William Lawrence 1790–1869* (Staplehurst: Spellmount, 1993).
Hathaway, E. (ed.), *A True Soldier Gentleman: The Memoirs of Lt. John Cooke 1791–1813* (Swanage: Shinglepicker, 2000).
Hawker, P., *Journal of a Regimental Officer during the Recent Campaign in Portugal and Spain under Lord Viscount Wellington* (London: Ken Trotman, 1981).
Hayter, A. (ed.), *The Backbone: Diaries of a Military Family in the Napoleonic Wars* (Edinburgh: Pentland Press, 1993).
Hayward, P. (ed.), *Surgeon Henry's Trifles: Events of a Military Life* (London: Chatto & Windus, 1970).
Henegan, R., *Seven Years Campaigning in the Peninsula and the Netherlands, from 1808 to 1815*, volume I (London: Henry Colburn, 1846).
Hibbert, C. (ed.), *The Wheatley Diary: A Journal and Sketchbook kept during the Peninsular War and the Waterloo Campaign* (Moreton-in-Marsh: Windrush Press, 1997).
Ingilby, W.B., *The Peninsular and Waterloo Journals of Lieutenant William Ingilby Royal Horse Artillery, 1810–15* (Godmanchester: Ken Trotman, 2016).
Jackson, B., *With Wellington's Staff at Waterloo: The Reminiscences of a Staff Officer During the Campaign of 1815 and with Napoleon on St Helena* (Leonaur, 2010).

Jones, H., 'Seven weeks' captivity in St Sebastian, in 1813', in W. Maxwell, *Peninsular Sketches; by Actors on the Scene*, volume II (Cambridge: Ken Trotman, 1998).
Knowles, R., *The War in the Peninsula: Some Letters of a Lancashire Officer* (Staplehurst: Spellmount, 2004).
[Leslie, C.], *Military Journal of Colonel Leslie* (Aberdeen: Aberdeen University Press, 1887).
Liddell-Hart, B.H., *The Letters of Private Wheeler 1809–1828* (Moreton-in-Marsh: Windrush Press, 1999).
MacCarthy, J.E.C., *Recollections of the Storming of the Castle of Badajoz by the Third Division* (Staplehurst: Spellmount, 2001).
Maempel, J.C., *Adventures of a Young Rifleman, in the French and English Armies, during the War in Spain and Portugal, from 1806 to 1816* (Leonaur, 2008).
Malcolm, J., *Reminiscences of a Campaign in the Pyrenees and South of France in 1814* (Cambridge: Ken Trotman, 1999).
Maxwell, H. (ed.), *The Creevey Papers*, volume I (London: John Murray, 1903).
Maxwell, W., *Peninsular Sketches; by Actors on the Scene* (Cambridge: Ken Trotman, 1998).
Memoirs of a Sergeant Late in the 43rd Light Infantry Regiment (London: John Mason, 1835).
Miller, B., *The Adventures of Serjeant Benjamin Miller Whilst Serving in the 4th Battalion of the Royal Regiment of Artillery 1796–1815* (Dallington: Naval & Military Press, 1999).
Mockler-Feryman, A.F. (ed.), *The Life of a Regimental Officer during the Great War 1793–1815: Compiled from the Correspondence of Colonel Samuel Rice* (London: William Blackwood, 1913).
Monick, S. (ed.), *Douglas's Tale of the Peninsula and Waterloo 1808–15* (London: Leo Cooper, 1997).
Monick, S. (ed.), *The Iberian and Waterloo Campaigns: The Letters of Lt James Hope (92nd (Highland) Regiment) 1811–1815* (Dallington: Naval & Military Press, 2000).
Morley, S., *Memoirs of a Sergeant of the 5th Regiment of Foot* (Godmanchester: Ken Trotman, 1999).
Muir, R. (ed.), *At Wellington's Right Hand: The Letters of Lieutenant-Colonel Sir Alexander Gordon, 1808–1815* (Phoenix Mill: Sutton, 2003).
Neale, A., *Letters from Portugal and Spain* (London: Phillips, 1809).
O'Keeffe, E. (ed.), *Narrative of the Eventful Life of Thomas Jackson, Militiaman and Coldstream Sergeant, 1803–15* (Solihull: Helion, 2018).
O'Neil, C., *The Military Adventures of Charles O'Neil* (Worcester, MA: Edward Livermore, 1851).

Pattison, F.H., *Personal Recollections of the Waterloo Campaign* (Upton: Gosling Press, 1992).
Pitt Lennox, W., *Fifty Years' Biographical Reminiscences*, 2 volumes (London: Hurst and Blackett, 1863).
Probert, R. (ed.), *Catherine Exley's Diary: The Life and Times of an Army Wife in the Peninsular War* (Kenilworth: Brandrum, 2014).
Reed, A., *Seven Years on the Peninsula: The Memoirs of Private Adam Reed, 47th (Lancashire) Foot 1806–17* (Godmanchester: Ken Trotman, 2012).
Reid, S. (ed.), *A Soldier of the Seventy-First from De la Plata to Waterloo 1806–1815 by Joseph Sinclair* (London: Frontline, 2010).
Robertson, I. (ed.), *The Exploits of Ensign Bakewell: With the Inniskillings in the Peninsula, 1810–1811; and in Paris, 1815* (London: Frontline, 2012).
Ross, H.D., *Memoir of Field-Marshal Sir Hew Dalrymple Ross* (Godmanchester: Ken Trotman, 2008).
Schaumann, A.L.F., *On the Road with Wellington* (London: Greenhill, 1999).
Scott, J., *Paris Revisited in 1815, by way of Brussels* (London: Longman, Hurst, Rees, Orme, and Brown, 1816).
Selby, J. (ed.), *The Napoleonic Wars: Thomas Morris* (Hamden: Archon Books, 1968).
Sherer, M., *Recollections of the Peninsula* (London: Longman, 1824).
Simmons, G., *A British Rifle Man* (London: A.C. Black, 1899).
Steevens, C., *With the 'Old & Bold' 1795 to 1818: The Reminiscences of an Officer of HM 20th Regiment During the Napoleonic Wars* (Leonaur, 2010).
Surtees, W., *Twenty-Five Years in the Rifle Brigade* (Edinburgh: Ballantyne and Company, 1833).
Swabey, W., *Diary of Campaigns in the Peninsula for the Years 1811, 12 and 13* (London: Ken Trotman, 1984).
Thompson, M.S. (ed.), *The Peninsular War Diary of Edmund Mulcaster RE, 1808–1810* (published by the editor, 2015).
Thompson, W.F.K. (ed.), *An Ensign in the Peninsular War: The Letters of John Aitchison* (London: Michael Joseph, 1994).
Tomkinson, W., *The Diary of a Cavalry Officer in the Peninsula and Waterloo Campaign 1809–1815* (London: S. Sonnenschein, 1894).
Vansittart, J. (ed.), *Surgeon James's Journal 1815* (London: Cassell, 1964).
Verner, W., *Reminiscences of William Verner (1782–1871) 7th Hussars* (London: Society for Army Historical Research, 1965).
Ward, W.C. (ed), Diaries and Letters of Madame D'Arblay (London: Frederick Warne and Co., 1892), volume III.

Wood, G., *The Subaltern Officer: A Narrative* (Godmanchester: Ken Trotman, 1986).

Secondary sources

Abel-Smith, B., *A History of the Nursing Profession* (London: Heinemann, 1960).
Ashforth, B.E. and G.E. Kreiner, '"How can you do it?": Dirty work and the challenge of constructing a positive identity', *Academy of Management Review* 24: 3 (1999), 413–34.
Bashford, A., *Purity and Pollution: Gender, Embodiment, and Victorian Medicine* (Basingstoke: Macmillan, 1998).
Beier, L.M., *Sufferers and Healers: The Experience of Illness in Seventeenth-Century England* (London: Routledge Kegan Paul, 1987).
Bolton, S. and C. Boyd, 'Trolley dolly or skilled emotion manager? Moving on from Hochschild's Managed Heart', *Work, Employment, and Society* 17: 2 (2003), 289–308.
Borsay, A., 'Nursing 1700–1830: Families, communities, institutions', A. Borsay and B. Hunter (eds), *Nursing and Midwifery in Britain since 1700* (Basingstoke: Palgrave, 2012).
Boulton, H.E., 'The Chester Infirmary', *Chester and North Wales Architectural Archaeological and Historical Society Journal* 47 (1960), 9–19.
Boulton, J., 'Welfare systems and the parish nurse in early modern London, 1650–1725', *Family and Community History* 10: 2 (2007), 127–51.
Bracken, P.J., 'Post-modernity and post-traumatic stress disorder', *Social Science and Medicine* 53: 6 (2001), 733–43.
Bradley, H., 'Across the Great Divide: The entry of men into "women's jobs"', in C.L. Williams (ed.), *Doing 'Women's Work': Men in Nontraditional Occupations* (Newbury Park, CA: Sage, 1993).
Brittain, O., 'Subjective experience and military masculinity at the beginning of the long eighteenth century, 1688–1714', *Journal for Eighteenth-Century Studies* 40: 2 (2017), 273–90.
Brockbank, W., *The History of Nursing at the Manchester Royal Infirmary 1752–1929* (Manchester: Manchester University Press, 1970).
Bullough, V.L. and B. Bullough, *The Care of the Sick: The Emergence of Modern Nursing* (New York: Prodist, 1978).
Butcher, E., 'War trauma and alcoholism in the early writings of Charlotte and Branwell Bronte', *Journal of Victorian Culture* 22: 4 (2017), 465–81.
Carpenter, M., 'The subordination of nurses in health care: Towards a social divisions approach', E. Riska and K. Wegar (eds), *Gender, Work and Medicine: Women and the Medical Division of Labour* (London: Sage, 1993).

Select bibliography 325

Carrara, B.S., C.A.A. Ventura, S.J. Bobbili, O.M.P. Jacobina, A. Khenti, and I.A. Costa Mendes, 'Stigma in health professionals towards people with mental illness: An integrative review', *Archives of Psychiatric Nursing* 33: 4 (2019), 311–18.

Carré, J., 'Hospital nurses in eighteenth-century Britain: Service without responsibility', I. Baudino and J. Carré (eds), *The Invisible Woman: Aspects of Women's Work in Eighteenth-Century Britain* (London: Routledge, 2005).

Charters, E., 'The caring fiscal-military state during the Seven Years War, 1756–1763', *Historical Journal* 52: 4 (2009), 921–41.

Clark, L., 'Sarah Harriet Burney: Traits of nature and families', *Lumen: Selected Proceedings from the Canadian Society for Eighteenth Century Studies* 19 (2000), 121–134.

Collins, S., 'Working with the psychological effects of trauma: Consequences for mental health-care workers – a literature review', *Journal of Psychiatric and Mental Health Nursing* 10: 4 (2003), 417–24.

Cottingham, M.D., R.J. Erickson, and J.M. Diefendorff, 'Examining men's status shield and status bonus: How gender frames the emotional labour and job satisfaction of nurses', *Sex Roles* 72: 7–8 (2015), 377–89.

Daly, G., '"Barbarity more suited to savages": British soldiers' views of Spanish and Portuguese violence', *War & Society* 35: 4 (2016), 242–58.

Dingwall, R., A.M. Rafferty, and C. Webster, *An Introduction to the Social History of Nursing* (London: Routledge, 1988).

Domingues-Gomez, E., 'Prevalence of secondary traumatic stress among emergency nurses', *Journal of Emergency Nursing* 35: 3 (2009), 199–204.

Evans, J., 'Men nurses: A historical and feminist perspective', *Journal of Advanced Nursing* 47: 3 (2004), 321–8.

Eyers, I. and T. Adams, 'Dementia care nursing, emotional labour and clinical supervision', T. Adams (ed.), *Dementia Care Nursing: Promoting Well-Being in People with Dementia and their Families* (Basingstoke: Palgrave Macmillan, 2007).

Field, J.F., 'Clandestine weddings at the Fleet prison, c.1710–1750: Who married there?', *Continuity and Change* 32: 3 (2017), 349–77.

Fissell, M., *Patients, Power, and the Poor in Eighteenth-Century Bristol* (Cambridge: Cambridge University Press, 1991).

Foyster, E., 'Boys will be boys? Manhood and aggression, 1660–1800', T. Hitchcock and M. Cohen (eds), *English Masculinities 1660–1800* (London: Longman, 1999).

Griffith, P. (ed.), *Modern Studies of the War in Spain and Portugal, 1808–1814* (London: Greenhill, 1999).

Harding, T., 'The construction of men who are nurses as gay', *Journal of Advanced Nursing* 60: 6 (2007), 636–44.
Hart, L., 'A ward of my own: Social organisation and identity among hospital domestics', P. Holden and J. Littlewood (eds), *Anthropology and Nursing* (London: Routledge, 1991).
Helmstadter, C., 'A third look at Sarah Gamp', *Canadian Bulletin of Medical History* 30: 2 (2013), 141–59.
Helmstadter, C. and J. Godden, *Nursing Before Nightingale 1815–1899* (Farnham: Routledge, 2011).
Henry, W., 'Women searchers of the dead in eighteenth- and nineteenth-century London', *Social History of Medicine* 29: 3 (2016), 445–66.
Hochschild, A.R., *The Managed Heart* (Berkeley, CA: University of California Press, 2012).
Howie, W.B., 'Complaints and complaint procedures in the eighteenth- and early nineteenth- century provincial hospitals in England', *Medical History* 25: 4 (1981), 345–62.
Hudson, G., 'Internal influences in the making of the English military hospital: The early eighteenth-century Greenwich', Geoffrey Hudson (ed.), *British Military and Naval Medicine 1600–1830* (Amsterdam: Rodopi, 2007).
Hughes, E.C., 'Work and the self', J.H. Rohrer and M. Sherif (eds), *Social Psychology at the Crossroads* (New York: Harper and Bros., 1951).
James, R.M., 'Health care in the Georgian household of Sir William and Lady Hannah East', *Historical Research* 82: 218 (2009), 694–714.
Jolley, M. and G. Brykczynska, *Nursing: Its Hidden Agendas* (Suffolk: St Edmundsbury Press, 1993).
Kennedy, C., *Narratives of the Revolutionary and Napoleonic Wars: Military and Civilian Experience* (Basingstoke: Palgrave Macmillan, 2013).
King, S., 'Nursing under the old Poor Law in midland and eastern England, 1780–1834', *Journal for the History of Medicine* 70: 4 (2014), 588–622.
Kopperman, P.E., 'Medical services in the British Army 1742–1783', *Journal of the History of Medicine* 34: 4 (1979), 428–55.
Lawrence, C.J., 'William Buchan: Medicine laid open', *Medical History* 19: 1 (1975), 20–35.
Lawson-Peebles, R., 'Style wars. The problems of writing military autobiography in the eighteenth century', A. Vernon (ed.), *Arms and the Self: War, the Military, and Autobiographical Writing* (Kent, OH: Kent State University Press, 2006).
Leong, E., *Recipes and Everyday Knowledge: Medicine, Science, and the Household in Early Modern England* (Chicago, IL: University of Chicago Press, 2018).
Lin, P.Y.C.E., 'Caring for the nation's families: British soldiers' and sailors' families and the state, 1793–1815', A. Forrest, K. Hagemann, and

J. Rendall (eds), *War, Society, and Culture, 1750–1850* (Basingstoke: Palgrave Macmillan, 2009).

Littlewood, J., 'Care and ambiguity: Towards a concept of nursing', P Holden and J. Littlewood (eds), *Anthropology and Nursing* (London: Routledge, 1991).

Mackintosh, C., 'A historical study of men in nursing', *Journal of Advanced Nursing* 26: 2 (1997), 232–6.

Mansell, C., 'Reconstructing the labour of care in early modern England', *Historical Journal* 67: 1 (2023), 1–21.

McAllister, M. and D.L. Brien, 'Narratives of the "not-so-good nurse": Rewriting nursing's virtue script', *Hecate* 41: 1–2 (2016), 79–97.

McLoughlin, G., *A Short History of the First Liverpool Infirmary 1749–1824* (London: Phillimore, 1978).

McMenemey, W.H., *History of Worcester Royal Infirmary* (London: Press Alliances, 1947).

McRorie Higgins, P., *Punish or Treat?: Medical Care in English Prisons 1770–1850* (Victoria, British Columbia: Trafford, 2007).

Moore, N., *The History of St Bartholomew's Hospital*, volumes I and II (London: Arthur Pearson, 1918).

Morgan, D., 'Theater of war. Combat, the military, and masculinities', H. Brod and M. Kaufman (eds), *Theorising Masculinities* (London: Sage, 1994).

Mortimer, B., 'Introduction', S. McGann and B. Mortimer (eds), *New Directions in Nursing History: International Perspectives* (London: Routledge, 2005).

Mortimer, I., *The Dying and the Doctors: The Medical Revolution in Seventeenth-Century England* (Woodbridge: Royal Historical Society, Boydell Press, 2009).

Munkhoff, R., 'Searchers of the dead: Authority, marginality, and the interpretation of plague in England, 1574–1665', *Gender & History* 11: 1 (1999), 1–29.

Nelson, S., 'The fork in the road: Nursing history versus the history of nursing?', *Nursing History Review* 10: 1 (2002), 175–88.

Neuendorf, M., *Emotions and the Making of Psychiatric Reform in Britain, c.1770–1820* (Cham: Springer Nature Switzerland, 2021).

Newton, H., *The Sick Child in Early Modern England, 1580–1720* (Oxford: Oxford University Press, 2012).

O'Lynn, C.E., 'History of men in nursing: A review', C.E. O'Lynn and R.E. Tranbarger (eds), *Men in Nursing: History, Challenges and Opportunities* (New York: Springer, 2007).

Ottaway, S., 'The elderly in the eighteenth-century workhouse', J. Reinarz and L. Schwarz (eds), *Medicine and the Workhouse* (Rochester, NY: University of Rochester Press, 2013).

Parry Jones, L., *The Trade in Lunacy: A Study of Private Madhouses in England in the Eighteenth and Nineteenth Centuries* (London: Routledge & Kegan Paul, 1972).

Pelling, M., *The Common Lot: Sickness, Medical Occupations, and the Urban Poor in Early Modern England* (London: Longman, 1998).

Peters, E., 'Trauma narratives of the English Civil War', *Journal for Early Modern Cultural Studies* 16: 1 (2016), 78–94.

Porter, R., *Mind-Forg'd Manacles: A History of Madness in England from the Restoration to the Regency* (London: Penguin, 1990).

Prosen, M., 'Nursing students' perception of gender-defined roles in nursing: A qualitative descriptive study', *BMC Nursing* 21: 104 (2022), 1–11.

Ramsey, N., *The Military Memoir and Romantic Literary Culture, 1780–1835* (Abingdon: Routledge, 2016).

Reinarz, J., *Birth of a Provincial Hospital* (Dugdale Society, 2003).

Reinarz, J., 'Learning to use their senses: Visitors to voluntary hospitals in eighteenth-century England', *Journal for Eighteenth Century Studies* 35: 4 (2012), 505–20.

Richardson, H., *English Hospitals, 1660–1948: A Survey of their Architecture and Design* (Swindon: Royal Commission on the Historical Monuments of England, 1998).

Rosenberg, C.E., 'Medical text and social context: Explaining William Buchan's *Domestic Medicine*', *Bulletin of the History of Medicine* 57: 1 (1983), 22–42.

Scarry, E., *The Body in Pain: The Making and Unmaking of the World* (Oxford: Oxford University Press, 1985).

Shaw, P., 'Longing for home: Robert Hamilton, nostalgia and the emotional life of the eighteenth-century soldier', *Journal for Eighteenth-Century Studies* 39: 1 (2016), 25–40.

Shepard, A., *Meanings of Manhood in Early Modern England* (Oxford: Oxford University Press, 2003).

Shepard, A., 'Crediting women in the early modern English economy', *History Workshop Journal* 79: 1 (2015), 1–24.

Shepard, A., 'Care', C. Macleod, A. Shepard, and M. Ågren (eds), *The Whole Economy: Work and Gender in Early Modern Europe* (Cambridge: Cambridge University Press, 2023).

Siena, K., 'Searchers of the dead in long eighteenth-century London', K. Kippen and L. Woods (eds), *Worth and Repute: Valuing Gender in Late Medieval and Early Modern Europe: Essays in honour of Barbara Todd* (Toronto: Centre for Reformation and Renaissance Studies, 2011).

Smith, L., 'The relative duties of man: Domestic medicine in England and France, ca. 1685–1740', *Journal of Family History* 31: 3 (2006), 237–56.

Smith, L.D., 'Behind closed doors; Lunatic asylum keepers, 1800–60', *Social History of Medicine* 1: 3 (1988), 301–27.
Smith, L.D., '"The keeper must himself be kept": Visitation and the lunatic asylum in England, 1750–1850', G. Mooney and J. Reinarz (eds), *Permeable Walls: Historical Perspectives on Hospital and Asylum Visiting* (Amsterdam: Rodopi, 2009).
Smith, P., *The Emotional Labour of Nursing* (Basingstoke: Macmillan, 1992).
Smith, P. and H. Cowie, 'Perspectives on emotional labour and bullying: Reviewing the role of emotions in nursing and healthcare', *International Journal of Work Organisation and Emotion* 3: 3 (2010), 227–36.
Smith, P. and M. Lorentzon, 'Comment: Is emotional labour ethical?', *Nursing Ethics* 12: 6 (2005), 638–42.
Spinney, E., 'Servants to the hospital and the state: Nurses in Plymouth and Haslar Naval Hospitals, 1775–1815', *Journal for Maritime Research* 20: 1 (2019), 1–17.
Spinney, E., 'Women's work: Nurses, orderlies and the gendered division of care in Revolutionary and Napoleonic era British army hospitals', *Nursing History Review* 31 (2023), 127–49.
Stobart, A., *Household Medicine in Seventeenth-Century England* (London: Bloomsbury, 2016).
Summers, A., 'The mysterious demise of Sarah Gamp: The domiciliary nurse and her detractors, *c.*1830–1860', *Victorian Studies* 32: 3 (1989), 365–86.
Taylor, D., 'Trauma and emotion in the battlefield correspondence of Andrew Mitchell (1708–1771)', *Emotions: History, Culture, Society* 2: 2 (2018), 292–311.
Thorpe, L., 'At the mercy of strange women: Plague nurses, marginality, and fear during the Great Plague of 1665', L. Hopkins and A. Norrie (eds), *Women on the Edge in Early Modern Europe* (Amsterdam: Amsterdam University Press, 2019).
Tosh, J., 'The old Adam and the new man: Emerging themes in the history of English masculinities, 1750–1850', T. Hitchcock and M. Cohen (eds), *English Masculinities 1660–1800* (London: Longman, 1999).
Townsend, K., 'Do production employees engage in emotional labour?', *Journal of Industrial Relations* 50: 1 (2008), 175–80.
Trembinski, D., 'Comparing premodern melancholy/mania and modern trauma: An argument in favor of historical experiences of trauma', *History of Psychology* 14: 1 (2011), 80–99.
Vernon, A. (ed.), *Arms and the Self: War, the Military, and Autobiographical Writing* (Kent, OH: Kent State University Press, 2006).
von Arni, E.G., 'Who cared? Military nursing during the English Civil Wars and Interregnum, 1642–60', G. Hudson (ed.), *British Military and Naval Medicine* (Amsterdam: Rodopi, 2007).

Wallis, P. and T. Pirohakul, 'Medical revolutions? The growth of medicine in England, 1660–1800', *Journal of Social History* 49: 3 (2016), 510–31.
Whittle, J., 'A critique of approaches to "domestic work": Women, work and the pre-industrial economy', *Past and Present* 243: 1 (2019), 35–70.
Williams, C., *The Staffordshire General Infirmary: A History of the Hospital from 1765* (Stafford: Mid Staffordshire General Hospital, 1992).
Williams, K., 'Ideologies of nursing: Their meanings and implications', R. Dingwall and J. McIntosh (eds), *Readings in the Sociology of Nursing* (Edinburgh: Churchill Livingstone, 1978).
Williams, P., 'Religion, respectability and the origins of the modern nurse', R. French and A. Wear (eds), *British Medicine in an Age of Reform* (London: Routledge, 1991).
Williams, S., 'Caring for the sick poor. Poor law nurses in Bedfordshire, c.1770–1834', P. Lane, N. Raven, and K.D.M. Snell (eds), *Women, Work and Wages in England, 1600–1850* (Woodbridge: Boydell, 2004).
Withey, A., *Physick and the Family: Health, Medicine and Care in Wales, 1600–1750* (Manchester: Manchester University Press, 2011).
Yeo, G., *Nursing at Barts: A History of Nursing Service and Nurse Education at St Bartholomew's Hospital, London* (Stroud: Alan Sutton, 1995).

Digitised sources

London Lives: www.londonlives.org for selected entries in Middlesex Justices' documents, St Thomas's Hospital minutes of the Court of Governors, St Thomas's Hospital Court and Committee minute books, and St Martins workhouse registers.
UK Parliamentary Papers (P.P.): https://parlipapers.proquest.com/parlipapers for:
  Journal of the House of Commons for 22 February 1763 (1763).
  Report from the Select Committee appointed to enquire into the State of Lunatics (1807).
  Report from the Commissioners on the Cold Bath Fields Prison (1809).
  Commissioners of Military Enquiry: Nineteenth Report (Military Hospitals) Appendix (1812).
  Report from the Committee on the State of the Gaols of the City of London (1814).
  Report from the Committee on Madhouses in England (1814–15).
  Report from the Committee on the King's Bench, Fleet, and Marshalsea Prisons (1815).
  Select Committee on Provisions for the Better Regulation of Madhouses in England: First Report (1815–16).

Report from the Committee on the Prisons within the City of London and Borough of Southwark, 1. Newgate (1818).
Second Report from the Committee on the Prisons within the City of London and Borough of Southwark, 2. Giltspur-Street Prison, 3. Whitecross-Street Prison, 4. Borough Compter, 5. Bridewell (1818).
A Return of the Number of Lunatics Confined in the different Gaols, Hospitals, and Lunatic Asylums (1819).
A Return of the Number of Houses Licensed for the Reception of Lunatics (1819).
Select Committee on State of Gaols, and Best Method of Providing for Reformation of Offenders (1819).
Royal Commission on State, Conduct, and Management of Fleet, Westminster and Marshalsea Prisons (1819).

Unpublished sources

Langtree, T., 'Notes on pre-Nightingale nursing: What it was and what it was not' (PhD thesis, James Cook University, 2020).

Nielsen, C., 'The Chelsea out-pensioners: Image and reality in eighteenth-century and early nineteenth-century social care' (PhD thesis, University of Newcastle, 2014).

Spinney, E., 'Naval and military nursing in the British Empire c.1763–1830' (PhD thesis, University of Saskatchewan, 2018).

Thorpe, L., '"In the middest of death": Medical responses to the Great Plague of 1665 with special reference to John Allin' (PhD thesis, Royal Holloway, University of London, 2017).

Index

Abell, Emily 228
Abel-Smith, Brian 3
accidents 61, 64–5, 146–7, 187, 266
Alleine family 45
almshouses 25, 131, 175–8
America/American 7, 35 n. 81, 44, 220, 228, 268, 280
amputation 280, 282
anti-nurse 27, 29, 57, 76, 220, 235–50, 265, 271, 275–7, 285, 311
apothecaries 42, 47–8, 58–9, 153, 159, 186–7, 222
Archer, Isaac 223
Army Medical Board 268
Ashforth, Blake 16–18, 248, 251
asylums 12, 22, 234–50, 311; *see also* Bethlem Hospital, York Asylum
Austen, Jane 41, 75
autonomy 55, 151, 199, 208, 228, 243–4, 250

Bamford, Samuel 54, 309
Barber, Francis 224
Bashford, Alison 18
Bath Infirmary 143, 162 n. 9
baths 150–1
Beatty, William 229–30

bedbugs 147
Begiato, Joanne 246
Berkshire 13
Bethlem Hospital 68, 235–6, 243–7
Birmingham Infirmary 133, 135–6, 139–40, 149–50, 154–5, 161
Boulton, Jeremy 8, 19
Borsay, Anne 4–5, 21, 23, 26, 131, 143, 153
Bristol 74, 138–9, 195, 236
Bristol Infirmary 133, 136
British Lying-In Hospital 199
Brownrigg, William 52
Brussels 29, 265, 288–95, 309, 311
Buchanan, John 148
Buchan, William 44–5, 52–3, 70–1, 74, 189, 313–4
burials 95, 113, 117, 139, 184–5, 188, 193, 197–8, 266, 280, 282
Burke, Edmund 75
Burnham, Robert 268
burns 64–5, 266
Burney, Charles 182, 204–8
Burney, Sarah Harriet 205–9, 310

Cappe, Catherine 224–5
Carré, Jacques 9
Catholics 20, 275, 277, 291–2

Index

Chester Infirmary 24, 135, 139–41, 150, 154
Clark, Alice 5
Cheselden, William 186–7, 191–2
Chester Infirmary 132–3, 144, 151
chamber pots 155–8, 161, 224, 247
Civil War (English) 19, 87, 267, 277–8, 285
Clark, Lorna 206
clothes 1, 43, 47–8, 66, 89, 95, 105–6, 110, 114, 153, 178, 186, 224, 241, 247, 266, 273, 280–1, 288
Collier family 58–60, 62, 74
compassion 29, 49, 106, 233, 267, 273, 275, 277, 279, 286
corpses 17, 43, 54, 59, 62, 74, 272
Courtney, Emma 71

Dalbiac, Susannah 272–4
Daly, Gavin 275, 277
D'Antonio, Patricia 21
D'Arblay, Frances (née Burney) 205, 289, 293
Darwin family 222
daughters 11, 15, 17, 48, 50, 62–5, 69, 118, 196, 202, 205, 207, 223–4, 272, 275, 289, 290
deaconesses *see* sisterhoods
Defoe, Daniel 1
Devis, Arthur 229–30
Devon and Exeter Infirmary 130, 133, 160
Dickens, Charles 3, 88, 311
dirty work 16–19, 91–2, 103–4, 111, 131, 145, 157, 161, 220, 244–8, 251, 279, 284, 311–12
disability 28, 63, 138, 175–9, 107, 181–3, 190, 209
Dorchester 45
Dorset 65

drunkenness 4, 51, 54, 61, 88–9, 91, 104–5, 107, 113, 120, 144–5, 175, 287, 295, 311
Dublin 57, 176, 196

East, Hannah 58, 72
Eaton, Charlotte (née Waldie) 291–3
effeminacy 221, 234, 246, 250
see also masculinity
embezzling 105, 201
emotion work 14, 23, 50–1, 64–5, 68, 71, 76, 164 n. 25, 204–9, 226–8, 241, 250, 283, 289, 292
enemas 59, 72–3, 75
enslaved people 50, 224–5
epidemics 8, 19, 22, 29, 63, 87
Equiano, Olaudah 225–6
Essex 223
Europe 7, 13, 44, 175, 267, 274, 278, 283
Evans, Joan 220
Exley, Catherine 280–1, 294

family/kin 2, 15–8, 21, 41, 47, 52, 55, 59–61, 63–4, 66–7, 75, 114–119, 177, 185, 204–5, 207, 220, 222–3, 225–6, 228, 241, 243–5, 251, 266, 272, 275, 288, 290, 312
fatigue 70–1, 146, 286
fees 45, 92–3, 103–4, 113, 156, 158, 161, 312
femininity 7, 16–17, 48–50, 52, 75, 221, 228, 235, 274, 310
fevers 44, 49, 58, 66, 74–5, 132, 138, 151, 190–1, 226, 233–4, 274, 281, 283
Field, Jacob 197
Fielding, Henry 249–50
Firmin, Thomas 12
first aid 65, 265–6, 274, 309

Fleet prison 194–5, 197, 234
Fliedner, Theodor 20
Fox, Sarah 62
France/French 15, 175, 179, 267–9, 275–7, 279, 281–3, 288
Freke, Elizabeth 62, 72
friends/friendship 45–7, 49, 51, 59, 63, 67, 74–5, 104, 113, 118, 156, 188, 202–3, 222–4, 226, 234, 243, 266, 275, 289, 292
Fry, Elizabeth 3, 20
Furneaux, Holly 274

Gamp, Sarah 3, 311
gaols 22, 158, 231, 258 n. 81
see also prisons
Garrick, David 205, 246
Gawthern, Abigail 58, 62, 74
Germany/German 265, 267, 276–7, 282–3, 288–9
Gibbon, Edward 63
Glasgow/Glaswegian 273–4, 282
Gloucester Infirmary 131, 133, 135, 137, 139–40, 143, 145, 147–8, 150, 152, 154, 156, 158–9, 222
Godden, Judith 3, 145, 159
gout 49, 58, 72, 189, 208
Grant, William 44
Greenwich Hospital 10, 176, 185, 190, 200, 208, 231
Grey family 15
Guy's Hospital 162 n. 8, 232, 236

Ham, Elizabeth 63, 65–6, 76
Hampshire 114
Harlow, Clarissa 45–6, 71
Harris, Walter 52
Haslar Hospital 10, 312
Hastings 58–60
Haverfordwest 2

Hays, Mary 71, 87, 89, 120
Helmstadter, Carol 3, 145, 159
Heroine of Matagorda *see* Reston, Agnes
Hochschild, Arlie 16, 18, 158
Holcroft, Thomas 226, 249
Holland, William 60, 62, 75, 223
Horsham 62
hospitals (military) 268, 278–83, 288–9
for civilian establishments *see* almshouses, asylums, and hospitals by name
Hôtel des Invalides 176, 179
Howard, John 141, 149, 154
Howie, William 130, 143, 145
Hoxton 67, 178, 237
Hudson, Geoff 10, 190, 312
Hughes, Everett 16–17, 248
humane/humanity 43, 59, 61–2, 71, 130, 224, 249, 266, 277, 289–90, 292–3
Hurst, Sarah 62–3

identity 6, 12, 15, 19, 48, 199, 208, 219–63, 310–11
infanticide 109–10, 120
infirmaries (provincial) 9, 21–22, 28, 43, 62, 92, 98, 103, 130–74, 176, 192, 214 n. 58, 222, 233, 235, 240, 246, 268, 279, 311–12; *see also* infirmaries by name
inquests 67, 69, 85 n. 134, 90, 146–7, 313
insanity 51, 67–9, 138, 178, 190, 220–1, 235–50
insomnia *see* nightwatching
Irish 13, 57, 99, 282

Jenner, Mark 155, 247
Johnson, Robert 44, 72
Johnson, Samuel 205, 224

Keats, John 226–8, 310
Kennedy, Catriona 272, 277, 285, 293
Kent 5, 13
Kilmainham Hospital 176, 196, 212 n. 35
kin *see* family
King, Steven 7, 9, 19
Kopperman, Paul 264, 280
Kreiner, Glen 16–18, 248, 251

Lamb, Charles 61, 67–9
Lamb, Mary 51, 63, 67–70, 76, 310
Lancashire 64, 259 n. 88
Langtree, Tanya 4, 6, 26
Larrey, Dominique 266
laundry 43, 91–2, 109, 141, 150, 247, 271, 278
Leeds Infirmary 130, 133, 136, 153
Leicester 236, 238
Leicester Infirmary 149
Lincoln County Hospital 159
Liverpool 138, 225
Liverpool Infirmary 131, 133, 135–7, 139–40, 142–3, 145–6, 152, 154, 158
London 3, 6, 8–13, 21, 23, 25, 27, 48, 54, 58–9, 87–129, 131, 137–8, 144, 146, 153, 159, 176, 185, 194, 205, 224, 232, 246, 312
London Lives 26, 88
lunacy *see* insanity
Lynn, John 272

Macdonald, John 224
Mackintosh, Carolyn 220
madhouses 51, 67, 69, 219, 233, 235–50
 see also asylums
Manchester Royal Infirmary 133, 136, 139–40, 155, 309

Mandeville, Bernard 175–6
Mansell, Charmian 313
many-to-many 21–2, 264, 266
many-to-one 21–2, 45, 221, 228
marriage 12, 47, 64, 109, 115, 118, 139, 143–4, 177, 180, 185, 193–200, 209, 244, 271, 273, 312
masculinity 16, 24, 179, 181, 219–63, 276–7, 310–11
 see also effeminacy
matrons 17, 21, 28, 90, 94, 96, 100–2, 105, 117, 137, 141, 143, 146, 150–4, 158, 176–7, 183, 185, 187–8, 200, 205, 207–8
Maynwaringe, Everard 55
medical students 107, 147
Metcalf, Urbane 240, 244–5, 247
midwives 94, 110, 280
Monro, Donald 278
monthly nursing 20, 54
Moore, Norman 97
Mortimer, Ian 5–7, 11, 19, 221
mothers 11, 17, 20, 41, 46–8, 51, 54, 58, 64–5, 67–8, 180, 205, 223, 227, 275, 282
murder 57, 67–9, 76, 82 n. 82, 111, 119, 201–2, 240, 281, 286

Nelson, Horatio 228–31, 248
Netherlands 267, 275, 277
Neuendorf, Mark 242
Nicklin, Susan 50–1, 55
Nightingale, Florence 3–4, 7, 15, 19–20, 29, 31 n. 23, 228, 244, 274, 290–1, 295
nightwatching 70–2, 152, 187
noise 145, 148, 244
non-conformists 117, 132, 224
Norfolk 13, 89
Norris, James 246

Northamptonshire 13
Norwich 141
Nottingham 138
nursery nursing 5, 21, 28, 53, 63–4

Old Bailey 26, 94, 100, 109, 111, 118
Old Poor Law *see* poor relief
one-to-many 21–2, 92, 221, 231
one-to-one 21–2, 180, 221, 223, 226, 281
opiates 151, 191, 206
Opie, Amelia 49
Ottaway, Susannah 190
Oxford 139, 178

pain 27, 55, 58, 74, 76, 189, 191, 277, 285, 289
palsy 148, 189, 208
Pelling, Margaret 3, 5, 7, 10–11, 16, 27, 157
pension 112, 114, 144, 175, 190, 199
Peterloo 4, 27, 309
physicians 14, 21, 42, 44, 48, 52–3, 59–60, 68, 70, 90, 132, 153, 178, 190, 227, 241, 265
Pilkington, Laetitia 54
plague 1–3, 4, 6, 8, 10, 18–19, 27–8, 41, 43, 50, 87, 272
Plymouth 10, 312
poor relief 7–11, 13, 25, 35 n. 72, 98, 144, 178, 180, 280 309
   see also workhouses
Porter, Agnes 48, 58, 69
Portugal/Portuguese 267, 272, 275–81, 285
poultices 58, 77 n. 8, 107, 136, 275
Prig, Betsy 88, 311
prisons 26, 55, 112, 158, 231–4, 251
   see also gaols, Fleet prison

professionalisation 4, 9–10, 13, 21–22, 47, 208, 228
Protestants 18–20, 87, 117, 132, 277

Quakers 13, 49, 62, 236, 243

race 13–15, 23, 49–50, 57, 224–5, 265, 271, 275
Radcliffe Infirmary (Oxford) 149
Refuge of the Destitute 112–13
Reinarz, Jonathan 135
Reston, Agnes (Heroine of Matagorda) 4, 273–4, 294
Retreat, The (York) 236
Richardson, Samuel 219–20, 250
risk 2, 6, 12, 14, 18, 24, 42–3, 52, 54–5, 57, 59, 66–7, 69–72, 74–5, 91, 98, 105, 112, 120, 131, 145, 149, 151–2, 161, 166 n. 53, 181, 192, 220, 222–3, 227–8, 235, 242–3, 247–8, 271, 276, 280, 283–6, 310
Royal Hospital Chelsea 21, 25, 28, 161, 175–218, 244, 265, 312
Royal Humane Society 266

Sabin, Linda 220
salaries *see* wages
Salisbury Infirmary 137, 171 n. 107
Salop Infirmary (Shrewsbury) 130, 132–3, 135–7, 139–40, 143–6, 151, 154–5, 159–60
Savile, Gertrude 61, 70, 74
Scarry, Elaine 292
searchers of the dead 6, 9–10, 14, 54, 109
separate spheres 51–2
servants 5, 15–16, 24, 43, 57–62, 64, 94, 105, 111, 139, 141–2, 150–1, 157, 182, 196–7, 219,

Index

222–4, 229, 231, 233, 242, 248, 250, 266, 283, 289–90, 311
settlement 8, 97–8, 114, 120, 141, 193
Severn, Joseph 226–8, 310
Shaw, Philip 285
Sheffield Infirmary 130, 133
Shrewsbury 146
  see also Salop Infirmary
Siena, Kevin 247
sisterhoods 18, 20, 291
sisters (as siblings) 11, 17, 58, 250
smallpox 8, 44, 53, 58–9, 62–3, 75, 148, 222–3
smell 145, 148–9, 155, 157, 192, 282
Smith, Leonard 233, 240–1, 244, 251
soldiers 22, 175–218, 242, 266–95
Somerset 65, 233
Spain/Spanish 264, 267, 275–7, 281–2
Spence, Craig 147
Spinney, Erin 4, 10, 19, 264, 279, 312
spinsters 6, 42, 63–9, 115–16, 194, 205, 226
Stafford Infirmary 24–5, 133, 137–45, 148, 150, 152
Stanley, Mary 3
status shield 16–17, 69, 106
St Bartholomew's Hospital (Barts) 9, 25, 28, 87–129, 137, 144, 146, 153, 156, 161, 185, 201–2, 204, 208, 214 n. 58, 232, 311–12
stigma 16–18, 27, 69, 157, 243–4, 247, 280, 311
Stoddart, Sarah 51
St Thomas's Hospital 24, 28, 87–8, 93, 95–6, 99, 105, 107, 113
suicide 74, 113, 147, 202, 227

Summers, Anne 3
surgeons 106–7, 130, 132, 149, 151, 153, 155, 186–7, 190–1, 222, 229, 231–2, 234, 265–6, 285, 289

Tanner, Thomas 44
Taunton 199
tenures 89, 96, 98–9, 100, 108, 131, 138–40, 142, 146, 154, 160–1, 176, 183, 185, 208
textiles 1, 92, 105–6, 110, 137, 167 n. 66, 192, 280, 311
theft 1, 27, 106, 113, 118
Thornton, Alice 266
Thorpe, Lara 6, 10–11
training 7, 9, 48–9, 91, 137, 157, 240, 311, 313
trauma 263 n. 141, 265, 284–7, 295, 310
Trembinski, Donna 284
Trench, Melesina 49, 71
Trimmer, Sarah 20, 46–8, 53–5, 72
Tryon, Thomas 14
tuberculosis 226–8

Unitarians *see* non-conformity

venereal disease/wards 44, 74, 89, 92–3, 103–4, 112, 114, 117, 138, 140, 146
Versluyson, Margaret 22
virtue script 38 n. 109, 69
vocation 47, 228, 231, 295, 310
von Arni, Eric Gruber 19, 277

Waddy, Jonathan 26
wages 6, 13, 25, 48, 93, 137–42, 145, 152, 159, 184, 186, 240, 244
war 22, 28, 57, 179, 264–308
Waterloo 29, 265, 267, 272, 288–95, 309

Weekes, Hampton 107
Weeton, Ellen (Nelly) 20, 63–5, 70, 76
wet nursing 5, 20, 53, 63, 74
Whittle, Jane 15
widows 6, 11–12, 115–16, 183, 185, 194–7, 198–9, 271–2
Wiesner, Merry 24
Wilde, Joseph 130, 153, 160
Williams, Samantha 8, 13, 221
wills 25, 116–17, 184–5, 202–4, 209
Wiltshire 13
Witt, Agnes 61, 223
wives 6, 11, 17, 42, 45, 52, 75, 81 n. 74, 115–6, 180, 183, 195–6, 198–9, 200, 203, 205, 209, 219, 222–3, 234, 250, 271–3, 275, 277–8, 280–1, 290

Woolley, Hannah 54
Worcester 98
Worcester Infirmary 133, 139–40, 144, 149, 152
Wordsworth, Dorothy 70, 74
workhouses 8–9, 22, 25, 89–90, 93, 98, 104, 137–8, 142, 146, 148, 155, 175, 187, 190, 201, 280, 309, 313; *see also* poor relief

Yeo, Geoffrey 96, 101
Yeovil 66
York Asylum 245
York Infirmary 133, 137
Yorkshire 280

www.ingramcontent.com/pod-product-compliance
Ingram Content Group UK Ltd.
Pitfield, Milton Keynes, MK11 3LW, UK
UKHW022014140225
455095UK00006B/38